NUTRITION

INTRODUCTION TO DISEASE PREVENTION

David Bissonnette RD. PhD

ST-JUDE NUTRITION MEDICAL COMMUNICATIONS LLC

Mankato, MN

First Published in 2014 by
St-Jude Nutrition Medical Communications
PO Box 5194
Mankato, MN, USA 56002
1st EDITION

© Copyright 2014 by
David Bissonnette
ISBN-13: 978-0-615-99280-8
ISBN-10: 0-615-99280-3

978-0-615-99280-8

Cover Image © TijanaM/shutterstock.com

Dedication

This book is dedicated to Jesus and his dear mother, Mary,
without whom, nothing would have been completed.

CONTENTS

FOREWORD

This is an introductory textbook on nutrition for health-care professionals; it is written in a way that invites students in dietetics, nutrition, nursing, health sciences, and medicine to think critically about nutrition within the field of medicine and public health. After all, it is precisely the increasing prevalence of obesity in the U.S., and all the secondary diseases that derive from it, such as heart disease and type-2 diabetes, that have set off alarm bells nationwide. Health professionals are warning that obesity and type-2 diabetes have reached epidemic proportions, affecting the lives of both the adults and the youth. If we remain unable to turn this thing around, it will, without a doubt, forcibly change the quality of life and the health of our nation. Since the early 1980s, we have been consuming an overabundance of food that has led to excessive intakes of fat, sugar and salt. Moreover, suboptimal fiber intake now threatens the gastrointestinal health of millions. We are now looking at a generation with food habits that are so impoverished, that they are threatening its very health.

As healthcare professionals, you are preparing to provide medical services of various types to a culture that has sickened itself with cheap processed foods and lifestyles of physical complaisance. The consequences are dire as great numbers of patients will be seeking help to manage heart disease, obesity, gastrointestinal diseases of various types, cancer, depression and type-2 diabetes; the financial cost to the system will be staggering and oppressive. These are the most significant diseases afflicting our society currently, and they will likely impact your life in some manner, either affecting you directly, or impacting family members and friends. They will also affect your careers as healthcare professionals, because of the onslaught of medical train wrecks that will be lining up for help in clinics and urgent cares all over the country. The tsunami has already it; you can ask any family physician, physician assistants, or nurse practitioner who has been working in the trenches for longer than 10 years. America is not just sick, but it is profoundly sick, and nutrition is at the epicenter of the disaster. And so it timely to be studying nutrition, as you will be introduced to many of the introductory concepts of nutrition and to the many diseases associated with diet. It is my hope that this textbook will provide you with a rich learning experience, and that you will go away, after completing this class, with a more in depth understanding of the role of nutrition in individual and public health.

This book comes with free access to one video on demand (VOD) documentary on obesity and diabetes, lasting 1 hour and 47 minutes. It explores the impact of nutrition on the obesity and diabetes crises in the United States. The promotional code to enter is FCS242; I invite to copy and paste this hyperlink and enter the promotional code for a free access to this documentary, which I produced, wrote and directed as a complement to this textbook. https://vimeo.com/ondemand/type2 diabeticnation.

Obesity and type II diabetes are currently driving healthcare costs and impacting American society at so many different levels. The documentary explores the prevalence, causes, assessment and the most current thinking in effective treatments, and so will be valuable in forming your critical thinking around these conditions. [A DIABETIC NATION: AN AMERICAN TRAGEDY The documentary promo code: FCS242]

Documentary website for video on demand: https://vimeo.com/ondemand/type2diabeticnation.

CHAPTER 1

NUTRITION FOR THE PREVENTION OF DISEASE

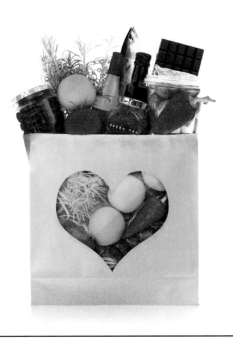

1.0. THE ROLE OF NUTRITION IN HEALTH

Preventative health care, centered on nutrition, is currently being promoted in the United States and Canada. The aging baby boomers are especially concerned with nutritional issues, as they now begin to battle chronic diseases that threaten this age group's desire for longevity and health. Osteoporosis, cardiovascular disease, and cancer are the very diseases that are concerning and costly to the health care system (Bissonnette, 2013).

Epidemiologists have been able to establish that diet and lifestyle are responsible for about 59% of cancer deaths in women and up to 45% in men (Anand, 2008). In teasing out the impact of diet alone, the American Cancer Society reports that nutritional factors alone account for one-third of cancer deaths in the U.S. Also, 70% of the incidences of cancer have been successfully tagged to dietary habits. So then, apart from smoking, diet and activity level, are the most modifiable determinants of cancer risk (Bissonnette, 2013). In establishing an association between disease and diet, researchers have empowered individuals to make good and healthy decisions that can greatly decrease disease risks; the reality though, is that the majority do not. In fact, some cancer incidences continue to grow at an alarming rate. The World Health Organization estimates that in 2001 there were 10 million cases of cancer worldwide; they expect the number to grow to almost 20 million cases per year over the next 20 years (WHO, 2001). The statistics are frightening, especially if one considers that 25% of Americans will likely be stricken by some form of cancer. So then, there is a strong incentive to find the elusive elixir and tackle the scourge head-on. Diet is central to everyone's life, but yet only a few appear to be concerned that they might be mismanaging their diet, and that the decision to do little could carry serious long term repercussions. Only a small number of consumers are ready to engage in new lifestyles that are more healthful, despite having access to a wealth of information via the internet, bookstores, and libraries. Many proponents of nutrition and health are attempting, through webpages, books and seminars, to popularize healthy nutrition practices and lifestyles. On the surface, though book and DVD sales appear to be good, there appears to be little change at the societal level. Why, all of sudden, is there a disconnect between food and health?

The idea that nutrition is preventative and even medicinal had been a foundation of Aristotelian medical theory. It argued that there were three origins of disease which impacted the humors of the body: first, excesses or deficiencies in diet, drink, or exercise; second, violent causes such as wounds, trauma, or extreme fatigue; and third, atmospheric conditions which could predispose the individual to disease (Bissonnette, 2013; Plato, 2005). Philosophers of the classical Greek period hypothesized that the body consisted in four humors, and that diseases arise from imbalances in these humors. It was the pre-Socratic philosopher, Empedocles of Agrigentum (500–430 BC), who proposed that the entire universe could be explained by the four elements of water, fire, earth and air; the notion of 4 elements was then adapted, by the practitioner of medicine, to a biological system based on 4 humors. There was a big picture of universal organization and symmetry that was drawn from this Empedoclean model which was seen as the root of all things (Maher, 2002). The four characteristics of these seasons were cold, hot, moist, and dry. Consistent with this idea of equilibrium, Plato, in the *Timaeus*, (Plato, 2005) describes the origins of disease from four perspectives: First, it could be an imbalance between four elements: fire, water, earth and air. It was understood that any excesses or deficiencies in these elements would result in changes in the cold, hot, moist, and dry properties of the body, thus leading invariably to disease. Plato then describes diseases of the "secondary formations" when there is insufficient food or drink to replenish the blood; the consequence is disease resulting from disturbances in marrow, bone, flesh, sinew, and blood. Conceptually, Plato writes of a decomposition or catabolic breakdown of flesh, and of blood changing to a black discharge in deficient diets. A third origin of disease is considered from breath, phlegm, and bile. Here Plato describes lung diseases and the transformation of body fluids during the disease processes as visible signs of the loss of body balance. Fourth, he accepts the notion that diseases can be caused by the soul and mind and stresses the importance of balance between mind and body for achieving health. And so nature and humans appeared to be intertwined, connected to the four seasons. These natural systems were based on the principles of balance and thus offered a rational structure that accommodated the belief that there were inherent dangers associated with excesses or clear deficiencies. Hippocrates derived maxims that were grounded in a common-sense understanding that the body needed a certain balance to be healthy. Hippocrates wrote, "Diseases that are generated by repletion are cured by depletion, and all which arise from depletion are cured by repletion; all which arises from exertion are cured by inactivity and all which arises from inactivity is cured by exertion" (Brothwell and Brothwell, 1969). Socrates believed that food played an essential role in replacing water and heat losses from the body. This was another concept of balance greatly advocated by the Greek masters.

The ancient Greek masters conceived such principles as "biological balance" and "codependency of mind and

bodily disease," strictly from rational thought and observations rather than from experimentation. Greek society forbade the dissection of animal and human remains which greatly limited their ability to conduct experimental investigations. Although their beliefs were somewhat rooted in some element of truth, insofar as there were homeostatic (equilibrium) mechanisms in the body, it is clear that their understanding of the pathophysiology of diseases was fundamentally flawed (Bissonnette, 2013).

It is clear that the Greeks understood nutrition to be an integral part of the individual and collective health, and that the body's balance was a central theme in human health. But it is surprising that this medical understanding of health extended to include the mind; and so they conceived that the mind and the body need to be in some kind of homeostasis for optimal health. Elizabeth Craik, a reputed British classics scholar, has written about Hippocratic balance. She has describes it as an equilibrium between physical conditioning and dietary elements (Craik, 1997). The physicians of the Greek period understood that balance for the individual was dependent on routines for eating frequencies and on types of foods that varied with seasons, customs, and geography. They promoted the belief that what we are, conditions what we should eat. In other words, our biological makeup commands our nutritional needs. This physical balance could be achieved by contrasting excesses with abstinence, and weight gain with subsequent weight loss.

Obesity in the classical Greek period was a known phenomenon, and so were the higher death rates among obese individuals. Obesity was described as an imbalance between calories consumed and exercise, or in other words from eating beyond the body's needs. Greek writings, consequently, refer to "Diaita" or regimented dieting, as a way of living complemented by exercise, baths, and emetics (Craik, 1997). And so, diet and food appear to be regarded as different in that diet fit within a strong therapeutic meaning, while nourishment or "trophe" was more akin to food (Bissonnette, 2013).

Diet, for the Hippocratic physician, had more to do with regimented austerity rather than with the enjoyment of attractive or good-tasting foods. Concoctions consisting of food and plant mixtures were purely medicinal in nature, and prescribed without any practical preparation or cooking guidelines. In the eyes of the Greek and Roman physicians, diets and medicines were of equal importance in containing or healing the diseases of the time. In Oribasios' *Medical Complications*,(Grant, 1995) Dieuches—a 3rd-century BC physician—understood the soporific properties of the poppy; he describes a poppy seed-based recipe for insomnia: "*It is sufficient to put into a pint and a half of the finest and ripest barley flour and half pints of milk and water, in the proportion of two-thirds of milk to one-third of water, and the head of a poppy that has been toasted; and after mixing in by the fire one tenth of an ounce of pounded figs, boil the ingredients together, and serve after cooking to the consistency of soup; it provides some respite and also sleep for those who are convalescent*"(Grant, 1995). Similarly, Hippocrates could displace the womb by using a mixture of cheese, barley, and poppy seeds. Flatulence and indigestion was also commonly treated using a plant called asafetida.

Consistent with the apparent medicinal wisdom of the Greeks, what we now recognize as nutritional deficiencies were fairly uncommon during the classical Greek period, and even during the Neolithic revolution (6000–2000 BC). These eras were characterized by the domestication of livestock and the cultivation of specific plants in order to ensure the provision of foodstuffs for a growing population. This was a turning point as the modern man began building fundamental dwellings and developing a hunting-fishing economy in addition to lithic technology (tools made of stone). Back in the Neolithic period, the human diet was founded on simple food habits, which consisted of a wide diversity of cereals, fish, domesticated animals, fruits, and vegetables. Tied with the domestication of animals was the consumption of goat and cow's milk, and milk products dating back to the Ur (2900 BC). Given the abundance of goats, archaeologists are of the opinion that ancient Greek society likely consumed mostly goat milk (Vickery, 1936). The Scythians, by contrast, who were a group of nomadic tribes that roamed the grassy steppes of Eurasia between 700 and 300 BC, drank reindeer and elk milk.

In Old Europe, archaeologists claim population health began to decline when nomadic groups transitioned to sedentism, and began planting crops and domesticating animals to feed the growing population (Richards, 2002). The greater food availability and a growing population became the vectors for an inevitable move toward urbanization. It is here that crowding conditions may have favored contagion and a more carbohydrate-based diet. Some scholars propose that, once the modern human began to consume porridge and breads in Europe, rice in Asia, and maize in the New World, human health and stature began to deteriorate. These same academics also tend also to idealize the Paleolithic diet, promoting, as it were, greater meat consumption as a pathway to optimal wealth. Others (Bissonnette, 2013) have argued that meat consumption, especially consumed in excess, remains a vector for poor long term health outcomes. The extent to which sedentism caused a decline in health is not clear however, for there still remain archeological vestiges of relatively good health among settled agrarian populations around the Aegean Sea. Although domestication of animals such sheep, swine, goats and cattle by the Aegean

people would have likely been practiced, it would appear that the meats were consumed only on special feasts (Maher, 2002). Also, proximity to the sea would have reasonably translated into a diet abundant in fish. In a similar way, Cycladic people of the Late and Early Bronze Age were great vertebrate fish consumers. In Neolithic times dependency on the sea is also supported by lasting vestiges of shells. This means that around 3000 BC the Greek family diet would have revolved around chickpeas, lentils, and bread, mixed with olive oil and goat cheese and served with wine (Kishlansky, 1991); there was little evidence of poor health.

Not long after the end of the Neolithic period, there is some evidence that nutritional deficiencies were known; an Egyptian medical treatise named the *Ebers papyrus* that dates back to 1600 BC contained a description of night blindness for which the recommended treatment was ox liver. A similar treatment was also found in Hippocrates' writings, in Roman texts as well as in Chinese literature dated AD 610. Other nutritional diseases like Beriberi, which resulted from thiamin deficiency, were also documented in China during a 9-month siege of the city of Tsai Chseng around AD 529. Thanks to pioneering work by Wald in the 1930s, we now understand that night vision requires the presence of vitamin A in the eye pigment, rhodopsin, and that liver is a rich source of that vitamin. Considering the abundance of fruits and vegetables, available to most hunting and collecting communities, it would have been quite unusual to find cases of vitamin C deficiency until after the Neolithic revolution. Hippocrates does document a condition involving the bleeding and ulceration of the gums, typical of scurvy (Brothwell and Brothwell, 1969).

Rickets, a disease resulting in the bowing of the long bones—the consequence of vitamin D deficiency— caused insufficient calcification of the bone matrix. It seemed to have occurred quite infrequently among the early populations of China and Scandinavia, as evidenced by archeological findings of the last century, which uncovered only a small number of slightly bowed long and pelvic bones. This was not an unexpected finding, given the abundant fish oils and vitamin D–rich fish consumed by these populations. In Neolithic times, there are vestiges of bowed tibias in Denmark. The frequency of bowed legs seems, however, to have increased in first and second century Rome because of poor child-rearing practices, which involved keeping the children indoors and away from the sun more than they should have. Overall, nutritional deficiencies were not widespread but episodic. Eating traditions of different peoples safeguarded the populations against the devastating consequences of poor nutrition, which could very effectively wipe out a country and even a civilization (Bissonnette, 2013).

Rickets = vitamin D deficiency

2.0. MALNUTRITION AND ITS IMPACT ON SOCIETY

It was the famines that catalysed human misery, at unprecedented levels, through hunger and deficiency diseases. Between the years 100 BC and AD 1910, for instance, China would have experienced more than 1,800 famines; the British Isles suffered from a total of 200 famines between the years AD 10 and 1850. Storms and frosts in addition to the military assaults by Hernando Cortés, which decimated 92% of the Aztec population, would have caused important food shortages among the Aztecs. Cortés' defeat of the Aztecs was so extensive that their labor-intensive agricultural system could not survive such an extensive slaughter of their workforce. Plant diseases were also responsible for major crop failures, such as rust disease in cereals; Aristotle (384–322 BC) recorded yearly variations of rust disease, which he attributed to warmth and moisture. Afterward, devastating famines ploughed through Europe from 1308 to 1332. Food was so scarce that people were forced to rely on dogs and cats to fill their cooking pots. When food became even more difficult to obtain, they ate dove excrement and even children (Kishlansky, 1991).

Mass hysteria drove crowds of hungry people to attack condemned prisoners in the gallows and hack away at their flesh. The numerous deaths that arose from these famines were often seen as provoked by the wrath of God or Satan. Hence, priests and witches were, in fact, perceived as the most effective healers because they claimed to know how to appease such a wrath by urging confessions and prayers. They also claimed to possess an empirical knowledge of sacred plants, which they used in medications (Nikiforuk, 1996). Following the famines, the population became very vulnerable to the plagues. The scourge of pneumonic and bubonic plagues visited the European continent, first between 1351 and 1358, wiping out roughly 24 million people, second in 1362, and again in 1369, when it killed primarily children (Nikiforuk, 1996).

The plague continued its infectious roaming, but with less virulence, for the following 100 years up to approximately 1469, killing about 13% of every new generation. The historical medieval documents that describe these times speak of intolerable levels of human suffering and fear. The plague made several visits before its final retreat from Europe in 1720, hitting Venice in 1575 and in 1630, killing one-third of its population. It then visited Marseille in 1720, decimating 80,000 people (**Figure 1.1**).

In the fifteenth century, following the most devastating period of the plague, European society was in a strong recovery phase; its resilience was aided by the Renaissance, which was a period during which numerous wars were gradually ending, and humanity was celebrating and exalting itself. During this post-plague recovery era, the survivors of the plague found it easier to get jobs because of a much smaller population base; the economy overall remained stagnant, as there was no population growth until the end of the 15th century. In fact, between the years 1350 to 1450, epidemics and plagues decimated the population every six years.

The periodic waves of unpredictable epidemics created psychological fear from which arose an ardent interest in meeting immediate rather than future needs. Luxury items were purchased by the rich and poor who

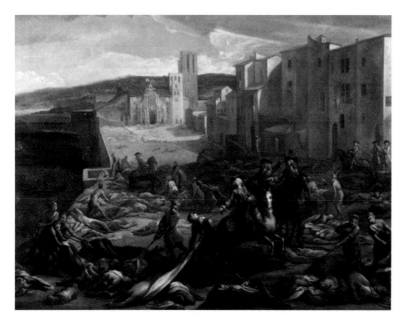

Figure 1.1. Michel Serre (1658-1733), *The Plague in Marseilles in 1721.* © DEA/G. DAGLI ORTI/ De Agostini Picture Library/ Getty Images.

espoused the 20th century's dictum of living for today. Agricultural production began to diversify, yielding specialty crops like sugar, saffron, fruits and wines; in addition, imported exotic goods from the Far East spilled over into the marketplace (Kishlansky, 1991). Once the population began to grow, early in the 16th century, so did the economy in response to increased demand. Life expectancy was improving and the population was healthier because of an improved diet that included greater varieties of foods. The agricultural surplus of grains in the late 15th century, in addition to better transportation and communication systems, improved the individual's access to food.

Cities grew as cohesive social and political centers, with the marketplace being at the epicenter of human activity. The cities were, however, made of dark and narrow streets that stunk of raw sewage, rotting foodstuff, and an overbearing stench emanating from animal slaughterhouses. Over the course of the 15th century, the marketplace became diversified in an unprecedented way: meat and dairy products were abundantly and frequently part of the diet. Consumption of such quantities of pork and lamb would not be seen again until the 19th century. Vegetables, however, were not found much in the diet of the lower classes, whereas sweet wines and citrus fruits were eaten by the rich to compensate for the lack of vegetables. Both an improved economy and diet contributed most significantly to population health.

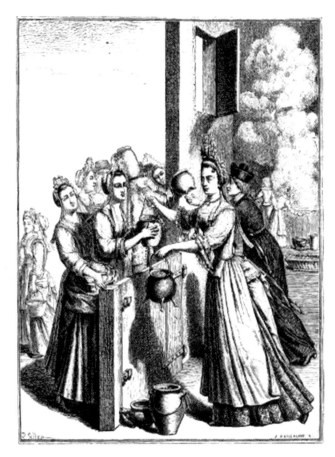

Figure 1.2. *Relief soup, in Paris, during the famine of 1709,* vintage engraved illustration. Magasin Pittoresque 1875 © Morphart Creation/Shutterstock.com.

2.1. Malnutrition during the 18th-Century Agricultural Revolution

At the beginning of the 18th century, Louis XIV drew France into a financial crisis of epic proportion, beginning in 1701 with his participation in the war of Spanish Succession, which was to last until 1714. The war became too costly to manage over time, leading to a debt so great, the monarch never recovered from it (Rowlands, 2009). It precipitated a financial crisis which destabilized the country's economy and military power; food prices significantly rose, causing wheat to accumulate in the numerous grain warehouses spread throughout the country. Louis XIV resisted the imposition of price ceilings on wheat and grain didn't reach the cities where human misery was growing quickly. Then in January 1709 record low temperatures of $-15C°$ engulfed France for several weeks, precipitating the famous famine of 1709 represented in this earlier period lithograph (**Figure 1.2**) (Miller, 1999; Rowlands, 2009).

The European population had begun to increase quite significantly by 1740 because of better housing and a greater availability of food. Agricultural output was increasing as a result of the Agricultural Revolution, which is considered one of the great turning points in human history Kishlansky, 1991). The paradox was that even though the food supply increased substantively, the population growth created a greater demand, driving prices upward but also causing wages to fall and therefore limiting the purchasing power of the population. The Agricultural Revolution led to the transformation of subsistence farming to commercial agriculture, thereby causing a consolidation of smaller estates into large plantations with better outputs to meet market conditions. Large fields were enclosed and dedicated to increasing the yield of single-crop production as opposed to a balance of commodities. This reorganization of the land led to the disintegration of the commons, and then to the buy-out of the middling-sized landholders. The resulting landless agrarian labor force ended up moving from farm to farm looking for work and food (Kishlansky, 1991). In the cities the plight of the poor was acute; general hospitals and other charitable organizations came to their aid. Even though widespread famines were no longer wiping out large populations—the last and most devastating famine in European history occurred in 1697, eradicating one-third of Finland's population—there was a persistent slow starvation and undernutrition in the population of that time (**Figure 1.3**).

It is estimated that between 10% and 15% of most societies were comprised of the truly starving poor; this represented about 20 million people, mostly situated in towns, who were suffering from hunger. Another 40% included those who were landless and jobless. Large masses were not dying, but the misery of individuals was certainly greater, as the prominence of hunger and of poor-quality diets were more rampant at the end of the 18th century than at the beginning. The nutritional quality of the diet during that time may have been the poorest in European history according to Robert Vial (1989). To be well nourished meant that there were enough calories in the form of bread and a full cooking pot of soup that usually contained vegetables. The modest families rarely saw excess calories in their diet, and the peasants' diet was even more deprived (Kishlansky, 1991). Mark Kishlansky (1991), in his book *Civilization in the West*, advances that the peasant usually ate very poorly. His diet consisted of small peas and cabbage during the summer and turnips, celery, and pumpkin during the winter. It was customary to dip the bread into the soup. The bread was usually made from a combination of rye, barley, and wheat. If there was work for the father, meat was consumed once a week, and there was generally lard available to enhance the taste of the soup. So it was understood that if the crock was generously filled with soup, and there was enough bread or potatoes, and occasionally some meat, then the people were eating well. This likely meant that the individual and the family could avoid important diseases, but such a diet was more intended as a survival strategy, rather than a means to achieving some kind of optimal health.

At the close of the 18th century and beginning of the 19th the Industrial Revolution began to take hold. People started to migrate in greater numbers from rural areas to the urban centers in search of the higher-paying factory jobs. As souls congregated in the cities, the ability of individuals and families to grow their own vegetables and fruits diminished greatly; they became reliant on the grocer's inventory. The consequence of this sociological trend resulted in significant dietary changes during the winter. The urbanite, unlike the rural dweller, had depleted his reserves of cabbage, leeks, and onions by early winter, leaving a diet limited to meat and bread until the spring. For that reason, scurvy outbreaks, occurring in the spring, attained near epidemic proportions, and were primarily centered in the cities. Physicians, with their medicines, were powerless at preventing the outbreaks or impeding their progress. The sparse diets, narrowly limited to starch,

bread, and tinned foods, and the frequent famines that devastated France in 1789, and between 1792 and 1795, caused overt physical manifestations of diseases. Although they were clearly observable by the medical doctors, they were nevertheless not preventable. Indeed, it was frequently presumed that nutritional diseases such as pellagra and scurvy were infectious.

2.2. Malnutrition during the 19th-Century Industrial Revolution

The problem of food scarcity still persisted in some regions near the end of the 18th century. The winter of 1793–94 was particularly difficult for the French who were still caught in the turmoil of the revolution; many towns were without bread, meat, butter, and vegetables. From the Industrial Revolution arose technological advances such as the stethoscope, electro-magnetism, the steam engine, and more sophisticated chemical assays. It brought the field of medicine into a new light; public opinion began to slowly change in favor of the physician, a shift that became more pronounced with the introduction of vaccinations in 1796.

However, despite these wondrous achievements in medicine and science, Europe was again reminded of the unpredictable and uncontrollable deadly forces of nature; a cholera pandemic began to strike the European continent in the early 1830s, creating terror among its population. A new generation was witnessing, dumbfounded and bewildered, medicine's incapacity to halt the scourge that struck both Paris in 1832 and the London district of Soho in 1854; 14,000 cases of cholera and 618 deaths were reported (Summers, 1989). The inefficaciousness of medical treatments and the vulnerability of man had suddenly become obvious once again. It took the relentless investigative work of the anesthetist John Snow to finally demonstrate the water-borne nature of the disease. His thorough epidemiological inquest tied the pandemic to a leaking cesspool that contaminated the drinking water of a well in what is now known as Broadwick Street in London (Summers, 1989).

As a result of this devastation, the government began to dedicate funds toward improving the physical environment of the poor in the cities; it enacted legislation directed at the implementation of public hygiene practices. Preventative medicine, at a public health level, had suddenly become more meaningful and beneficial to the people than facilitating physician-based treatments at an individual level. Equally important was the work of an English reformer by the name of Sir Edwin Chadwick who instituted the national system of public health in England. He helped dispel the belief that it

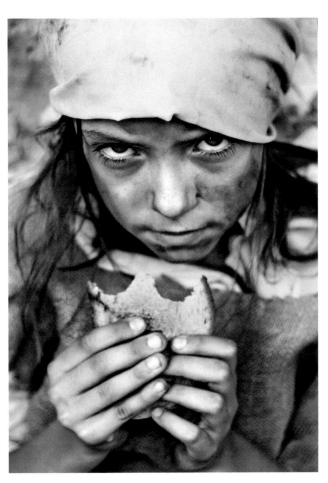

Figure 1.3. A portrait of a poor beggar child with a piece of bread in her hands. © NinaMalyna/Shutterstock.com.

was the moral fiber of the poor that was making them ill and clearly demonstrated instead that it was the impoverished environment in which the poor were living that was making them sick. He almost single-handedly convinced the English Parliament to implement a sophisticated network of sewers that helped significantly decrease death rates.

Chadwick revolutionized public health in Britain by implementing a school meals program, a School Medical Service (1907) and the National Insurance Act (1911), thus providing free medical services to much of the working class. These reforms eventually led to full social security in Britain by 1948. The cholera epidemic ended both because of dramatic improvements in public hygiene and because of the lower class's greater purchasing power, The labor class now worked long hours in factories and brought home larger incomes. It was, in truth, the overall improved living conditions of the people that caused disease and death rates to plummet, and not any single medical intervention (Summers, 1989; Margotta, 1996). The greater incomes meant that complete families

had greater access to milk, potatoes, and meats for consumption. The improved availability of food ensured that a broader population base was well fed and resistant to infections (Summers, 1989; Margotta, 1996).

There was, however, a problem with the purity of food supply both in Europe and in the U.S. that needed to be managed promptly. By 1880, greater urbanization took place with more rural farm workers gravitating to the cities for work. This coincided with technological advancements that permitted the establishment of large-scale urban manufacturing. Food production changed dramatically to accommodate the large population base, now conglomerating in the cities. It was in this context that numerous food vendors began popping up everywhere to make money. The industrial production and distribution scale of milk prompted deceptive practices among some farmers and dairy producers. They would frequently dilute milk with water in order to artificially and deceptively boost volumes, thus increasing sales. Unfortunately, the incidence of food poisonings jumped noticeably as volume rather than quality became the priority. Several historians claim that there was a public uneasiness surrounding the consumption of manufactured food because of the perceived deceptions wielded by many of the food distributors. According to Petrick, "the urbanizing process made acquiring and consuming all manners of food (from meat to milk to apples, flour and canned goods) an anxiety-provoking process, especially for the women who were largely responsible for purchasing and cooking the family's meals" (Petrick, 2011).

The first U.S. regulation of the food industry began when President Abraham Lincoln founded the U.S. Department of Agriculture (USDA) through an act of Congress in 1862. But it was the USDA's Division of Chemistry that was assigned the task, under the leadership of chief chemist of Dr. Harvey W. Wiley, of controlling food adulteration at the national level by establishing food processing standards. He campaigned strongly in support of passing the **Pure Food & Drug Act**, which was often referred to as the Wiley Act (Wiley, 1929). The Division of Chemistry soon was renamed the **Bureau of Chemistry** under the tutelage of Charles M. Whetherill in 1901. The federal government's goal with this act was to monitor the purity of the food supply, which, at that point, was a welcomed involvement as many impurities were contaminating the U.S. food supply. In fact, it was not uncommon in the 1800s to find pieces of metal, sand, rock, and organic material—such as bugs and rotting and diseased meat—in food products.

The period of 1870 to 1930 favored the development of the canning industry, which gradually contributed toward making the food supply safer; but there were problems or birthing pains, as it were, associated with canning at such a wide scale. For instance, chemists early on discovered that by adding small doses of sodium benzoate to food, they could extend the holding time of vegetables significantly after harvest, thus allowing year-round canning to take place. The Bureau of Chemistry's Harvey Wiley found, however, that even in small doses, sodium benzoate caused some gastrointestinal distress (Wiley, 1929). Also, acid foods such as tomatoes would cause the lead solder in cans to leach into tomatoes, thus increasing the risk of lead poisoning. The young and the elderly, according to historians, would commonly succumb to food-borne illnesses; it was dangerous to eat as there were no preparation standards governing the industry until the Pure Food and Drug Act of 1906. It has been argued that infant mortality during that time was elevated because of food-borne illnesses. Indeed, poor canning practices put the public at risk of botulism poisoning. Even as the 20th century began, scandals of food adulteration and chemical contaminations frequently made newspaper headlines.

In England, during that same time period, the problem of food adulteration was a reality as well, and it was finally exposed by Thomas Accum's book titled *Treatise on the Adulteration of Foods and Culinary Poisons*, published in 1820. As a chemist, Accum was able to accurately describe practices that shocked the nation. He documented the popular use of alum in wheat flour, in addition to lead and copper salts in beer brewing. Although he was run out of the country by food industry leaders for his scathing description of the food industry, other books followed that were equally condemning of food manufacturing practices.

In Europe, between 1880 and 1914, the food supply and food production were undergoing important changes that were concentrically driven by the nutrient paradigm and the hope for safe food. In the late 19th century, the discovery of vitamins fueled a new and deeper understanding of food, first from the scientific perspective, second in terms of the business of manufacturing and marketing foods, and third at the political level. It is here that legally binding government regulatory systems were set up to ensure consumer health and prevent fraud.[10] The nutrient paradigm propelled efforts toward nutrient-based standardizations and regaining the consumer's trust, which had been lost since the food adulteration scandals of the early 1800s. Petrick makes the case that the problem was very pervasive. She writes, "more and more American consumers, particularly women, really believed that foodstuffs could bring illness and death into their homes evidenced by their willingness to pay higher prices for special sanitary packaging, like glass bottles and tin cans"(Petrick, 2011).

The H.J. Heinz Company, founded in 1876, was one of the first companies in the late 19th century, along with National Biscuit Company (NABISCO), Quaker Oats, Kellogg's, and the Campbell Food company, to introduce very high-quality food preparation standards that the public was craving for. Their pricing was often twice that of unbranded foods, but the public, perturbed by the industry's nefarious practices, was willing to pay for pure products. Hence began the powerful U.S. food corporations that were soon going to establish a world presence. Advances in technology during the 1800s permitted the food industry to reach higher standards of quality and food safety.

A pure food supply was not a dream of unreachable idealism. It was becoming enforceable with the railway expansion across the continental U.S., which, thanks to electricity, now used refrigeration cars. Indeed, these innovative changes ensured year-round safe transportation of meat and other perishable foods. By the late 1800s, however, food manufacturing had attained such a sophisticated level of processing—most of it aimed at feeding pure food to a large population base—that many food ingredients were devoid of nutrients. In the U.S., there was a delayed awakening to the reality that a pure food supply could not be the complete answer to population health.

In the background of all these innovative changes was the 19th-century Health Reform Movement. Fueled by Sylvester Graham's writings and speeches, the Health Reform Movement by the 1830s was decrying the modernization of the food supply. Graham, in his *Treatise on Bread and Bread-Making,* encouraged his readers to purchase the best unrefined flour, in order to make homemade bread baked in their own ovens. In a time of vanishing self-sufficiency, writes Stephen Nissenbaum (1980), it was a call to return to traditional bread-making that fell pretty much on deaf ears. The American household was changing rapidly at the turn of the 19th century; it transitioned from a production unit—85% of manufactured goods were generated from the household in 1800—to a purchasing unit by 1830, with furniture, clothes, and food primarily bought outside the home. The dramatic decline in household self-sufficiency within a generation translated into a more commercial dependence on food. Between 1850 and 1900, writes Bobrow-Strain (2007) in *Kills the Body Twelve Ways,*the number of commercial bakeries increased 700 percent, causing homemade bread to drop from 80% to a mere 6% of all bread produced in the U.S. by 1920 (Bobrow-Strain, 2007). The white sliced bread saved valuable time, was shelf-stable, and was safe. Bobrow-Strain writes: "In an age obsessed with concerns about purity, hygiene, and sanitation, the new loaves were engineered to appear streamlined, sparkling clean, and whiter than white. After decades of enduring a reputation for filth, contamination, and foot dragging around pure-food legislation, commercial bakers had turned purity into their greatest selling point"(Bobrow-Strain, 2007).

In the cities the establishment of stores and shops facilitated access to ready-made white wheat-raised yeast breads, pastries, and cakes stabilized with preservatives such as alum, ammonia, sulphate of zinc, and even sulphate of copper (Nissenbaum, 1980). The pretty white cakes and breads were attractive and tasty, but the commercialization appeared to have been at the expense of pure ingredients.

2.3. Malnutrition and Food Impurity in the 20th Century

Interest in nutrition in the earlier part of the 20th century was quite high, as malnutrition was rampant around the U.S. Experts now believe that because Americans were consuming over 50% of their calories as white bread by the 1930s—a consequence of 1917 war rationing habits combined with the Great Depression's cheap food budgeting—malnutrition became a prominent problem in the U.S. Indeed, many U.S. soldiers were not fit enough to enter a war—one-third of those rejected for active duty were malnourished—let alone bring such a war to closure. The situation became so alarming that the Food and Nutrition Board of the National Academy of Sciences sponsored the National Nutrition Conference for Defense in 1941, as a forum to study strategies that could turn the malnutrition around. By the late 1930s and early 1940s epidemiologists unearthed a surprisingly elevated 75% prevalence of riboflavin deficiency among low-income high school kids; 65% prevalence of scurvy or near scurvy among government administration workers; and a 54% prevalence of preclinical vitamin A deficiency among low-income whites and blacks. In a New York City community health center that serviced low-income high school students, malnutrition was identified in 37% of students by 1938, writes Bobrow-Strain in his bestseller *White Bread (Bobrow-Strain, 2013)*. Malnutrition was rampantly affecting children and adults throughout the country because of a serious failure of public health nutrition programs. It was the recognition of this failure to realign the dietary habits of Americans, throughout the 1930s with healthy eating principles that galvanized support for a major shift in eating practices. The goal was to alter the population's preference for white bread in favor of brown whole wheat. But the public would not budge; it held on to its beloved white bread, like a shipwrecked mariner to its buoy. It was clear that in 1941 the U.S.'s intention to join the war effort was driving the resolve to eradicate malnutrition

nationwide one way or the other. Public health nutrition education programs and advertising could not get the masses to abandon their white impoverished bread. It became evident that the government could not impose new and healthy eating practices on the population. Such dietary shifts could only come from the inner soul of a people. That kind of change was not about to take place despite the fact that national security was at risk.

The white flour was so heavily processed around 1911—the consequence of the roller mills and the bleach treatments—that no nutrient in the flour could survive. As early as 1910, Harvey W Wiley, the head of the Food and Drug Administration (FDA), fought ardently against the practice of bleaching flour—a processing method that utilized nitrogen trichloride.[17] Even after he successfully got the practice of bleaching flour banned by a Supreme Court decision in and around 1911, Dr. Wiley was ousted from his position in 1912; the ban on bleaching was then bypassed by an overriding administrative decision. Dr. Wiley later described the bleached flour in a 1914 issue of *Good Housekeeping* as "white and waxy as the face of a corpse," according to a 1954 article by James Rorty in the *National Police Gazette* (Wiley, 1929).

Nitrogen trichloride continued to be used in flour right up to 1948 when British nutritionist Lord Mellanby conducted a series of well-controlled experiments on dogs in which running fits of epilepsy-like behaviors were noted in dogs fed trichloride-bleach bread. American nutritionists, wanting to verify the findings, were able to duplicate the same worrisome outcomes in guinea pigs, rats, monkeys, and rabbits. The FDA then banned nitrogen trichloride as a bleaching agent after 40 years of use. Not long after, despite protests by U.S. Army nutritionists, the FDA approved chlorine dioxide as a new bleaching agent. It is surprising that, despite the Supreme Court ban on bleach back in 1911, the practice of bleaching flour still continued and is currently permitted today.

The processing of the American food supply had become so extensive between 1900 and 1940 that there were reported cases of malnutrition even among U.S. Army recruits. It is in this context that the USDA issued the second version of the food guide in 1921 with specific quantities from each food group recommended to be purchased on a weekly basis. By 1923 a modified version of the guide was published to assist the nontraditional families with greater than five members. In the 1930s the harsh economic realities of the 1929 crash and the ensuing jump in food prices translated into hardship accessing good, wholesome, and affordable food. Numerous soup lines were set up to feed the many hungry unemployed men and their families

As early as the 1920s there was suspicion among food reformists that something wasn't right. Benjamin

R Jacobs, a nutritional biochemist who worked for the Bureau of Chemistry (now the FDA), which came under the control of the USDA by the 1920s, recorded the loss of nutrients in flour processing and began experimenting on methods of enrichment. To address the growing prevalence of malnutrition showing up among the masses of unemployed, Hazel Stiebeling, a USDA food economist, devised a new food guide in 1933, consisting of 12 food groups (Stiebeling, and Ward, 1933). This third official USDA food guide lasted until the end of the 1930s. One of the noteworthy features of this guide was that flour and cereals were encouraged to be eaten as desired. Again, the goal was to steer weekly purchases of foods in a way that would cover the nutritional requirements of families (Stiebeling, and Ward, 1933). However, this food guide may have misdirected the American population to liberally consume processed cereals and bleached flours that were devoid of nutrient content. Did the adoption of this food guide directly cause malnutrition to become rampant throughout the U.S.? It is hard to say, but it most certainly did not help matters. During the Depression access to protective foods such as milk, butter, tomatoes, citrus fruits, leafy, green, and yellow vegetables, and eggs was rather difficult. Stiebeling (1939), estimated at the time that the U.S. diet needed to contain 20% more milk, 15% more butter, about 70% more tomatoes and citrus, a 100% increase in vegetables, and finally a 35% jump in egg intake in order to reclassify it as *nutritionally good*. Evidently, the extent to which the American diet was suboptimal in the 1930s must have

been significant and worrisome enough for home economist Margaret Reid to write about what she labeled as "a hidden hunger that threatens to lower the zest for living and to sap the productive capacity of workers and the stamina of the armed forces" (Reid, 1943).

In the U.S., the meat industry, whether at the level of slaughterhouses or packing plants, was unsanitary and dangerous. Immigrant workers gravitated there because the work was so repugnant that the industry had trouble hiring U.S.-born workers (**Figure 1.4**). However, in 1906, author Upton Sinclair wrote *The Jungle*, a novel that gave a scathing depiction of the meatpacking industry as it existed in the U.S. at the beginning of the twentieth century. Sinclair recounts the abuses of the paid slave laborers, who worked long hours in such filthy working conditions that meatpacking became known as the most dangerous occupation in the U.S. *The Jungle* shocked the U.S. public with its vivid description of the filth of packing and slaughter houses. Even today that reputation still remains, according to Eric Schlosser's *Fast Food Nation*. Sinclair describes horrific scenes of workers accidently falling into meat grinders only to have their remains incorporated into the meat products and shipped to merchants for distribution in stores. Though he initially mistrusted Sinclair's depiction of the meat industry, President Theodor Roosevelt became convinced of the accuracy of Sinclair's description after he sent trusted Labor Commissioner Charles P. Neill and social worker James Bronson Reynolds to conduct surprise audits of the American meatpacking industry. Even with the schedule of audit visits leaked to the plants ahead

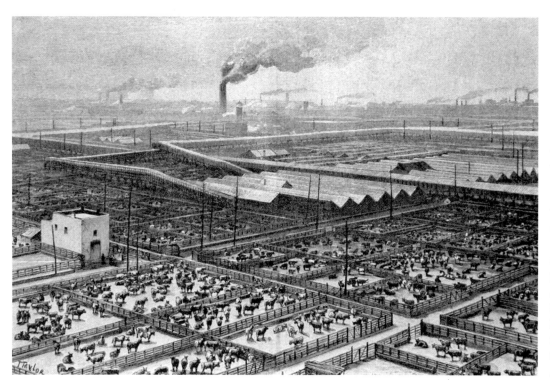

Figure 1.4.
Central slaughterhouse in Chicago. Engraving was by Maynar, from picture by painter Taylor. Published in magazine Niva, publishing house A.F. Marx, St. Petersburg, Russia, 1893 © Oleg Golovnev/ Shutterstock .com.

of time—plants had time at least to do some cleaning—the Neil-Reynold's report to the president confirmed that Upton Sinclair had indeed written an accurate portrayal of the industry.[11] As a result, President Roosevelt presented the report to Congress in 1906, which, along with public pressure arising from Sinclair's novel, facilitated the enactment of the **Federal Meat Inspection Act (FMIA)** and the **Pure Food and Drug Act** in 1906 (USDA).

The idea of achieving a pure food supply did not address whether it was permissible to use substitutes or additives in food. However, the new science and technology that was emerging from the chemical advances of the late 18th century and from the Industrial Revolution of the 19th century provided business with the ability to develop a wider assortment of cheaper foods in the U.S. and abroad.

Three things were occurring that hinted that this pure American food was scandalously compromised nutritionally. First, by the 1930s and 1940s, as the U.S. continued to manufacture and market cheap processed foods, food chemists were identifying sizable amounts of food products that were nutritionally deficient. Because of the vitamin era that had commenced by the early 20th century, there was a growing understanding that the nutritional quality of the food was paramount for individual and population health. Meanwhile numerous cases of malnutrition were popping up everywhere as the U.S. reliance on bleached white bread continued to grow (Bobrow-Strain, 2013). Second, the FDA in the U.S. and Health and Welfare in Canada began proposing a number of bills that would regulate the food industry, which by the 1930s had begun to increasingly refine food, removing important concentrations of nutrients and non-nutrients. One of the bills was intended to force the food industry to add some of those nutrients back, to "enrich" the foods they were producing. The bill was defeated in the U.S., but producers began enriching flour and cereals voluntarily after World War II. Even today, enrichment is not forced. In Canada, regulatory policies for the enrichment of processed flour were first past in 1964, requiring that all flour be enriched with thiamin, riboflavin, niacin, and iron. Third, as the 1950s, 1960s, and 1970s began to unfold, there was a sense that synthesized vitamins could be used by the food and pharmaceutical industries to mimic and surpass the quality of breast milk and food in general.

2.4. Nutrition and Chronic Disease in the 21th Century

2.4.1. The Prevalence of Chronic Disease in the U.S.

According to the CDC, the U.S.'s national health expenditure grew between 1980 and 2010 from $256 billion to $2.6 trillion, a jump that is so extraordinarily large that it defies the imagination (CDC, 2011).

In just 30 years, health care costs increased 915% in the United States, saddling the population with a cost burden that is currently at 16.4% of the national income. Moreover, there is something more disturbing taking place that many do not yet fully comprehend (CDC, 2011). A closer examination of health costs in 2010 reveals that slightly more than 50% of total health care expenditure originated from hospital care and physician/clinical services (Martin, 2010). Concomitantly, employer-sponsored insurance health coverage premiums for families rose 113%, which further oppressed industry and business with daunting expenses. Coincidentally, the prevalence of chronic diseases such as heart disease, diabetes, and cancer grew at such an alarming rate that the CDC now estimates that as much as 75% of the total health care costs are tied to chronic diseases (CMMS, 2012).

Since the 1980s, the most significant contributor to the epidemic of chronic diseases now observed in American society has been the surprising surge in obesity. Obesity is indeed at the source of conditions like hypertension, atherosclerosis, gallbladder disease, sleep apnea, type II diabetes, and depression, yet physicians will rarely address it. This is because it is a public health problem, but only 3.2% of the national health expenditure is dedicated to government-sponsored public health. The popular opinion that our current financial health care woes are the result of expensive insurance premiums may not be the complete truth. Often forgotten in the discussion is precisely the incredible rise in chronic diseases that is driving health care costs upwards. Indeed, the nature of the diseases with which we are afflicted is costly to manage and physically compromising.

In the last 20 years, health care costs have increased in tandem with the complexity of the illnesses of regular patients seen in family practice.

2.4.2. The Causes and Prevention of Chronic Disease.

In the 1970s a more complex and significant epidemiological problem of overeating and poor quality food consumption began to emerge. Scientists identified four key dietary components that, when eaten in excess, were considered deleterious to human health: saturated fat, cholesterol, fat, and sodium. It was, however, the Senate Select Committee on Nutrition and Human Needs (1977), headed by Senator George McGovern in 1977, that introduced the Dietary Goals for the United States. They represented a dramatic shift that focused on dietary excesses as opposed to the nutrient deficiencies that ravaged American society throughout the 1930s

(Bobrow-Strain, 2013). The public was given quantitative dietary guidance aimed at keeping dietary carbohydrates to between 55% and 60% of calories, cholesterol (which was entirely animal-based) at <300 mg per day, maintaining total fat at <30% of calories, saturated fat low, sugar at <15% of calories, and finally salt at <3 g per day. The main reason was that higher risks of obesity, diabetes, heart disease, and stroke had been tied to high fat, sugar, saturated fat, and cholesterol intakes, whereas the ingestion of high salt got tagged to hypertension. Recommendations were also made to lower salt, sugar, and meat intake specifically, in order to decrease fat and saturated fat. These dietary goals met with much resistance from a food industry that did not take kindly to the recommendation to eat less. Notably, the National Dairy Council, the Salt Institute, the United Egg Producers, the American National Cattlemen's Association, and the National Livestock and Meat Board reacted violently to the goal of eating less meat and eggs. Moreover, the American Medical Association insisted that medical issues needed to be managed by the physicians and not the government. Finally, the scientific community was not convinced that there existed sufficient data to support the cut-off goals. The pressure by the food industry was powerful and noticeably influenced the committee to sanitize the guidelines in order to ensure the support of the meat and egg industries. Marion Nestle (2002), author of *Food Politics*, argues that the wording was

significantly amended to reflect a more positive slant on meat consumption. Hence, the initial recommendation to decrease meat ingestion was changed to "decrease consumption of animal fat, and choose meats, poultry, and fish which will reduce saturated fat intake." This was a positive slant that the meat industry could live with, but it poorly reflected the scientific findings that tied many cancers to populations that consume abundant meat. The meat industry insisted that the committee destroy all copies of the original report. McGovern was voted out of office not long after, and the industry made it very clear to bureaucrats never to challenge meat consumption again, writes Marian Nestle (2002).

Despite the forceful hand of industry in manipulating the outcomes of the guidelines, a deleterious label did nevertheless get pinned on red meat, eggs, and whole milk—the public intuitively knew it needed to cut back on fats, and that generally meant meat. Indeed, these dietary components were enshrined into the "foods to avoid" category of every dietitian's therapeutic pamphlet for the treatment of cardiovascular disease. Consequently, red meat and butter consumption did eventually decline over time leading to a drop in saturated fat intake, whereas poultry and fish intake increased. This shift in eating patterns should have caused the incidence of heart disease to decline in the population, if not for the nefarious trans-fats, generated from all the margarines and shortenings that flooded the marketplace in

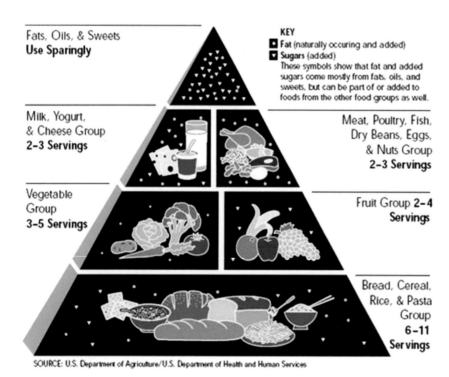

SOURCE: U.S. Department of Agriculture/U.S. Department of Health and Human Services

Figure 1.5. USDA Food Guide Pyramid.

response to the bad press given to animal fat as early as the 1980s. The true nefarious atherogenicity of the trans-fats emerged with vengeance 13 years later, when Willett and his colleagues[29] from Harvard confirmed in 1993 that trans-fats did cause LDL cholesterol to increase, HDL cholesterol (good cholesterol) to drop, and markers of inflammation to increase. The Harvard group was following up on suspicions, raised by Welsh researchers (Thomas et al. 1981), that trans-fats might contribute to ischemic heart disease.

Meanwhile, in 1979 two main events of significance occurred in the nutrition world. First, the USDA formulated a new food guide that was comprised of five food groups (**Figure 1.5**) with an additional group (fats, sweets, and alcoholic beverages) added to the top of the pyramid. This was an important departure from the classic role of the food guide, which was to optimize the nutrition quality of the diet. This new guide was more pragmatic in that it clearly identified, for the first time, overeating as a significant problem and pointed the finger at a culprit food group that needed to be consumed sparingly. Because of the controversy that emerged from the 1977 Dietary Goals for the U.S., a task force sponsored by the American Society of Clinical Nutrition (1979), was established to bring scientific credence to the recommendations. It became evident from many nutrition research studies that excessive salt, fat, and sugar intakes led to chronic diseases. The findings of this task force were released by the Department of Health, Education and Welfare, now the Department of Health and Human Services (DHHS); for the first time, strong scientific evidence supported the importance of reducing excessive calories, fat, cholesterol, salt, and sugar in the diet in order to diminish the risk of diseases. The Surgeon General of the United States included the findings of this task force in his 1979 Healthy People Report, which concluded that it was indeed possible to lower disease rates by adopting healthy dietary practices. From this report, the 1980 Dietary Guidelines for Americans was published; again it encountered considerable opposition, especially from the food industry, who opposed the extrapolations that were made in order to formulate practical ways to create a healthful diet. Consequently, a Dietary Guidelines Advisory Committee was formed to provide scientific validity to these recommendations. When the 1985 Dietary Guidelines for Americans were issued 5 years later, there was very little opposition from the medical community and the food industry. It just was no longer debatable that dietary intakes, at the population level, needed to be modified. Davis and Saltos point out that the 1985 Guidelines resembled those of 1980, except that "Some changes were made to provide guidance about nutrition topics that became more prominent

after 1980, such as following unsafe weight-loss diets, using large dose supplements, and drinking of alcoholic beverages by pregnant women" (Davis and Saltos, 1999).

The Surgeon General's 1988 Report on Nutrition and Health emphasized the importance of embracing new dietary trends as a way of quelling the disturbing rise in chronic disease. Davis and Saltos write: "Recommendations in the report promoted a dietary pattern that emphasized consumption of vegetables, fruits, and whole-grain products foods rich in complex carbohydrates and fiber and of fish, poultry without skin, lean meats, and low-fat dairy products selected to reduce consumption of total fat, saturated fat, and cholesterol" (Davis and Saltos, 1999). Then, in 1989, the National Research Council's Food and Nutrition Board reiterated the Council's Diet and Health Report that stressed the importance of decreasing total fat and saturated fat intakes to maintain a low risk of contracting chronic diseases and some cancers. The report quantified specific limits on fat, notably: <30% calories as total fat; <10% calories for saturated fat; and <300 mg for dietary cholesterol. Also, there was an emphasis to consume a minimum of five servings per day of fruits and vegetables and at least six servings per day of breads, cereals or legumes. The USDA, in concert with the National Cancer Institute, the Produce for Better Health Foundation, CDC, and the American Cancer Society, attempted in 1991 to popularize fruits and vegetables by instituting a nationwide Eat 5 a Day nutrition education campaign (**Figure 1.6**).

The program was an almost complete failure, as it did not manage to budge the population from its dislike of fruits and vegetables. Meanwhile, for the very first

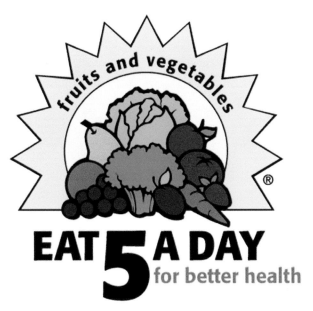

Figure 1.6. The Eat 5 a Day nutrition campaign.

time, the 1990 Dietary Guidelines for American, jointly produced by DHHS and the USDA, formulated a numerical goal for saturated fat, <10% of calories, and reiterated the previously established total fat cut-off, <30% of calories. As early as 1988, the USDA began work to graphically represent the food guide, which since 1985 was known only in USDA publications as *A Pattern for Daily Food Choices*. The decision to use the *Food Pyramid* in 1992 (**Figure 1.5**), as a visual reference to healthy eating in the U.S., was applauded as a strategic public health move that could ideally convey that breads and cereals in addition to fruits and vegetables needed to be prominent in the diet (Davis and Saltos, 1999; Frazao, 1999). The pyramid was also supportive of the Eat 5 a Day campaign (**Figure 1.6**), which, when broken down, translated into a recommended minimum of three vegetables and two fruits every day. But the pyramid situated all fats at the tip of the pyramid, thereby intimating that all fats should be minimally consumed. This was consistent with the low-fat strategies for the management of weight loss and heart disease, popular in diets. The limitation was that, even at that time, it was known that omega-3 fats were beneficial and that omega-9 monounsaturated fats, like olive oil, appeared to provide substantive health benefits. In the end, the scientific consensus was that all fats were not equal. In 2005, the pyramid was completely revised

again (**Figure 1.7**), but this time, the emphasis was placed on balancing between exercise and food.

A new webpage was attached to the guide from which, more detailed servings could be obtained (Davis and Saltos, 1999; Frazao, 1999). However, there were several problems that were conveyed by this rather vague but colorful pyramid. First, it appeared to intimate that exercise allows consumers to walk right over the pyramid, and eat whatever they want; second, the elongated pyramid strips did not communicate very well that some food groups need to be consumed in greater proportion than others. Here again, the government deflected any harm away from the meat industry by creating a purple strip that appeared only slightly smaller in size to that of vegetables. The research leading up to the 2005 publication of the pyramid did not convincingly demonstrate that red meat was linked to colorectal cancer. At best, conclusions from the 1997 review by the World Cancer Research Fund could only indicate a possible association between red meat and colorectal cancer; they concluded that red meat intake should be less than 3 oz-wt per day. Other reviews found moderate links. Murtaugh (2004) pointed out, in a 2004 commentary, that up until that time, the data did not differentiate between the impact of regular consumption of large versus small and infrequent quantities of red meat in relations to colorectal

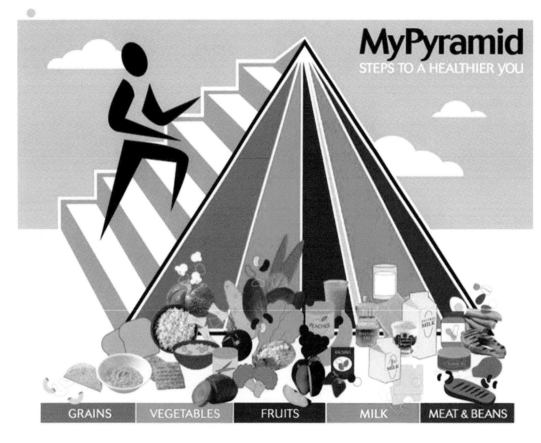

Figure 1.7. The New USDA food pyramid.

cancer incidences. Prior to 2005 however, the research did imply that total fat and, in particular, animal fat in addition to processed, salted, cured or smoked meats, subject to high temperature treatments and nitrite compounds, were tied to rectal cancer. In truth, the most convincing studies were the large-scale prospective Nurses' Health and U.S. Professional Men's cohorts. The data were studied by Walter Willett and his team from Harvard in the early to mid-1990s and showed a significant association between colon cancer and red meat specifically (Giovannucci et al. 1994; Willett et al. 1990). The implications were worrisome and difficult to contest as they clearly implicated long-term red meat consumption to cancer.

What wasn't clearly established was whether small amounts of meat consumption were considered a risk and whether red meat's impact was related more to a displacement of protective cruciferous vegetables out of the diet, rather than to an intrinsic problem with red meat (Murtaugh, 2004). Indeed Trustwell (2002) points out that, early in the new millennium, red meat was equivocally associated with cancer depending on exposure, quantities consumed and whether meat was lean or fatty. Not even the data linking cured and processed meats to cancer was convincing. In 2011, the USDA came up with the MYPLATE food guide (**Figure 1.8**) in answer to the criticism that the 2005 pyramid created too much confusion (Davis & Saltos, 1999; Frazao, 1999). So, in this more recent version, a familiar dinner plate usurps a pyramid. Here, the consumer more easily understands

that the goal is to match the MyPlate image, in which fruits and vegetables makeup 50% of the plate, grains represent 25%, and protein foods, roughly 25%.

According to the Willett team (Pan et al 2012) from Harvard, there is substantial evidence now showing significant risk of diabetes, cardiovascular disease, and cancers with red meat intake. Analyzing data from both the Health Professionals Follow-up Study (HPFS) and the Nurses' Health Study (NHS), Willett and colleagues (Pan et al. 2012) were able to show that both processed and unprocessed red meat intake was associated with a greater overall mortality. This more recent 2006 data showed that the risk of mortality noticeably and significantly declined when fish, nuts, poultry, legumes, and low-fat dairy replaced red meat. Close to 38,000 men and 83,000 women were followed in the two prospective cohorts, and dietary information was compounded over time to measure the effect of long-term intake. It appears that the stronger evidence emerging since 2005, which disapprovingly waved an accusatory finger at processed and unprocessed red meats, caused the USDA to design the MyPlate image so as to emphasize protein foods rather than meat. The MyPlate website offers the consumer the opportunity to generate a Daily Food Plan or a Daily Food Plan Worksheet based on age and approximate calorie requirements. For instance, an individual 18 years or older who requires 2,400 kcal/day, can click the website located at www.ChooseMyPlate.gov to create a food plan consisting of the following daily servings from each of the food groups:

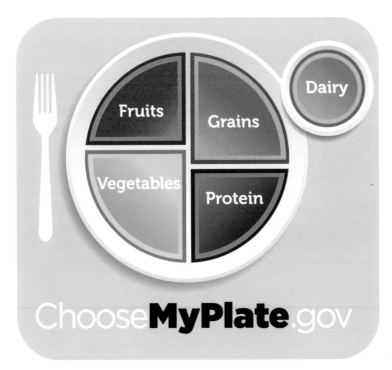

Figure 1.8. The MyPlate food guide.

GRAINS: 8 oz equivalent/day
VEGETABLES: 3 cups equivalent/day
FRUITS: 2 cups equivalent/day
DAIRY: 3 cups equivalent/day
PROTEIN FOODS: 6.5 oz equivalent/day

The Daily Food Plan Worksheet allows the consumer to enter the foods consumed and the daily food choices from each of the groups. In addition, physical activities can be documented in addition to the total daily time commitment. The goal is 150 minutes per week. The next interesting option is called the **Super-Tracker** which consists of a food tracker and a physical activity tracker. The food tracker allows the consumer to measure calories and serving equivalents from each of the food groups, which are graphically displayed in the form of histograms. This newer food guide is meant to be more interactive, but only time will tell if it will be efficacious in abating the obesity crisis and its many derived secondary diseases.

NOTE

1. Significant sections of this chapter have been copied from chapter 2 of the textbook: IT'S ALL ABOUT NUTRITION: Saving the Health of Americans, and blended into this chapter with the permission of the copyright holder © David Bissonnette

REFERENCES

1. American Cancer Society. (2002). Cancer Prevention and Early Detection, facts and figures 2002. Available at http://www.cancer.org/downloads/STT/CPED2002.pdf.
2. American Society of Clinical Nutrition (1979) Task Force. The evidence relating six dietary factors to the nation's health. *American Journal of Clinical Nutrition* (Supplement); 32:2621-2748.
3. Anand, P., et al. (2008). Cancer Is a Preventable Disease That Requires Major Lifestyle Changes. *Pharmaceutical Research* 25 (9): 2097–2116.
4. Bissonnette. D.J. (2013). It's All About Nutrition: Saving the Health of Americans. New York: University Press of America, 217pp
5. Bobrow-Strain, A. (2013) White Bread: A Social History of the Store-Bought Loaf. Beacon Press, Boston, pp: 272.
6. Bobrow-Strain, A. (2007) Kills A Body Twelve Ways: Bread Fears and the Politics of What to Eat Gastronomica: The Journal of Food and Culture; 7(3): 45-52 retrieved August 8, 2013 from: http://comenius.susqu.edu/biol/312/killsabodytwelveways.pdf.
7. Brothwell, D and Brothwell, P. (1969) Ancient Peoples and Places Food in Antiquity: A Survey of the Diet of Early People. Thames and Hudson, London 248 pp.
8. Carrick, P. (2001) Medical Ethics in the Ancient World. Washington, DC: Georgetown University Press. 108pp.
9. Cartwright, C. Origins and History of Homeopathy. Available at http://www.oxford-omeopathy.org.uk/home-opathy-origins-history.htm.
10. Centers for Medicare and Medicaid Services, Office of the Actuary, National Health Statistics Group. *National Health Care Expenditures Data.* January 2012.
11. Centers for Disease Control and Prevention. Rising Health Care Costs Are Unsustainable. April 2011. Retrieved December 30, 2013 from: http://www.cdc.gov/workplacehealthpromotion/businesscase/reasons/rising.html.
12. Craik, E. Hippocratic diaita (1995). In: Wilkins, J., Harvey, D., and Dobson, M.(Eds) Food in Antiquity. University of Exeter Press, Exeter UK. p: 353-350.
13. Craik, E. (1997). "Diet, Diaita and Dietetics." In: *The Greek World.* A. Powell, (ed.).pp.387-402.London: Routledge.
14. Davis, C. and Saltos, E. (1999) Dietary Recommendations and How they have Changed Over Time. In: America's Eating Habits: Changes and Consequences. Frazao, E (Ed) USDA Economic Research Service, Washington, DC. USDA. Agriculture Information Bulletin No. (AIB-750): 33-50.
15. Frazao, E. (1999) America's Eating Habits: Changes and Consequences. USDA Economic Research Service. USDA. Agriculture Information Bulletin No. (AIB-750) 494 pp, May Retrieved Sept 10, 2013 from: http://www.ers.usda.gov/publications/aib-agricultural-information-bulletin/aib750.aspx.
16. Frericks, RR. Broad Street Pump Outbreak. UCLA Department of Epidemiology, School of Public Health website. Available at http://www.ph.ucla.edu/epi/snow/broad streetpump.html.
17. Giovannucci E, Rimm EB, Stampfer MJ, Colditz GA, Ascherio A & Willett WC (1994): Intake of fat, meat and fiber in relation to risk of colon cancer in men. Cancer Res. 54, 2390 – 2397.
18. Grant, M. (1995) Oribasios and Medical Dietetics or the Three Ps. In: Wilkins, J., Harvey, D., and Dobson, M.(Eds) Food in Antiquity. University of Exeter Press, Exeter UK, p: 371-379.
19. Kishlansky, M., Geary, P., and O'Brien, P. (1991). *Civilization in the West.* New York: HarperCollins, p. 1021.
20. Maher, M. (2002) The Odyssey of the Ancient Greek Diet. Totem: The University of Western Ontario Journal of Anthropology 10(1):7-13.
21. Margotta, R. (1996). *The Hamlyn History of Medicine,* ed. Paul Lewis. London: Institute of Neurology.
22. Martin AB et al. (2012). Growth in US Health Spending Remained Slow in 2010; Health Share of Gross Domestic Product was Unchanged from 2009. *Health Affairs.*
23. Miller, Judith A. (1999). *Mastering the Market: The State and the Grain-Trade in Northern France, 1700–1860.* Cambridge, UK: The Press Syndicate of the University of Cambridge.
24. Milner, J. A. (2000) Functional Foods: The US perspective. *American Journal of Clinical Nutrition* 71(6):1654s–1659s.

25. Murtaugh, MA (2004) Meat Consumption and the Risk of Colon and Rectal Cancer. Current Medical Literature: Clinical Nutrition; Vol. 13 Issue 4, p61.

26. Nestle, M. (2002) Food Politics: How the Food Industry Influences Nutrition & Health. Berkeley, CA, University of California Press, 457pp.

27. Nikiforuk, A. (1996) The Fourth Horseman: A Short History of Plagues, Scourges and Emerging Viruses. Toronto: Penguin Group. 262pp.

28. Nissenbaum, S. (1980) Sex, Diet, and Debility in Jacksonian America. Chicago: The Dorsey press. American Society and Culture: The Dorsey Collection, 198pp

29. Pan A, Sun Q, Bernstein AM, Schulze MB, Manson JE, Stampfer MJ, Willett WC, Hu FB: (2012) Red meat consumption and mortality: results from 2 prospective cohort studies. *Arch Intern Med* 172:555-563.

30. Peterson, M. S. (1965). Establishing a modern food industry: The resources of the technical literature. In: *Food Technology the World Over.* Vol 2, ed. M. S. Peterson and D. K. Tressler. Westport, CT: AVI Publishing, pp. 3–37.

31. Petrick, G. B. (2011). 'Purity as life': H.J. Heinz, religious sentiment, and the beginning of the industrial diet. *History and Technology* 27(1): 37–64

32. Plato. Critias and Timaeus (2005). Chicago: Acheron Press.

33. Popkin, B., & Nielson, A. (2003). The World's Increased Intake of Sugar. *Nutrition Research Newsletter* 22 (12):7.

34. Reid, MG. (1943) Food for the People. New York, John Wiley & Sons, 653pp

35. Richards, M.P. (2002) A Brief Review of the Archeological Evidence for Palaeolithic and Neolithic Subsistence European Journal of Clinical Nutrition 56.

36. Rowlands, G. (2009) France 1709: Le Crunch. *History Today* 59(2). Available at http://www.historytoday.com/guy-rowlands/france-1709–le-crunch.

37. Stiebeling, HK. (1939) Better Nutrition as a National Goal: The Problem, Year Book of Agriculture p 380.

38. Stiebeling, H.K. and M. Ward.(1933) *Diets at Four Levels of Nutrition Content and Cost.* U.S. Department of Agriculture, Circ. No. 296, 59 pp.

39. Summers, Judith. *Soho — A History of London's Most Colourful Neighborhood,* Bloomsbury, London, 1989, pp. 113-117.

40. Suzuki, N. (2010) Popular Health Movement and Diet Reform in 19th Century America *The Japanese Journal of American Studies* 21:111–137

41. Thomas LH, Jones PR, Winter JA, Smith H. (1981) Hydrogenated oils and fats: the presence of chemically-modified

42. Trustwell, AS. (2002) Meat Consumption and Cancer of the Large Bowel. European Journal of Clinical Nutrition 56, Suppl 1, S19–S24.

43. U.S. Senate Select Committee on Nutrition and Human Needs. (1977) Dietary Goals for the United States, 2nd ed. Washington, DC, U.S. Government Printing Office.

44. USDA Food Safety & Inspection Service. FSIS History. Available at http://www.fsis.usda.gov/wps/portal/informational/aboutfsis/history.

45. Vial, R. (1989) Moeurs, santé et maladies en 1789; Societe des editions Londreys, Paris, pp.327.

46. Vickery, K.F. (1936) Food in Early Greece. University of Illinois, 97 pp.

47. Wiley, HW. (1929). The History of a Crime Against the Food Law. Milwaukee, WI, Lee Foundation for Nutritional Research, 413pp

48. Willett WC, Stampfer MJ, Colditz GA, Rosner BA & Speizer FE (1990): Relation of meat, fat and fiber intake to the risk of colon cancer in a prospective study among women. New Engl. J. Med. 232, 1664 –1672.

49. World Health Organization (2001) Cancer Strategy [Online] Available: retrieved August 2012 http://www.who.int/ncd/cancer/strategy.htm.

50. World Health Organization. (2001). Cancer Strategy. Available at http://www.who.int/ncd/cancer/strategy.htm.

51. Wynder, E. L., and Gori, G. B. (1977). Contributions of the environment to cancer incidence: an epidemiologic exercise. *J Natl Cancer Inst* 58: 825–32.

CHAPTER 2

KEY NUTRITION CONCEPTS AND CALCULATIONS

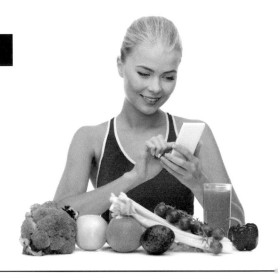

2.1. PRINCIPLES OF HEALTHY EATING

2.1.1. Population Dietary Guidelines to Achieving Health.

Nutrition research, consisting of long-term prospective studies, often lasting several decades, has concluded that nutrition plays a key role in the prevention of chronic diseases. In fact, it is currently believed that dietary and lifestyle modifications can prevent or at least minimize the development of chronic diseases derived from being obese or overweight, which, according to 2008 statistics, cost $147 billion per year to manage. This is because obesity leads to a vast array of costly chronic conditions that significantly affect quality of life, notably cardiovascular disease, hypertension, type 2 diabetes, sleep apnea, gastrointestinal diseases (diverticulosis, gallbladder), degenerative disorders (arthritis), asthma, and some cancers. Therefore early intervention programs are encouraged in obesity and overweight prevention, as dietary preferences and habits are more strongly established during infancy and childhood. In the last 10 years type 2 diabetes has become a worrisome epidemic, now affecting 8% of adult Americans; if the current trend is not changed, type 2 diabetes is forecasted to afflict 33% of adult Americans by 2050.

It is somewhat reassuring to note that changes in lifestyle do wield a tremendous impact in the prevention of some cancers. Although overall cancer incidence has declined in recent years, cancer nevertheless claimed more lives in individuals younger than 85 years old than heart disease. In fact between 14% and 20% of all cancer deaths are tied to overweight and obesity. The overall dietary trend to reduce total fat intake has shown some benefit, notably the reduction in the incidences of breast and ovarian cancers.

In the year 2000, the U.S. Department of Health and Human Services (HHS) put forth the Healthy People 2010 guidelines to help people reduce the risk of lifestyle-related disease. Unfortunately, it made very little progress toward this goal. So here we are again with the Healthy People 2020 trying to decrease chronic disease caused by diet and overweight. Healthy People 2010 guidelines recommend these key goals to reduce death rates from the most significant threats:

1. Attaining high-quality, longer lives free of preventable disease, disability, injury, and premature death.
2. Achieving health equity, eliminating disparities, and improving the health of all groups.
3. Creating social and physical environments that promote good health for all.

4. Promoting quality of life, healthy development, and healthy behaviors across all life stages. (HHS, www. healthypeople.gov)

These new recommendations recognize the role of not only diet and exercise but also the policies and environments in schools, work sites, health care organizations, and communities that encourage or discourage healthy behaviors. All these environments need to have policies and practices that are influential in managing healthy body weights in the population (Healthy People 2020, Overview). In fact, nutrition and weight status are among the top 42 topics that are addressed in Healthy People 2020.

The Healthy People 2020 define a healthy diet as respecting these three precepts:

1. Consume a variety of nutrient-dense foods within and across the food groups, especially whole grains, fruits, vegetables, low-fat or fat-free milk or milk products, and lean meats and other protein sources.
2. Limit the intake of saturated and *trans* fats, cholesterol, added sugars, sodium (salt), and alcohol.
3. Limit caloric intake to meet caloric needs. (*Dietary Guidelines for Americans*; U.S. Department of Health and Human Services [DHHS], 2005)

The *Dietary Guidelines for Americans* (DGAs), formulated every 5 years by the USDA and HHS, are meant to identify the key dietary and lifestyle issues that need to be addressed for population disease reduction. They represent the practical ways of achieving part of the Healthy People goals. The 2010 DGAs revolve around two major concepts: The first is that calorie balance needs to be maintained in order to ensure that healthy weights are achieved over the long term. The second is that nutrient-dense foods and beverages need to be regularly consumed in order to optimize health in the population. The DGAs are based on two food patterns: the USDA Food Patterns that are described in the food pyramid or the MyPlate figure and their vegetarian adaptations, and the DASH (Dietary Approaches to Stop Hypertension). There are four main recommendations to help the U.S. population achieve long-term health and well-being by following these eating patterns:

1. Reduce the prevalence of overweight and obesity by reducing overall calorie intake and increasing physical activity.
2. Consume more plant-based foods, seafood, and fat-free or low fat dairy products.
3. Significantly reduce the intake of foods containing added sugars and solid fats.

4. Meet the 2008 Physical Activity Guidelines for Americans. (*Dietary Guidelines for Americans*; U.S. Department of Agriculture [USDA], 2010)

The importance of regular exercise cannot be overstated in these public health goals, as it is now recognized that regular vigorous exercises are associated with a 30% decline in colon cancers, which is the third greatest cause of cancer death in the U.S.

There is good evidence to suggest that weight management practices should revolve around consuming the recommended macronutrient distribution ranges for the three macronutrients. Maintaining low total fat intake and relatively high carbohydrate intake is one of the key strategies to ensure modest weight loss over time. The more efficacious strategies for significant weight reduction always include a notable investment in moderate to strenuous exercise on a regular basis. But first, the focus of this discussion will be on the main macronutrients.

2.1.2. Carbohydrates

Carbohydrates can be structurally organized into simple sugars consisting in monosaccharides (glucose, fructose, galactose), disaccharides (sucrose, lactose, maltose), trioses (glycerose), tetroses (erythrose), and pentoses (ribose). Each disaccharide consists of two monosaccharides linked together by a glycosidic bond (Figure 2.1). The chemical structure in Figure 2.1 illustrates how glucose linked to fructose through a glycosidic bond creates sucrose, otherwise known as table sugar. Similarly, when galactose combines with glucose there is a formation of lactose, which is the main sugar in milk. And when two glucose monosaccharides are linked, maltose is formed; this sugar is used extensively by the food industry as an additive to beverages, beer, cereals, pasta, and a variety of other processed food products requiring slight sweetening. There are in addition more complex carbohydrates called oligosaccharides (cellulose), consisting of 3 to 10 monosaccharides, or polysaccharides (starch or glycogen) entailing more than 10 monosaccharides.

Starches are divided into either **amylose** or **amylopectin** (Figure 2.2). Amylose consists of unbranched glucose molecules linearly connected by glycosidic α (1-4) bonds. Only about 21% of starches consist of amylose, whereas between 75% to 83% of starches are made up of amylopectin. Indeed, potato, rice, and wheat, which are abundantly consumed in the U.S., are elevated in amylopectin, whereas the foods elevated in amylose tend to be referred to as *resistant starches*. Foods such as starchy fruits (banana) and vegetables (parsnips), beans, and legumes (soybeans, kidney beans, navy beans, lentils)

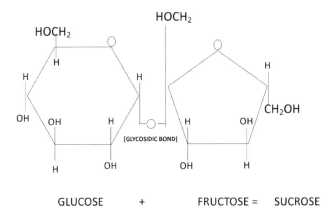

Figure 2.1. Chemical structure of sucrose.

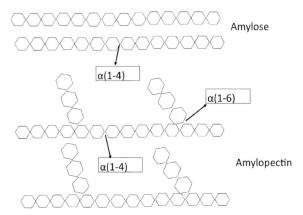

Figure 2.2. Dietary starches.

tend to be elevated in the resistant starch called amylose. Amylopectin is a branched starch consisting of both the linear glycosidic α (1-4) and the branched ß (1-6) bonds (Figure 2.2). Because of the extensive branching, it is easier for enzymes to digest the amylopectin, thus leading to a greater glucose release into the blood compared with amylose, which has no branching. The Recommended Dietary Allowance (RDA) for carbohydrates is 130 g per day for adults and is derived from the smallest amount that is required for adequate brain nourishment and to prevent ketosis. Ketone production—resulting in ketosis or rise of ketones in the blood—occurs from an incomplete metabolism of fat because of inadequate carbohydrate intake.

Cellulose is an indigestible plant starch made up of glucose molecules linked together by ß (1-4) bonds that are nonhydrolysable by the amylase enzyme; this is because the amylase enzyme can only hydrolyze α (1-4) glycosidic bonds. Cellulose is most abundantly found in legumes, which represent an excellent source of fiber. Most of the North American diet consists of starches (60%), whereas 30% is made up of sucrose and 10% consists of lactose. (Keim et al., 2006).

The Acceptable Macronutrient Distribution Range (AMDR) was established by the USDA in order to give guidance for dietary planning for three specific purposes: (1) to ensure a low prevalence of chronic disease in the population, (2) to ensure the adequate intake of essential nutrients by the population, and (3) to encourage adequate energy intake to sustain physical activity and weight maintenance (NAS, 2005c). The premise of these recommendations is grounded in the understanding that any significant deviance in the proportion of macronutrients consumed regularly by a population can lead to a higher prevalence of chronic disease. Consequently, epidemiologists have concluded that the AMDR for carbohydrates needs to be between 45% and 65% of energy needs or

DRI calories in order to ensure adequate fiber, sugar, and complex starch intake and energy. In practical terms this translates into between 225 g and 325 g of carbohydrates on a 2,000 kcal diet. (NAS, 2005b)

It has been shown that when **added sugar** represents more than 25% of total calories required, there is a concomitant decline in the nutrient quality of the diet. Indeed, studies demonstrate that a mean added sugar intake of 26.7% of total energy leads to lower intakes of vitamins A, C, B_{12}, folate, calcium, phosphorus, magnesium, and iron. (NAS, 2005b) An ideal recommended amount of added sugar has not been established, but a maximal amount of 25% of calories is accepted as tolerable. Added sugar has been identified as the sugar added to food during processing and includes, glucose, dextrose, sucrose, fructose, high fructose corn syrup, corn syrup, molasses, syrups, maltose, and lactose. Similarly, when **total sugar** is <25% of DRI calories, there is no apparent reduction of any nutrients in the diet (NAS, 2005b).

To ensure gastrointestinal health and prevent cardiovascular disease it is imperative that the majority of carbohydrates come from complex starches like whole grain starches and fruits and vegetables. No RDA has been established for fiber but there is an adequate intake (AI) value determined to be 14 g of fiber per 1,000 kcal for women, which equates to 25 g per day, and 38 g for adult men, which also equates to 25 g per day. The position paper of the American Dietetic Association on the health implications of fiber is in agreement with this AI. These recommendations are in stark contrast with the mean 15 g per day usually consumed by U.S. adults. The health benefits of fiber are clearly stated in the position paper: "Many fiber sources, including cereal bran, psyllium seed husk, methylcellulose, and a mixed high-fiber diet, increase stool weight, thereby promoting normal laxation. Stool weight continues to increase as fiber intake increases, but the added fiber tends to normalize defecation frequency to one bowel movement daily and gastrointestinal transit time to 2 to 4 days."

Dietary fiber helps prevent chronic disease over the long term in several ways. First, **soluble fiber** captures cholesterol and bile and evacuates them through the stool, thus helping in the control of blood cholesterol. Second, soluble fiber captures environmental toxins that have contaminated our food, thus reducing exposure time to the enterocytes of the gastrointestinal wall because of the rapid transit time of stool loaded with fiber. This reduced transit time means that carcinogens in foods have a reduced exposure to the lining cells of the intestine, thus minimizing the chance of DNA mutations that can eventually lead to cancer. Third and finally, **insoluble fiber** facilitates a more rapid movement of stool through the colon (large intestine). It is well recognized that high-fiber diets can decrease the overall risk of colon cancer in the population (Keim et al. 2006).

2.1.3. Proteins

Proteins make up the structural components of cells, hormones, and enzymes. They consist of amino acids—there are 20 amino acids in all—which are made up of an amino-N group (NH3), a carboxyl-carbon group (COOH), and a side chain (R), responsible for the distinct identity of each amino acid. (See Figure 2.3.)

It is the nitrogen specifically that distinguishes proteins from the other macronutrients. Amino acids are categorized as indispensable, dispensable, or conditionally indispensable. There are a total of nine indispensable amino acids, represented in Table 2.1. *Indispensable* means that all of the nine amino acids must be contained in the dietary protein in order to be used in the structural synthesis of body proteins in the form of muscle, collagen, and various organs. *Conditionally indispensable* means that the amino acids are indispensable only in certain individuals, like premature infants or individuals with certain conditions like metabolic abnormalities resulting from trauma or disease. In neonates, for instance, the transformative action of enzymes may be subdued or compromised enough to slow the synthesis of cysteine from methionine, thus making cysteine conditionally indispensable. In catabolic states, glutamine synthesis may also be limited, thus necessitating the inclusion of

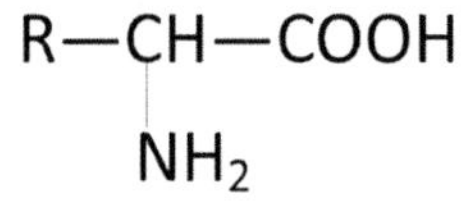

$$R—CH—COOH$$
$$NH_2$$

Figure 2.3. Chemical structure of an amino acid.

TABLE 2.1. The Dispensable and Indispensable Amino Acids

Indispensable	Conditionally Indispensable	Dispensable
Leucine	Arginine	Alanine
Isoleucine	Cysteine	Aspartic Acid
Valine	Glutamine	Asparagine
Threonine	Glycine	Glutamic acid
Lysine	Proline	Serine
Histidine	Tyrosine	
Methionine		
Phenylalanine		
Tryptophane		

glutamine in the nutritional support of ICU patients. The *dispensable* amino acids (alanine, aspartic acid, asparagine, glutamic acid, and serine) can be endogenously synthesized and are not required from the diet.

Proteins come in various lengths and complexity. Two amino acids linked together by a peptide bond are called a dipeptide; three amino acids linked together by peptide bonds are called tripeptide; and more than three amino acids linked together are called polypeptides. The skeletal muscle, representing 43% of the total protein in the body, is the most abundant protein structure. Skin and blood each contain 15% of protein, while visceral protein found in the liver, heart, and spleen accounts for 10% of total body protein. The most abundant proteins in the body can thus be identified as **actin, myosin, collagen,** and **hemoglobin.** After fats, proteins are the second largest energy reserve in the entire body. In malnutrition, it is specifically the noncollagen proteins that become vulnerable to catabolism resulting in protein erosion.

Proteins of **high biological value** come from animals and contain all nine indispensable amino acids. Proteins of lower biological value, originating from plants, are either limited or low in some indispensable amino acids. For instance, the protein in bread, pasta, and rice is of poor biological value and cannot be used to synthesize bodily protein structures such as muscle. Vegetable protein, as a rule, is considered protein of lower biological value. This means that vegans, who only consume vegetables, legumes, and grains in their diet, must apply the vegetarian principle of **protein complementarity** in order consume all the nine essential amino acids in sufficient amounts to allow protein synthesis to take place in the body. Lysine is the amino acid that is limited in grains whereas methionine is the one limited in legumes. When both legumes and grains are combined together they complement each other's limiting amino acid, thus providing all nine essential amino acids.

While qualitatively, the amino acid makeup of the diet is important, the quantity of protein consumed plays a paramount role in meeting the nutritional needs of individuals. Consequently, protein requirements can be established very accurately using the body weight or, less accurately, using caloric requirements. Body weight serves as a reliable standard, as it better reflects individual needs. Reliable nitrogen balance studies have confirmed the RDA for the adult body equals 0.8 g per kg body weight (BWT) of protein for normal maintenance; for a 70-kg person requiring 2,500 kcal per day this represents 9% of DRI calories. The WHO reports that 97.5% of the population appears to require 0.83 g protein per kg body weight per day. Justifiably then, it can be advanced that 10% of DRI calories represents a reasonable estimation of minimal protein requirements. The DGAs (2010) recommend that dietary protein intake be between 10% and 35% of total caloric intake. The WHO stresses that protein intakes should not exceed 1.5 g per kg BWT. This amount represents 16.8% of DRI calories for a 70-kg person requiring 2,500 kcal/day. Most individuals do not benefit from ingesting more than 1.33 g per kg BWT in terms of gaining additional protein mass during heavy exercise. For a 70-kg person requiring 2500 kcal per day, this translates into 15% of calories. Most adults, according to the WHO, will likely meet their protein requirements by consuming between 10% and 15% of DRI calories.

2.1.4. Lipids

Lipids encompass a broad assortment of compounds that include triglycerides, phospholipids, and sterols, all playing roles in the structure of cells and the makeup of hormones. Fats in the form of triglycerides represent 95% of all lipids consumed in the diet, and they are a significant source of energy for the body. Structurally, 90% of the triglyceride consists of fatty acids, and the other 10% is made up of glycerol, which is the 3-carbon backbone to the triglyceride (see Figure 2.4). A fatty acid attaches to each of the hydroxyl (OH) ends of the glycerol molecule to form a triglyceride.

Fatty acids are carbon chains of varied lengths ranging between 2 and 26 carbons, all recognizable by the

C—OH

C—OH

C—OH

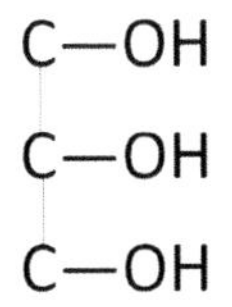

Figure 2.4. Glycerol molecule—the backbone of the triglyceride molecule.

methyl end (CH3-) and the carboxyl group (-COOH) at the other end of the chain (Jones & Kubow, 2006).

$$CH3==CH—CH==CH—CH—COOH$$

These fatty acids can be in the form of saturated fatty acids, cis-polyunsaturated (n-6 or n-3) fatty acids, cis-monounsaturated (n-9) fatty acids, or trans fatty acids.

Saturated: CH3—CH—CH—CH—COOH

Polyunsaturated: CH3—CH==CH==CH—COOH

Structurally, the polyunsaturated fats have two or more double bonds; they tend to be of vegetable origin and in a liquid state at room temperature. The two exceptions are coconut and palm oils, which are saturated despite being of vegetable origin. Saturated fats have no double bonds and will be a hard consistency at room temperature. It is these fatty acids that are the main substrate for the absorption of fat-soluble vitamins (A, D, E, and K). In other words, without fats, humans and mammals in general would not be able to absorb fat-soluble vitamins.

Each gram of fat (fatty acid) contains 9 kcal, or more than twice the energy found in either protein or carbohydrates. There is no RDA or AI for fat, nor is there a tolerable upper intake level (UL) because of insufficient data. There is, however, an AMDR for the healthy consumption of fat that varies between 20% and 35% of DRI calories. Studies have found that fat intakes of 42% to 50% of calories have been associated with prothrombodic blood markers and coagulation factors. And while in a diet-crazed society total fat intake appears to be the main concern for weight loss purposes, the quality of the fat holds an equal if not superior position of importance.

The idea that fat played a critical role in animal growth and development was proposed by German nutritional scientist H. Aron in 1918. It wasn't clear whether it was the absence of fatty acids or of the vitamins solubilized in them that was responsible for compromised growth. It took until 1929 before George and Mildred Burr—two nutritional biochemists from the Department of Botany at the University of Minnesota—showed that fats were essential for the normal growth of rats, independent of vitamin content. When fed a fat-free diet, rats began showing symptoms of scaly skin, tail necrosis, impaired growth and fertility, and increased death rates. However, one of the rat groups was treated with a 20% lard diet, which reversed the symptoms; the lard consisted of 10% linoleic acid. It was this work and other studies that confirmed the notion of essential fatty acid deficiencies. Other studies demonstrated that it was specifically the **linoleic (C18:2n-6)** and **α-linolenic**

Dietary Fat Content Comparisons

	Saturated Fat	Poly-unsaturated Fat / Linoleic Acid	Alpha-Linolenic Acid	Mono-unsaturated Fat
Canola oil	7	11		61
Flaxseed oil	10	48		26
Safflower oil	10		Trace	14
Sunflower oil	12		1	16
Corn oil	13		1	29
Olive oil	15	1		75
Soybean oil	15		8	23
Peanut oil	19		Trace	48
Cottonseed oil	27		Trace	19
Lard	43		1	47
Beef tallow	48		1	49
Palm oil	51		Trace	39
Butterfat	68		1	28
Coconut oil	91			7

Legend:
Saturated Fat
Poly-unsaturated Fat
Linoleic Acid
Alpha-Linolenic Acid
Mono-unsaturated Fat

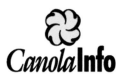

CanolaInfo

CanolaInfo 306.387.6610   www.canolainfo.org   canolainfo@canolainfo.org

Figure 2.5. Dietary fat content comparisons of different types of oils. Used with permission from the Canola Council of Canada. ©2007, CanolaInfo.

acids (C18:3n3) that were finally recognized as essential. This meant that individuals have to consume fatty acids via the diet in order to acquire their nutritional and physiological benefits. This was confirmed in 1958 when infant formula lacking fatty acids led to essential fatty acid deficiency in human infants.

There is currently not enough data to develop an RDA for the fatty acids. Consequently an AI was derived from the mean intake of a community that showed no signs of deficiency (NAS, 2005e). The AI for linoleic acid was determined to be 17 g per /day for young men and 12 g per day for young women. The AMDR for linoleic acid is 5% to 10% of DRI calories. The AI for α-linolenic (n-3) acid is 1.6 g per day for men and 1.1 g per day for women. There is also an AMDR for α-linolenic acid: 0.6%–1.2% of DRI calories. Most of the oils consumed in the U.S. are polyunsaturated oils such corn, soy, and sunflower seed oils (Figure 2.5). They are mostly composed of linoleic acid. Maintaining the intake of linoleic within 5% to 10% of DRI calories is a worthy objective, as there is some concern that exceeding the 10% cut-off may create a pro-oxidant and pro-inflammatory environment that could dispose the body to develop chronic diseases such as cardiovascular disease and cancer. The DGAs caution the population to consume less than 10% (<10%) of DRI calories in the form of saturated fat. This is because excess saturated fat in the diet has been associated with increased risk of heart disease.

Monounsaturated fats (MUFAs) are of the omega-9 (n-9) classification, chemically represented by no more than one unsaturated bond:

$$CH3—CH—CH==CH—CH—CH—COOH$$

Although not considered essential in the diet, MUFAs have been found to decrease the risk of heart disease. Current intakes of MUFAs in the U.S. are estimated to be between 12% and 13% of energy intake, and roughly 50% comes from animal meat fat such as beef tallow and lard (Figure 2.5). Clinical trials have shown that ingesting 17%–33% percent of calories as MUFAs reduced risk factors; individuals who experienced therapeutic benefits ingested even 33%–50% of total energy as MUFAs.

Taking these studies into account, from a minimalist approach it can be argued that a healthy diet should not contain less than 11% of DRI calories as MUFAs, even though no official RDA, AI, or AMDR for MUFAs currently exists. Here is the basic rationale: Given that saturated fats should be <10% of DRI calories, and that polyunsaturated fats (mostly made of omega-6 linoleic acid) should remain between 5% and 10% of DRI calories, this leaves 11% of DRI calories coming from the omega-9 MUFAs. If MUFA intake is suboptimal (<11%

DRI calories), then, in order to meet 30% of energy in the form of fat, the rest of the fatty acids must be supplied from either saturated fats, polyunsaturated fats, or both. This is not desirable given the importance of keeping the pro-oxidant n-6 fats between 5% and 10% of DRI calories (USDA, Chapter 11). The oils with the highest content of MUFA fats are olive, peanut, and canola oils (Figure 2.5).

These findings were confirmed by the 1986 Seven Countries study, which reported that with higher intakes of monounsaturated fats, there was a significant decline in mortality rates from coronary heart disease (USDA, Chapter 11). A meta-analysis conducted on several feeding trials has concluded that overall MUFAs appear to modestly decrease LDLs and increase HDLs. A number of studies published since the early 1990s also report that monounsaturated fat intake—oleic acid specifically—offers good protection against cancers of the breast, colon, and possibly the prostate. Although some study findings have been equivocal about oleic acid's protective role against cancer, there is convincing evidence that olive oil consumption—rich in oleic acid—protects against breast cancer specifically (USDA, Chapter 11).

2.2. DETERMING THE DIETARY REFERENCE INTAKES (DRIS)

In the United States, the Institute of Medicine (IOM), one of the arms of the National Academy of Sciences, works to establish dietary guidelines. Specifically, the IOM's Food and Nutrition Board (FNB) has established specific dietary reference intakes (DRIs) for macronutrients in order to ensure long-term population health. The DRIs consist of a set of recommended intakes for various nutrients that fused together the U.S. Recommended Dietary Allowance and the Canadian Recommended Nutrient Intakes (RNIs). The joint effort was coordinated by Standing Committee on the Scientific Evaluation of Dietary Reference Intakes (DRIs) of the FNB in collaboration with Health Canada. (See Figure 2.6.)

To determine the DRIs, the FNB gathered together several key nutritional markers: the Recommended Dietary Allowances (RDAs, the adequate intakes (AIs), the estimated average requirements (EARs), and the tolerable upper intake levels (ULs). Each of these levels represents a different type of nutritional measurement, which will be defined in the following sections.

Establishing the RDA. The Recommended Dietary Allowance (RDA) refers to dietary nutrient intake levels that need to be ingested by the individual to achieve an adequate intake of the specific nutrient. In that sense, a nutrient's RDA is the *minimum* intake goal deemed

necessary, over a prolonged period, to meet the nutritional needs of an individual for that nutrient; it is not an optimal level to attain but rather the minimal intake for good health for most people. The FNB defines the RDA as "the average daily dietary nutrient intake level sufficient to meet the nutrient requirement of nearly all (97 to 98 percent) healthy individuals in a particular life stage and gender group" (Chapter 1, FNB).

The RDA is determined first by establishing the EAR of that nutrient. The variability of nutrient needs is determined between individuals and then a standard deviation is calculated. The RDA is then established by adding 2 standard deviations to the EAR as indicated in equation 2.1:

(2.1) RDA = EAR + (2 × *SD* requirement)

If the data are insufficient to calculate a standard deviation, then a standard 10% coefficient of variability (CV) is determined. In this case the RDA would be established using equation (2.2):

(2.2) RDA = EAR + 2 (0.1 × EAR) = 1.2 × EAR

Establishing the EAR. The estimate average requirement (EAR) is defined by the FNB as "the average daily nutrient intake level estimated to meet the requirement of half (50%) the healthy individuals in a particular life stage and gender group." From a practical perspective the EAR does not represent the nutrient needs of an individual and thus cannot be used as a specific goal to be achieved by an individual. Rather, the EAR is intended to estimate the nutrient needs of a population, and in that sense any randomly selected individual would have a 50:50 chance that the EAR matches their true requirement of a specific nutrient. The EAR can only be used as a standard with which a mean population intake could be compared. Similarly, it can be used in order to plan the diet of a group. A government can use the EAR to establish agricultural policies for a nation or determine food relief strategies for a population affected by famine. Also, defining the size and makeup of a food relief basket, for those on social assistance, would be done using the EAR.

Establishing the AI. Adequate intake levels (AIs) are defined by the FNB as "the recommended average daily intake level based on observed or experimentally determined approximations or estimates of nutrient intake by a group (or groups) of apparently healthy people that are assumed to be adequate—used when an RDA cannot be determined." The RDA sometimes cannot be determined because of limitations in scientific methodology; therefore estimations are made based on sound observations. Researchers will identify a healthy population in

DIETARY REFERENCE INTAKES (DRIs)

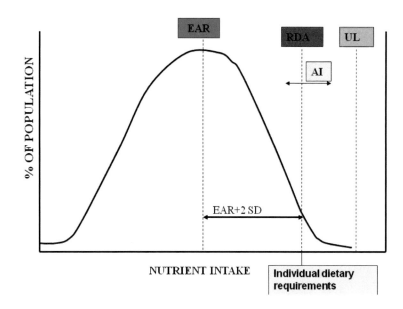

Figure 2.6. Dietary reference intakes (DRIs).

which no underlying nutritional deficiency diseases are observable. Next, they conduct a random dietary assessment of a large sample of the population in order to measure the median nutrient intake. The FNB affirms that the AI is expected to meet or surpass the amount deemed necessary for normal growth, the maintenance of good health, and adequate blood circulating nutrients concentrations. However, because the AI is much less accurately derived than the RDA, there is the possibility the AI may overshoot an individual's true RDA. Hence, when using AIs in individual counseling, much more caution must be used.

Establishing the UL. The tolerable upper intake level (UL) is the highest cut-off below which the majority of the population runs no risk of experiencing nutrient toxicity. The UL is not to be considered as an intake goal; rather it is the *top* level at which an individual' nutrient intake can be considered safe without fear of toxicity. It is noteworthy that the risk of toxicity increases exponentially the more a person exceeds the UL. The need to establish a UL arose with the extensive food fortification that has taken place since the 1990s and the widespread use of nutrient supplements.

2.3. MEANINGFUL CALCULATION CONCEPTS

When making nutritional calculations, there are several definitions to keep in mind. First, there are two broad categories of nutrients: *Macronutrients* consist of carbohydrates, protein, and fat, and *micronutrients* consist of vitamins, minerals, and microminerals. (A third category is water, which must be consumed daily in order to maintain a water level of 50%–70% of the total body weight).

There is, in addition, a very distinct category called the *non-nutrient components* of food. These components are not considered essential for life since their absence from the diet does not cause specific deficiency symptoms. However, these non-nutrients include a broad spectrum of phytochemicals that shield the biological system from known chronic diseases like many types of cancers and heart disease. It is not surprising, then, that simple diets consisting of varied fruits, vegetables, breads, and cereal products, which contain these non-nutrients, consumed in abundance with dairy and little meat, are consistent with good health.

Making nutritional calculations also requires familiarity with measurement units. Measuring food intake, body energy requirements, and body composition are key to determining levels of macro- and micronutrients in a population. In the U.S., we use the English-based "customary units" of pounds, ounces, feet, and so on. Researchers outside the U.S. (and sometimes in the U.S. as well) present these levels in metric measurements. Table 2.2 presents the important metric conversions that are necessary to convert customary units into metric units.

Accuracy in conversion is crucial in making key assessments of food intake, body energy requirements, and body composition. Many of the formulas in the nutritional and medical sciences use metric weights in kilograms, height in either meters or centimeters, and fluid measurements in milliliters and grams. This becomes relevant when estimating food and fluid intake and prescribing infusion rates of medicines and nutrients in the area of nutritional support and critical care medicine. For instance, protein prescriptions can be given according to body weight. A patient weighing 175 lb who is not obese can be given protein as 1.2 g per kg body weight. How many grams can this patient receive? First, the person's body weight must be converted to kilograms. How is that done? Table 2.2 indicates that 1 lb = 0.454 kg. So multiply the weight in pounds by 0.454 kg: the patient weighs 79.45 kg. If you are prescribing 1.2 g protein per kg body weight, then his target protein intake will be 95.34 g or (rounded down) 95 g of protein.

Another important calculation is the estimation of resting energy needs and total energy needs (this includes physical activities). These energy requirements are estimated using height in centimeters or meters and weight in kilograms. Hence, if a 35-year-old man, 5 feet 10 inches tall and weighing 250 lb, is seen in outpatient clinic for weight loss, the dietitian will have to calculate the patient's energy needs—at his current weight—in order to determine how many calories he normally requires for weight maintenance. In the initial consultation, the goal is to assess the patient's current dietary practices and compare the estimated caloric or energy intake with the recommended intake. The patient's weight will need to be converted to kilograms (250 lb × 0.454 kg/lb =113.5 kg). His height in centimeters will need to be established (70 inches × 2.54 cm/inch = 177.8 cm). In order to determine the resting energy expenditure (REE), these values are then inserted into a gender-specific formula, along with his age, in order to determine REE. This is the amount of calories needed to maintain a stable weight while lying in the supine (laying-down) position. The preferred formula for non-hospitalized patients is the Mifflin equation:

TABLE 2.2. Metric Conversion Table

US Customary Units	Metric Units
1 lb (16 oz weight)	454 g (0.454 kg)
1 oz (weight)	28 g
1 oz (fluid measure)	30 ml
2.2 lb	1 kg
1 inch	2.54 cm = 0.0254 m
1 measuring cup	240 ml
1 tablespoon	15 ml
1 foot = 12 inches	30.48 cm

REE for Men = $[10 \times$ (weight in kg) $+ 6.25 \times$ (height in cm)$] - [(5 \times A$ (age) $- 5)]$

REE for Women = $[10 \times$ (weight in kg) $+ 6.25 \times$ (height in cm)$] - [(5 \times A$ (age) $+ 161)]$

In order to establish this man's REE, it would be necessary to enter his weight in kilograms (113.5 kg), his height in centimeters (177.8 cm), and his age in years (35 years) into the formula above, to get this:

REE = $[(10 \times 113.5$ kg$) + (6.25 \times 177.8$ cm$)] - [(5 \times 35) - 5] = (1135 + 1111.25) - 170 = 2,076$ kcal

The patient's REE would be documented as 2,076 kcal per day. This resting energy level normally represents 60%–75% of total energy expenditure (TEE). The thermic effect of food equals 10% of TEE, and exercise generally ranges between 15% and 30% of TEE (McArdle et al., 2013). A person who exercises above the norm would be closer to an REE of 60% whereas one with exercise levels below the norm would have an REE closer to 75%. The next step would involve multiplying the REE by an activity factor based on whether the patient is generally (a) sedentary, (b) mildly active, (c) moderately active, (d) very active, or (e) extremely active (see Table 2.3).

Shirley Gerrior and colleagues propose two sets of formulas based on gender that can help establish the TEE without having to first establish the REE.

FOCUS BOX 2.1

EXERCISE 1: It's important to be able to convert units from one measurement system to another accurately and with ease. Study Table 2.1 and then test yourself. If a patient weighs 198 lb and his height is 5 feet 10 inches, determine his weight in kilograms and his height in centimeters.
Answer 1: Weight in kilograms = 198 lb × 0.454 kg/lb = 89.89 kg. Height in centimeters = 5 feet 10 inches = 70 inches. 70 inches × 2.54 cm/inch = 177.8 cm or 1.78 m.
EXERCISE 2: If a person consumes 3 cups of milk in a day, how many milliliters does he consume?
Answer 2: 1 cup = 240 ml. 3 cups = 720 ml (or 0.72 liters).

For men:

TEE = $[864 - (9.72 \times age_{years})] + [PA \times ((14.2 \times wt_{kg}) + (503 \times ht_{meters}))]$

For women:

TEE = $[387 - (7.31 \times age_{years})] + [PA \times ((10.9 \times wt_{kg}) + (660.7 \times ht_{meters}))]$

TABLE 2.3. Activity Factors (AF) for Different Levels of Activity for the Determination of Total Daily Energy Needs

Activity Level	Activity Factor Male	Activity Factor Female
Sedentary	1.0	1.00
Mildly active	1.12	1.14
Active	1.27	1.27
Very active	1.54	1.45
Extremely active	2.20	2.00

Gerrior S, et al. (2006). *Prev Chronic Dis.* [serial online] 3(4):1–4. Available at http://www.cdc.gov/pcd/issues/2006/oct/06_0034.htm.

Using the previous case of the 35-year-old, 250-lb man, it would now be possible to estimate his total energy expenditure if we determine that he is "active." The completed equation would then be expressed as follows:

TEE = $[864 - (9.72 \times 35)] + [1.27 \times ((14.2 \times 113.5 kg) + (5.03 \times 1.78 m))]$

It is possible to simplify the expression of the above equation:

TEE = $[500] + [1.27 \times (1612 + 9.02)]$
TEE = $500 + 2059 = 2559$ kcal/day

Thus 2560 (rounded up from 2559) represents the total energy expenditure (TEE) of the 250-lb, 35-year-old active male. It would good to practice using this formula and the Mifflin equation for determining REE.

2.3. ORGANIZING NUTRIENTS

Table 2.4 introduces an organized system of nutrient classifications: macronutrients, micronutrients, and water. Note that the caloric value of food comes only from the macronutrients and alcohol.

```
CARBOHYDRATES: 4 kcal/g
PROTEIN: 4 kcal/g
FAT: 9 kcal/g
ALCOHOL: 7 kcal/g
```

Dieticians and others need to be able to competently convert grams (g) of macronutrients into calories (kcal). For example, a patient who is prescribed 300 g of carbohydrates needs to be ingesting 1,200 carbohydrate kcal (300 g × 4 kcal/g). In a similar fashion, 100 g of protein intake is equivalent to 400 kcal of protein (100 g × 4 kcal/g). Finally a patient who consumes 65 g of fat daily is taking in a total of 585 kcal/day (65 g × 9 kcal/g).

2.3.1. Principle of a Diet Prescription

Using the patient's total energy requirements, a dietitian can assign a specific percent of those calories to carbohydrates, protein, and fat. Afterward, the goal is to convert those calories to grams of carbohydrates, protein, and fat. The final step is to assign servings of foods that match up with the macronutrient assignment.

Let's look at an example. Mr. Johnson's DRI for calories is 3,545 kcal per day. The dietitian assigns a percent of the total calories to carbohydrates consistent with DRGs for Americans, somewhere between 45% and 65% of DRI calories. She decides to calculate 60% of calories as carbohydrates; this means about 532 g of carbohydrates (3,545 kcal × 0.60, divided by 4 kcal/g). Similarly, she prescribes 15% of DRI calories to protein, which is consistent with the recommended DRG range (10%–35% of DRI calories); this translates into 133 g of protein per day (3,545 kcal × 0.15, divided by 4 kcal/g). And finally, the dietitian assigns 25% of the calories to fat. The dietician recommends that one-quarter of all daily energy intakes come from fat (DRGs recommend 20%–35%); this means the patient would consume a total of 98.5 g of fat (3545 kcal × 0.25, divided by 9kcal/g). It is important that the percent values add up to 100% (60% + 15% + 25%). In summary then, the patient's complete dietary prescription is outlined here:

```
CARBOHYDRATES: 532 g
PROTEIN: 133 g
FAT: 99 g
```

Table 2.4 provides a broad understanding of the requirements for nutrients. Water-soluble vitamins are needed on daily basis because they are not stored extensively in the body. Fat-soluble vitamin requirements, on the other hand, are based on monthly needs, as the body reserve for these vitamins tends to be more significant since they are stored in organs—most notably the liver—and adipose tissue.

The importance of water cannot be overstated as it is directly tied to blood volume and blood pressure. Insufficient volume of water consumed translates into less blood volume and pressure and consequently a lower rate of oxygen reaching the tissue. Lower oxygen rates can lead to dizziness and fatigue. This makes sense if you consider that water makes up between 50% and 70% of a normal body weight. The body water reserve is divided between the extracellular and intracellular fluids, and it therefore plays a critical role in facilitating the movement of anions and cations in and out of the cells. The standard fluid prescription is based on energy requirements and as such will vary depending on whether a person is sedentary, active, or very active. Additionally, fluid need is tied to whether the environment is temperature-controlled or hot. A temperate environment will necessitate 1.0 ml per kcal. When the temperature is warm to hot, the fluid prescription will vary between 1.0 and 1.5 ml per kcal. In practical terms, this means that a male athlete training outdoors in 85F° weather, and who requires 3,400 kcal per day, may need to ingest a total daily fluid load of up to 5.1 liters (3,400 kcal × 1.5 = 5,100 ml).

TABLE 2.4. Macronutrients and Micronutrients

Nutrient Class	Definition	Function
1.0 MACRONUTRIENTS	Large molecular structures of carbon, oxygen, and hydrogen	They provide energy.
Carbohydrates	Complex starches, simple sugars, and fiber	They provide a rapid source of calories: 4 kcal/g; they are the only source of fiber with recommended intake of 14 g/1,000 kcal.
Proteins	Molecularly made up of amino acids, which consist of nitrogen, oxygen, carbon, and hydrogen	They are essential for building muscle and cell structures linked to organs and vascular network; they provide energy: 4 kcal/g.
Fats	A broad category of lipids consisting of triglycerides, phospholipids, and sterols	They ensure neurological development and absorption of fat-soluble vitamins; provide 9 kcal/g and essential fatty acids: linolenic (omega-3) and linoleic (omega-6) fatty acids.
2.0 MICRONUTRIENTS	Small organic compounds	They are required from the diet in small amounts in order to ensure proper biological functions.
Fat-soluble vitamins	Vitamins A, E, D, K	They require fat for absorption and storage; requirements are given in monthly amounts.
Water-soluble vitamins	Vitamins making up B complex and C	They require an aqueous environment for absorption and are not stored; requirements are given in daily amounts.
Major minerals	Ca, P, Mg, Na, K	Requirements are given in daily amounts.
Microminerals	Fe, Cu, Cr, Zn, F	Requirements are given in daily amounts.
3.0 WATER	1.0–1.5 ml/kcal	50–70% of the body is made up of water.

REFERENCES

1. Bissonnette DJ. (2013). *It's All About Nutrition: Saving the Health of Americans.* Lanham, MD: University Press of America.

2. Burr GO, Burr MM. (1929). A new deficiency disease produced by the rigid exclusion of fat from the diet. *J Biol Chem.* 82:345–367.

3. Gerrior S, et al. (2006). An easy approach to calculate estimated energy requirements. *Prev Chronic Dis.* [serial online] 3(4):1–4. Available at http://www.cdc.gov/pcd/issues/2006/oct/06_0034.htm.

4. Healthy People 2020. Nutrition and Weight Status. Available at http://www.healthypeople.gov/2020/topicsobjectives2020/overview.aspx?topicid=29#one.

5. Johnson PK, Sabate J. (2006). Nutritional implications of vegetarian diets. In: Shils ME, Shike M, Ross AC, Caballero B, Cousins RJ, eds. *Modern Nutrition in Health and Disease.* 10th ed. Philadelphia: Lippincott Williams & Wilkins; 1638–1654.

6. Jones PJH, Kubow S. (2006). Lipids, sterols and their metabolites. In: *Modern Nutrition in Health and Disease,* 10th ed., ed. Shils ME, Shike M, Ross AC, Caballero B, Cousins RJ. Philadelphia: Lippincott Williams & Wilkins, pp. 92–135.

7. Keim NL, Levin RJ, Havel PJ. (2006). Carbohydrates. In: Shils ME, Shike M, Ross AC, Caballero B, Cousins RJ, eds. *Modern Nutrition in Health and Disease.* 10th ed. Philadelphia: Lippincott Williams & Wilkins; 62–82.

8. Lupton, JR, Trumbo PR. (2006). Dietary fiber. In: Shils ME, Shike M, Ross AC, Caballero B, Cousins RJ, eds. *Modern Nutrition in Health and Disease.* 10th ed. Philadelphia: Lippincott Williams & Wilkins; 83–91.

9. Mathews DE. (2006). Proteins and amino acids. In: Shils ME, Shike M, Ross AC, Caballero B, Cousins RJ, eds. *Modern Nutrition in Health and Disease.* 10th ed. Philadelphia: Lippincott Williams & Wilkins; 23–61.

10. Mifflin MD, et al. (1990) A new predictive equation for resting energy expenditure in healthy individuals. *Am J Clin Nutr.* 51:241–247.

11. National Academy of Sciences (NAS), Institute of Medicine, Food and Nutrition Board. (2005a). Dietary Reference Intakes for Energy, Carbohydrate, Fiber, Fat, Fatty Acids, Cholesterol, Protein, and Amino Acids (Macronutrients). Chapter 1: Introduction to Dietary Reference Intakes. Available at http://www.nal.usda.gov/fnic/DRI//DRI_Energy/21-37.pdf.

12. National Academy of Sciences (NAS), Institute of Medicine, Food and Nutrition Board. (2005b). Dietary Reference Intakes for Energy, Carbohydrate, Fiber, Fat, Fatty Acids, Cholesterol, Protein, and Amino Acids (Macronutrients). Chapter 11: Macronutrients and Healthful Diets. Available at http://www.nal.usda.gov/fnic/DRI//DRI_Energy/769-879.pdf.

13. National Academy of Sciences (NAS), Institute of Medicine, Food and Nutrition Board. (2005c). Dietary Reference Intakes for Energy, Carbohydrate, Fiber, Fat, Fatty Acids, Cholesterol, Protein, and Amino Acids (Macronutrients). Chapter 13: Applications of Dietary Reference Intakes for Macronutrients. Available at http://www.nal.usda.gov/fnic/DRI//DRI_Energy/936-967.pdf.

14. National Academy of Sciences (NAS), Institute of Medicine, Food and Nutrition Board. (2005d). Dietary Reference Intakes for Energy, Carbohydrate, Fiber, Fat, Fatty Acids, Cholesterol, Protein, and Amino Acids (Macronutrients). Chapter 10: Proteins and Amino Acids. Available at http://www.nal.usda.gov/fnic/DRI//DRI_Energy/589-768.pdf.

15. National Academy of Sciences (NAS), Institute of Medicine, Food and Nutrition Board. (2005e). Dietary Reference Intakes for Energy, Carbohydrate, Fiber, Fat, Fatty Acids, Cholesterol, Protein, and Amino Acids (Macronutrients). Chapter 8: Dietary Fat: Total Fat & Fatty Acids Available at http://www.nal.usda.gov/fnic/DRI//DRI_Energy/422-541.pdf.

16. Academy of Nutrition and Dietetics. (2008). Position Paper of the Academy of Nutrition and Dietetics—Health Implications of Dietary Fiber. *JADA* 108(10):1716–1731. Available at http://www.eatright.org/About/Content.aspx?id=8355.

17. Academy of Nutrition and Dietetics. (2013). Position Paper of the Academy of Nutrition and Dietetics: The Role of Nutrition in Health Promotion and Chronic Disease Prevention. *J Acad Nutr Diet.* 113:972–979. Available at http://www.eatright.org/About/Content.aspx?id=8381.

18. U.S. Department of Agriculture, U.S. Department of Health and Human Services. (2010). *Dietary Guidelines for Americans, 2010.* 7th ed. Washington, DC: U.S. Government Printing Office.

19. U.S. Department of Health and Human Services. HealthyPeople.gov. Available at http://www.healthypeople.gov/2020/default.aspx.

20. U.S. Department of Health and Human Services (DHHS) and U.S. Department of Agriculture (USDA). (2005). *Dietary Guidelines for Americans.* 6th ed. Washington, DC: U.S. Government Printing Office.

21. WHO. (n.d.). Dietary Recommendations/Nutritional Requirements. Available at http://www.who.int/nutrition/topics/nutrecomm/en/.

22. WHO. (2002). WHO Technical Report Series 935. Protein and Amino Acid Requirements in Human Nutrition. Report of a Joint WHO/FAO/UNU Expert Consultation. Geneva: United Nations University.

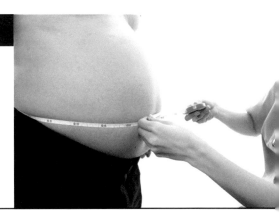

CHAPTER 3

THE PROBLEM OF OBESITY

3.1. THE PREVALENCE OF OBESITY IN THE U.S.

The prevalence of obesity is central to the discussion of public health in the U.S. because of the numerous secondary diseases that arise from it. Obesity is an epidemic in this country and has attained pandemic status worldwide. NIH surveillance data documented that 67% of adults ≥20 years of age were either overweight or obese and that as many as 34% of adults were obese (Ogden et al., 2006). Epidemiologists predict that, if left unchecked, the obesity prevalence will grow to 47% of the U.S. adult population by 2030 (Kelly et al., 2008). More troubling were the findings that 31.7% of children and adolescents (2–19 years old) were also overweight or obese. When these data are stratified, disturbing statistics begin to emerge that carry dire repercussions at a national level. Indeed, between 1988 and 2008 the prevalence of obesity in children (6–11 years old) jumped an astounding 400%—going from 4% to 20% in three decades (Roger et al., 2012), which is the cause of much alarm sociologically as well as medically. This has translated in a dramatic surge in health care problems throughout the U.S. According to the CDC, national health expenditure between 1980 and 2010 grew from $256 billion to $2.6 trillion per year, a jump that is so

extraordinarily large that it defies the imagination (Astrup et al., 2004). What has gone wrong?

The obesity problem is not limited to the U.S. For example, the number of overweight adults in China (18.6%) is growing at a rate that is alarming enough to cause epidemiologists to warn of a public health problem. In fact, the pervasiveness of both the obese and overweight adult Chinese has increased 49.3% between 1992 and 2002, going from roughly 14.6% in 1993 to 21.8% in 2002.

3.2. THE CAUSES OF OBESITY

The Harvard School of Public Health identifies three leading factors that are fueling the obesity crisis worldwide (Harvard School of Public Health, 2012): first, the food environment; second, the built environment; and third, new technologies.

3.2.1. The Food Environment

Countries that are stricken with economic hardship, unemployment, and poverty experience decreased food availability. In developing countries, land is often owned by large agribusiness companies and used to produce cash crops like sugar destined for export rather than food crops intended to sustain the local population. A dedication to large-scale production of cash crops, in addition to lowering the quantity and quality of the food supply available to local farmers, makes crops like sugar very cheap for nations that import it. This translates into greater consumption of soft drinks, vegetable oils, meats, and dairy products according to Barry Popkin. The increased caloric density of the world's diet is responsible for important increases in obesity, specifically in countries like Mexico, China, and India.

In the U.S. the problem of obesity is continuing to be a concern. One particular area of worry is the effect of diet and obesity on pregnancy. The National Health and Nutrition Examination Survey (NHANES) (Ogden et al., 2006) found that between 1999 and 2002, 26% of women of reproductive age considered themselves overweight, and 29% claimed to be obese. In total, then, 55% of adult women between the ages of 18 and 40 were potentially beginning their pregnancy already suffering from a weight management problem that could impact the fetus directly (Ogden et al., 2006). This would have increased the risks of neural tube defects, spontaneous miscarriage, preterm delivery, and neonatal respiratory distress. Moreover, when a woman is obese and depositing fat in the abdominal area, she is also producing more atherogenic lipoproteins in the blood in addition to excess adipocytokines and free radicals. These compounds threaten the integrity of the vascular lining and other cells. During pregnancy it is unclear to what extent these nefarious byproducts of obesity make their way past the placenta and affect the baby directly. We do know that medical practitioners are increasingly treating mothers who begin their pregnancies overweight or obese. They must manage these women by prescribing calorie-controlled diets aimed at limiting the total weight gain, in addition to the rate of weight gain over the duration of the pregnancy.

3.2.2. The Built Environment

The urbanization of America has led to the disappearance of agricultural communities and their replacement by malls and other retail and residential spaces. As rural farm workers gravitated to the urban centers for better-paying factory jobs, they required cars to shop and work. This has led to a decrease in overall energy expenditure. Walking has become less of a necessity of daily living, and demanding physical labor has been replaced by desk work in the financial, service, and information markets.

The global effect of built environments on weight was confirmed by a study of obesity in China. Sara

Bleich, a research scientist with the Harvard Initiative for Global Health, in attempting to comprehend the complex issues involved in worldwide obesity, concluded that "Results indicate that the increase in caloric intake is associated with technological innovations such as reduced food prices, as well as changing socio-demographic factors, such as increased urbanization and increased female labor force participation" (Bleich et al., 2007).

3.2.3. Medical Issues

Genetic and epigenetic changes and metabolic anomalies can also contribute to obesity. Metabolic abnormalities or chromosomal defects can alter the basal energy levels of the body, change the propensity to store fat, or even affect the satiety signals that control appetite. These conditions together affect only 1% of the population, however, and therefore cannot be considered as influential in the current U.S. obesity epidemic.

There are genetic abnormalities responsible for unusual weight gain and fat deposits, but for the sake of keeping the text relevant to an introductory course in nutrition, I will only mention four. The first is called **Prader-Willi syndrome (PWS)**. This is a rare congenital condition that originates from a defect in the father's chromosome, causing mental retardation, hypogonadism, hypotonic muscles, short stature, and an insatiable appetite leading to obesity early in life. Patients with PWS have an average height that varies between 4 feet 11 inches and 5 feet 1 inch. These children, if left unsupervised, can eat constantly and gain frightful amounts of weight. This form of chromosomal abnormality, which occurs at a frequency of 1 in every 15,000 to 30,000 births, causes these children to eat and store fat more readily because of a disturbance in the signals sent to the satiety center of the brain. The average weight for people with PWS is 176 lb for females and 216 lb for males. (A variation on PWS in which the chromosomal anomaly occurs on a specific maternal chromosome is called Angleman's syndrome and is characterized by a more severe mental retardation but without any obesity.)

The second genetically based obesity condition is **Bardet-Biedl syndrome**. It is recognizable by the symptoms of retinal degeneration, mental retardation, obesity, polydactyly (additional fingers), and hypogenitalism.

The third genetic abnormality that leads to obesity is called **Alstrom-Hallgren syndrome**. This third condition bears many similarities to Bardet-Biedl syndrome in that it is also characteristically identified by obesity and blindness. To help distinguish the two, additional symptoms have been tagged to Alstrom-Hallgren syndrome:

deafness, diabetes mellitus, and the absence of mental retardation. (Bray, 1998; Bissonnette, 2013)

Finally, the fourth genetic condition, which was identified by Friedman in 1994 in the obese ob/ob mouse and subsequently observed in obese cousins of Pakistani descent in 1997, has been identified as **leptin deficiency** (Farooqi and O'Rahilly, 2009). In leptin deficiency, mutations to the gene responsible for encoding leptin leads to hyperphagia (overeating), a severe form of obesity (morbid obesity), hypogonadism, and a compromised immune system. Obese individuals who lack the adipose tissue–derived protein leptin are unable to utilize the body's normal homeostatic mechanism that recognizes increasing adipose tissue as feedback to shut off the hunger signal. Therefore leptin-deficient patients have a persistent uncontrollable appetite that causes them to eat insatiably without experiencing the soothing effects of being full. When patients with this disorder are treated with leptin, their appetites normalize and they lose weight (Farooqi and O'Rahilly, 2009).

The genetic disposition for obesity (apart from specific disorders) began to be studied seriously in the eighteenth and nineteenth centuries. As genetics evolved during the twentieth century, with the important discoveries of Francis H. C. Crick (1916–2004) and James D. Watson (1928–), the notion of a single obesity gene—known as a Mendelian transmission—came into the discussion. Dr. Claude Bouchard, while he was professor at Laval University in Quebec, did phenomenal work in the 1988 Quebec Family Study. His team tracked family ties to obesity and was successful in differentiating between the impact of the environment and genetics (Bouchard et al., 1988; Bouchard, 1997). In reviewing the 1991 Norway and 1998 Quebec studies, he was able to quantify the heritability of obesity to between 25% and 40% of inter-individual differences in BMI and body fat. Bouchard concludes: "Thus the genetic heritability of the obesity phenotypes accounts for 25–40% of the age- and gender-adjusted phenotypic variances." In other words, family ties appear to increase the risk of a young child becoming obese.

Other studies have confirmed the correlation between obese children and obese parents. One study of obese children showed that 30% had two obese parents (though Bouchard clarifies that between 25% and 35% of obese individuals came from families with normal weight parents). Other research from the 1990s calculate that the risk of becoming obese increases two- to threefold if there is obesity in the family and that the risk increases further with the severity of the obesity.

What is unclear, however, is whether this is because of an "obesity gene" or simply family culture in terms of eating and exercise habits. No studies so far have been able to confirm a Mendelian transmission that could explain familial obesity. The Bouchard studies were able to quantify that 60%–75% of obesity variances between individuals were not genetically based but rather were tied to the environment in a broad sense—everything from accessibility to fast foods, grocery stores, and fresh and affordable produce to single-parent families with low incomes and poor eating habits, right down to individual and family food preferences, in addition to low physical activities. In other words, it appears that the genes load the gun, but that it is the environment that pulls the trigger.

3.2.4. Satiety Mechanisms

The cause of obesity does appear to be greatly influence by the calories we consume versus the calories we expend in physical activity. Given that we live in an environment that has conditioned us to lower physical activity (Bissonnette, 2013), the question really boils down to why our satiety mechanism does not kick in to preserve us from overeating. In order to answer this question, it is best to review the two main mechanisms involved in appetite regulation.

First, there is the **homeostatic mechanism** that is centrally regulated by the arcuate nucleus located in the hypothalamus. This central nervous system regulatory mechanism depends on a long-term signaling mechanism involving insulin and leptin and on a short-term episodic signaling involving ghrelin, peptide YY, cholecystokinin, and glucagon-like peptide. The interaction of these two systems informs the brain about energy stores and the variance in the flow of nutrients in relations to eating. In practical terms this means that when body fat reserves go down, leptin—a hormone secreted from adipocytes—also declines in the blood, thus stimulating the hypothalamus's appetite center. In contrast, when leptin increases from a greater number or size of adipose tissue, the appetite center is less stimulated; the desire for food is kept in check. Insulin is a hormone secreted in response to the ingestion of carbohydrates and protein. When excess carbohydrates are consumed, the ß cells of the pancreas secrete more insulin, thereby facilitating greater absorption of glucose into the cells and possibly greater fat synthesis in the case of excess glucose. With greater adiposity there is a tendency toward insulin insensitivity, leading to a metabolic condition called **insulin resistance**, which is usually seen as high insulin. Insulin concentrations in this condition remain elevated but lose their effectiveness in facilitating glucose access to cells. Consequently, blood glucose remains elevated (hyperglycemia), and so does blood insulin. Interestingly, in normal weight individuals, when insulin is maintained low—normally seen in response to low carbohydrate intake—this facilitates the signaling for the breakdown of fat (lipolysis). However, in insulin resistance, the persistence in elevated insulin may actually prevent the lipolysis or the breakdown of fat. This could be responsible for trapping individuals in chronic obesity or fatness. Also it is believed that in the **adipo-insular axis**, insulin stimulates the release of leptin from white adipose tissue, thus controlling appetite (Perry and Wang, 2012).

This signaling process maintains body reserves of fat relatively constant and, in theory, at a healthy level. In situations of chronic obesity, it is not clear whether the body develops a new homeostasis that is set at a higher weight and at a greater adiposity. If this is the case, then understandably the body's homeostatic mechanism would work in favor of maintaining this new normal, albeit at a greater weight and with more body fat.

The short-term episodic signaling system responds to the short-term consumption of food. Hence, when the stomach is empty, the ghrelin hormone is secreted from the stomach to alert the brain that it needs to eat; hunger is thus great when ghrelin levels in the blood are elevated. Cholecystokinin is the first gut hormone to be released from the GI tract. Within 15 minutes of initiating the ingestion of a meal, this hormone acts by reducing the appetite (Perry and Wang, 2012). Similarly, glucagon-like peptide (GLP-1) is also released from both the small intestine and the colon in response to number of calories ingested. The peripheral administration of GLP-1 or GLP-1 receptor agonists has clear anorexigenic effect, or suppression of appetite. Their action appears to reduced gastric acid secretion and gastric emptying. There is growing evidence that in obese individuals there is a delay in the release of GLP-1, which in turn delays appetite suppression after ingesting food. **Oxyntomodulin** is the more recently discovered gut hormone capable of suppressing the appetite. With a similar precursor as GLP-1, this hormone is secreted concomitantly with GLP-1 in proportion to the calories consumed at a meal.

The second process of appetite regulations comes from a cortico-limbic neural network that stimulates the hedonic center of the brain, otherwise known as the pleasure center, located in the frontal lobe (American Dietetic Association [ADA], 2009). The neural network receives signals from endocannabinoids, serotonin, and dopamine. This is where the pleasantness, the liking, and the wanting of a food get tagged to food palatability. It is a strong driving force behind our desire to eat certain foods, and it can lead to significant weight gain if there is an inappropriate sensitization of the hedonic system to unhealthy foods (ADA, 2009). It is well recognized that the draw to consuming specific foods is linked to our desire experience the pleasure sensations of that food. How often have we claimed, at the end of a gargantuan Thanksgiving meal, that we simply could not eat another bite, but changed our mind quickly when the pumpkin pie was served. Our memory of how delicious that pie is and our desire for pleasure become strong motivators to eat, even though we may have an abundance of adipose tissue; in this case the desire for pleasure overrides the long-term homeostatic mechanism involving leptin. Researchers are now using terminology like "addiction" to describe this kind of relationship to food, principally because of a **dopaminergic dysfunction** evidenced by a notable decline in the number of dopamine receptors in the striatum of the brain. The relationship with obesity is such that the more obese an individual, the lower the number of dopamine receptors.

There are two hypotheses that have been postulated to explain this anomaly: First, those addicted to foods experience a high degree of pleasure from food because of abundant release of dopamine associated with specific highly flavorful foods. Second, normal amounts of food do not provide enough rewards to the hedonic system because of the lower number of receptors. The need for pleasure rewards therefore incentivizes greater food intake (Yarnell et al., 2013).

3.3. OBESITY TREATMENTS

3.3.1. Popular Weight Loss Methods

Diet Restrictions. The most popular form of obesity treatment is dietary restriction. The rationale is founded on the principle that if calories or energy is restricted, then body weight will decline at a rate that is proportional to the degree that energy is limited. The classic and generally accepted approach is to prescribe a low-fat diet that restricts calories by 500–1,000 kcal per day in order to cause 1–2 lb weight loss per week. Medically, there are significant improvements in heart disease risk factors with as little as 5%–10% weight loss.

Since the 1970s numerous weight loss diets have come in and out of vogue. Very low calorie diets (VLCDs), popular for their rapid rate of weight loss, prescribed an intake of only 300–800 kcal per day fortified with a complete arsenal of micronutrients containing 100% of the RDA. This kind of diet is not generally consistent with long-term health, as energy is too restrictive to accommodate normal and sustainable eating behavior. VLCDs afforded 3–5 lb of weight loss per week, but a high likelihood of regaining most of the weight. VLCDs are not advised for people with BMIs <30 but are now frequently prescribed for patients preparing to undergo gastric bypass surgery.

There were also low calorie diets (LCDs) that recommended 1000–1,600 kcal per day. These diets generally offered adequate nutrition quality but insufficient energy for some individuals (Weight Control Information Network 2014). Many recent diets (Atkins, Pritikin, Scarsdale, Weight Watchers) are LCDs and offer meal plans that contained the specified amount of calories. However, overall, these diets have not been successful in maintaining weight loss over the long term (1–5 years). Often the weight regain surpassed the amount of weight that was initially lost, and the dieter ended up heavier than before. Tracy Mann and colleagues (2007) found between 33% and 67% regained more weight than lost.

The documentary *Obesity in America: A National Crisis* (Bissonnette, 2009) does a complete review of diet restrictions as treatment modality. Ma et al. (2007) did a comprehensive review of the most popular diets since the 1970s. They rated diets on their overall nutritional content and ability to lead to long-term, sustainable weight reduction, measured on a scale they called the alternative healthy eating index. Dean Ornish and Weight Watchers diets achieved high scores of 92.3% and 82% diet quality, respectively. The other diets investigated in the review were classified as suboptimal since they extensively manipulated macronutrients and did not propose reasonable and healthy ways of eating that were sustainable. The problem with many diets is that they restrict calories too far below the normal energy needs for weight maintenance. It is not uncommon for an obese individual requiring 3,800 kcal per day to be placed on a low-carbohydrate diet of 1,500 kcal per day with only 20 g per day of carbohydrates. The patient will indeed lose weight along with body protein in the initial phase of the diet because he is experiencing the equivalent of starvation.

The type of dietary strategy that is fixated on extensive caloric restriction is in clear opposition with the position paper of the American Dietetic Association (2009) on weight management. The ADA's position clearly states the importance of long-term sustainable weight loss, healthful eating practices that are enduring, and physical activity: "successful weight management to improve overall health for adults require[s] a lifelong commitment to healthful lifestyle behaviors emphasizing sustainable and enjoyable eating practices and daily physical activity."

Physiologically, there are a few things that happen to the body when it is placed on very restrictive or very low calorie diets (VLCD) or an LCD that restricts carbohydrates. First, the body begins to produce **ketone bodies** in order to continue to nourish the brain despite the low glucose availability. The ketones also have an anorexic effect, thus cutting the appetite and helping the dieter to more easily control food intake, at least in the short term. This occurs because glycogen reserves in the liver—used for glucose homeostasis in the blood—become depleted within 12–14 hours of fasting or being on such a low-carbohydrate diet. The quantity of carbohydrates is too low to favor fat oxidation.

One of the key concepts of fat metabolism is that **fat burns in the flame of carbohydrate metabolism**. In other words, carbohydrates are necessary to provide the metabolites needed for oxaloacetate to be formed in the tricarboxilic acid (TCA) cycle. This formation of **oxaloacetate** is important for the continued function of the TCA cycle, located in the mitochondria of the cell; this is the site of fat, protein, and carbohydrate oxidation. The TCA cycle along with the electron-transport chain, located in the mitochondrial membrane, are the main sites of ATP production. If there is insufficient energy produced (ATP) because body fat is not properly metabolized, ketone production is evidence that fat is not getting oxidized.

The second thing that happens in this kind of highly restrictive caloric diet is that the body attempts to recapture the lost weight as part of a survival mechanism aimed at maintaining homeostasis. It does this by causing an increase in appetite. Leptin, a hormone generated from the fat cells of the body, signals the hypothalamus about the body fat reserves. When body fat reserves have declined, circulating leptin concentrations will also be low, thus signaling an appetite response from the hypothalamus and a recovery of lost body fat. Similarly, when adipose tissue is abundant, circulating leptin will be more elevated, thus producing a loss of appetite. Also, as part of the homeostatic mechanism, ghrelin, a stomach hormone that lets the brain know that it needs food when it is empty, encourages the dieter to seek food to satisfy his hunger. The combined effect of low leptin and elevated ghrelin can make binging difficult to resist. This why these highly restrictive calorie diets often lead to ravenous appetites, uncontrollable eating, and significant weight regain.

The third thing that happens when a person is on a VLCD is that the dieter experiences cravings because of the habituation of the brain's hedonic center to high taste sensations through chronic consumption of fast foods and snack foods high in salt, sugar, and fat. This becomes an even greater problem in obese children who have been brought up on highly processed with highly addictive flavors. The more subtle taste of fresh fruits and vegetables cannot compete with the sensational flavors and aromas that have been developed in processed foods. How can an apple compete with a hamburger, a banana split, or a milkshake? The answer is that it can't. The child remains attached to an impoverished food supply that stimulates high taste sensations while providing virtually no nutritional quality.

This is an inappropriate sensitization of the hedonic system that can have dire consequences for the child brought up on junk food. It explains how teenagers can consume up to 1,000 kcal per day in soft drinks alone. This kind of deviant food consumption displaces nutritional foods such as milk, vegetables, and fruits out of the daily menu. Here then lies the problem. An obese patient will not have any kind of ability to appreciate the nutritious menu proposed by, say, a dietitian in an outpatient clinic for healthy weight loss. Although children do not fully understand the importance of healthy weights, teenagers do. Yet an obese teenager's taste habituation enslaves him into seeking repeat acquisition behavior. He knows what he likes, and what he likes supplants what is healthy. The reality is that compliance to healthy eating standards will not take place until later in adulthood. This is a very difficult situation that makes resolving the obesity crisis that much more difficult to contend with.

Pharmacotherapy. The use of anorectic agents to suppress appetite became a popular treatment modality in the late 1990s and early in the 2000s. Appetite was viewed as the enemy, and therapies tried to eliminate or limit the appetite so that the struggle to keep calories in check was more manageable. Sibutramine and Orlistat were two drugs that received FDA approval for long-term clinical management of obesity in the early 2000s. Studies were done in both adults and children, and the results were predictable: While the subjects took the drugs daily, weight loss was regular and significant. When the drugs were discontinued, weight regain was observed in almost all of the subjects. A 2002 meta-analysis by Haddock et al. demonstrated that no one medication showed clear superiority in treatment effect over another. Interestingly, prolonged therapy after 6 months did not coincide with continued or greater weight loss. In fact, more of a plateau appears to occur at the 6-month mark, with no evidence of benefit occurring afterward.

Sibutramine—a mixed serotonin, norepinephrine, and dopamine reuptake inhibitor—was banned by the FDA in 2010 because of concerns it led to higher risks of stroke and cardiovascular events (Yarnell et al., 2013). Orlistat is the only remaining drug that has been approved to treat obesity for up to 1 year. It works by inhibiting fat absorption and has only been able to afford a mean 6.5 lb of weight loss at the end of a year. The Yarnell team, after reviewing the overall effectiveness of drug therapy in weight loss, concluded that "Despite their use, these pharmaceuticals for obesity have failed to produce significant, enduring weight loss and at best have provided only modest, short-term benefit." They argued that because food addiction is now being discussed as

meaningful player in the obesity crisis, "the role of behavior modification can be highlighted in conjunction with pharmacological interventions, for the treatment of food addictions."

3.3.2. The Most Effective Obesity Treatments

Exercise. While the longstanding strategies of weight loss diets have not produced the desired results in the majority of the population, research still shows that total daily or weekly caloric deficits are necessary for weight loss. Studies have shown that long-term weight loss is achieved with programs that include physical activity.

Very few studies have included sufficient amounts of exercise to even permit a 5% loss of body weight from exercise alone. The time commitment to physical activity must be quite large in order to cause substantive weight loss by increasing energy expenditure alone. Using doubly labeled water, Schoeller and colleagues (1997) demonstrated that in order to maintain weight loss, individuals need to commit to expending between 11 and 12 kcal per kg per day in physical activity beyond normal daily expenditure. This represents a surprisingly elevated amount of energy that few people have the time to commit to. For instance, a 183-lb (83-kg) individual would have to expend approximately 955 kcal per day, 7 days per week, in order to maintain weight loss. This represents a 2.5-hour commitment at the gym every day. Realistically, few would be able to free up that much time in a day.

The National Weight Loss Registry currently tracks 10,000 people—80% of participants are women—who have lost on average 66 lb and kept it off for a mean of 5.5 years. On average, Registry members report expending 2,684 kcal per week from exercise alone—the equivalent of walking 4 miles per day seven days a week (ADA, 2009). A more recent visit to the Registry's website shows that about 90% of the subjects participate in at least 1 hour of daily exercise—the most popular activity being walking. This would equate to expending 1,800–2,100 kcal per week or roughly 300 kcal per day for just this additional walking. In addition, 62% of participants watched less than 10 hours of TV per week. The point here is that the commitment to physical activity must be significant in order to derive any clear benefits, but so must be the decision to minimize sedentary activities like computers, television, and gaming.

The current 2010 *Dietary Guidelines for Americans* now includes the Federal Physical Activity Guidelines for Americans that were issued in late 2008 and recommend between 150 and 300 minutes per week of moderate aerobic exercise. Many individuals require much more than that, but 150–300 minutes is certainly a good place to start.

Behavioral Intervention. Behavior modification was an approach that became popular in the late 1980s. Now it's more aptly called cognitive behavioral therapy, and its goal is to identify cues that set off or trigger inappropriate eating habits. The principle is based on the notion that small but consistent changes in behavior are more enduring than large and dramatic shifts in behavior. This approach utilizes food and exercise monitoring, extensive record keeping, problem solving, and nutrition education in an attempt to restructure the individual's knowledge base, way of thinking, and ultimately behavior. It strongly advocates going beyond weight scales and weight losses and instead emphasizes that health and fitness come with changes in lifestyles anchored in behavioral modification.

The ADA's Nutrition Counseling work group has been, for several years, monitoring the effectiveness of self-monitoring for weight loss in the adult population. Right now the evidence is limited that behavioral modification and behavioral therapy are effective; results over the long term show that weight loss is modest and weight regain occurs frequently. The PREMIER, Diabetes Prevention Program, Finnish Diabetes Prevention, and Look-AHEAD studies have shown significant changes in body weight and in risk indicators of heart disease and cardiovascular disease in those groups subject to lifestyle modification strategies (ADA, 2009). The Diabetes Prevention Program, in particular, demonstrated that behavioral modification was even more efficacious at causing weight loss over the long term than general recommendations and pharmacotherapy. Yarnell et al. (2013) recognize that psychotherapy can be helpful in managing co-morbid psychiatric disorders such as depression, anxiety, loneliness, boredom, anger, and interpersonal conflict that lead to dysfunctional eating such as binging and to significant weight gain and obesity.

Bariatric Surgeries. There is a class of obesity called morbid obesity that has grown a startling 400% between 1983 and 2000. Morbid obesity refers to individuals who are at least 100 lb over their healthy weight and who carry a high degree of morbidity or sickness that is far more serious than plain obesity. Morbid obesity is diagnosed when the body mass index (BMI) is >40 but less than 50. Remarkably the rate of increase of those who were super obese, defined as having a BMI >50, during that same time interval was 500%. Using data from the Behavioral Risk Factor Surveillance System, Sturm and Hattori (2013) measured a 70% increase in the prevalence of morbid obesity between 2000 and 2010, with the rate of increase slowing down since 2005. As it stands

right now, 6.6% of the adult population is classified as morbidly obese, about 15.5 million people (Sturm and Hattori, 2013).

Bariatric surgical interventions have been traditionally reserved for individuals with BMIs >40 who have not been successful in trying less invasive weight loss methods. The surgery has also been performed on individuals with BMIs between 35 and 40 if they also suffer from diabetes, hypertension, or sleep apnea. Bariatric surgeries have been shown to be the most effective therapy in terms of initiating significant and sustainable weight loss. There are a number of types of bariatric surgery: gastric bypass, adjustable gastric band, gastroplasty, biliopancreatic diversion, and gastric sleeve. These procedures have been successful in facilitating excess weight loss that varies between 47.5% and 70% (ADA, 2009).

There are, however, problems with bariatric surgery. Although on average, bariatric surgery causes an overall mean initial weight loss of 88 lb, between 20% and 30% of patients experience complications that are responsible for nutrient deficiencies and long-term health problems reported upon follow-up. Moreover, there is a troubling regain of lost weight in about 20%–34% of surgeries (Yarnell et al., 2013). Results remain more impressive than weight loss diets, but surgery doesn't address the fact that compulsive eating is a behavioral problem that is not completely solved with a smaller stomach pouch. Patients who have become morbidly obese have chronically consumed calories that have significantly exceeded their body's requirements. If a person puts on 25 extra pounds at the end of a year, but does nothing to attempt to lose this weight, this person risks becoming morbidly obese after 4–5 years. On a daily basis, this translates into an extra 240 kcal per day above the normal requirement. Add in a noticeable drop in physical activity, and additional pounds are added on more quickly.

The human cost associated with this form of gigantic bodily distortion goes beyond measure. At this point, the propensity to fall and fracture limbs increases, and the motivation to do exercise drops dramatically; fatigue and chronic pain become prominent complaints. Hence patients are not likely to comply with new healthy dietary directives, nor are they prone to initiate exercise regimes that are rigorous enough to cause significant energy expenditure. Surgery, then, is seen as a life-saving intervention.

3.4. NUTRITIONAL ASSESSMENT

It is crucial to establish a prognosis when a patient first begins treatment for weight loss and attendant health problems. A poor prognosis would be given if the patient had a high risk of complications or a low probability of complying with medical or dietetic directives. By contrast, a good prognosis signifies a good chance that the patient will comply with medical or therapeutic directives and a good chance of recovering from the disease or condition, in this case obesity and some of the secondary diseases such as insulin resistance and hypertension. In the treatment of obesity, a good prognosis would be assigned to an obese patient who is motivated to lose weight and who in all likelihood will successfully lose at least 10% of the initial body weight; this is sufficient to decrease several risk factors secondary to obesity such as hypertension, hyperlipidemia, and hyperglycemia.

A prognosis can best be formulated by interviewing the patient and documenting key relevant issues in the body composition, medical history, psychological profile, and nutritional information.

3.4.1. Body Composition.

The first step in establishing a prognosis involves determining the patient's body composition using **anthropometric** measurements. There are four anthropometric measures that are frequently used: height, weight, body mass index (BMI), and waist circumference. These tools help the clinician or dietitian determine if the body is disproportionally large or small relative to a standard norm. The BMI has been stratified to more objectively identify those who are overweight or obese. This identification is not based on appearance but rather on disease risk. A BMI of 25–29.9 indicates overweight, a BMI of 30–34.9 indicates obesity class-1, a BMI of 35–39.9 indicates obesity class-2, a BMI of 40–50 indicates morbid obesity, and a BMI greater than 50 is termed super obesity (National Institutes of Health [NIH], 2000; Sturm and Hattori, 2013). The higher the BMIs above the normal range of 18.5–24.9, the greater the risk of heart disease.

The waist circumference is a fast method to predict whether a patient is at risk of metabolic syndrome. If the waist circumference is greater than 40 inches and 35 inches, for men and women respectively, there is a high risk of morbidities (hypertension, type 2 diabetes, and hyperlipidemias) and mortality independent of the BMI measurement. The NIH's Heart, Blood, and Lung Institute method of determining waist circumference consists of placing the measuring tape at the superior border of the iliac crest and wrapping it around the waist. This measurement is directly associated with abdominal fat build-up, which is more atherogenic than fat deposits in other anatomical locations.

Total body fat is also very valuable as an accurate risk assessor; however, there was little data before 2000 linking body fat to health risks. Gallagher and colleagues (2000) successfully linked BMIs to body fat percentages. Establishing percent body fat in patients is important because someone could be overweight because of increased muscle mass; this individual would not be at risk even though his BMI might be high. On the other hand if the patient has a percent body fat greater than the norm, determined by either skinfold measurements, bioelectrical impedance measurement, or BodPod, then he is truly classified as over fat. Both Gallagher and colleagues and the U.S. Army Body Composition Program (2013; AR 600-9) identified healthy body fat levels of roughly 8%–24% for most men and 20%–35% for most women.

TABLE 3.1. Healthy Body Fat Percent in Whites, African Americans, and Asians

	Healthy BMI	% Body Fat
Men	18.5–24.9	8–23%
Women	18.5–24.9	20–35%

Gallagher et al. (2000). *AJCN.* 72(3):694–701.

3.4.2. Medical History

The second step in determining a prognosis is the medical history. Medical history is vital for determining if there are any endocrine, neurological, or genetic causes of obesity. Here it would be pertinent to identify the age of onset of the obesity and the family weight history specific to both parents and grandparents. Also pertinent is the history of medications used and their purposes. Next it would be useful to document the obesity-related disorders that have been flagged such as hypertension, hyperlipidemias, sleep apnea, and gallbladder disease. The metabolic and degenerative characteristics of the obesity should also be noted. It would be useful to document the severity of the obesity based on BMI, percent body fat, anatomical traits, degenerative features, and the extent of physical disabilities linked to the obesity in addition to the neoplastic complications.

3.4.3. Psychological Evaluation

The third step in determining a prognosis is a psychological evaluation. The clinician should interview the patient and also look for medical signs of any of the following issues: suicidal ideation, drug use, binge eating, bulimia, depression, post-traumatic stress disorder, or any kind of addictive behavior.

3.4.4. Nutritional Evaluation

The fourth and final step in determining a prognosis is a nutritional evaluation. At this step it is important to consider the patient's weight history by documenting the age of onset of obesity, the maximal weight maintained as an adult, the lowest weight achieved, the duration of weight loss, and the specific weight loss method used. It would be pertinent to note the various weight loss diets followed as a teenager and as an adult. There a several that can be identified: fasting, very low calorie diets, low calorie diets, dieting and exercise in combination, appetite suppressant medication, bariatric surgery, behavior modification, psychiatric counseling, and liposuction.

The goal here is to understand to what extent the patient has had a history of yo-yo dieting and whether he or she has engaged in abusive dieting practices. Abusive practices, especially when the patient is young, can predispose the patient to compulsive food behaviors that endure into adulthood. It would be relevant for the dietitian or clinician to identify any behaviors symptomatic of disordered eating. At this point the primary care physician would need to be alerted so that a psychological consult could be issued.

The next step involves an assessment of the patient's dietary patterns. Using a **24-hour recall, usual food intake,** or **food frequency questionnaire (FFQ)**, the dietitian can document the patient's usual daily meal patterns looking for skipped meals, determining snacking practices, and establishing the largest and smallest meals consumed daily. Using the usual food intake measure, the dietitian can get an idea of the nutritional quality of the diet and approximate total calories consumed. It is vital that the clinician know the approximate calories consumed on a daily basis and compare it the patients estimated total energy expenditure (TEE).

The FFQ is an excellent method of assessing the quality and variety of food consumed on a regular basis. For instance, the FFQ can help answer the question: Does my patient consume enough fruits and vegetable? The dietitian will document the weekly frequency with which the patient consumed vegetables from the cruciferous family (broccoli, cabbage, brussels sprouts, cauliflower, broccoflower, turnip, kale). This class of vegetable is a good source of **vitamin C**, **soluble fiber,** and **phytochemicals** that are protective against heart disease and many types of cancers. A computer-generated nutrient profile, indicating elevated vitamin A content, is considered an excellent surrogate for a rich and colorful vegetable intake. This is because ß-carotene, a carotenoid abundantly found in orange and dark green vegetables, is a precursor to **vitamin A**. It also is an antioxidant that plays a protective role against oxidative stress.

In the North American context, there are a select number of nutrients that are medically pertinent in obesity cases, as they tend to be either suboptimal in the diet or excessive and thus affect health in an important way. Those nutrients that are excessive and significantly increase the risk of cardiovascular disease (CVD) and metabolic syndrome are saturated fats and trans-fatty acids. They need to be replaced by monounsaturated fats and omega-3 fats (Willett et al., 2006). Paradoxically, despite the abundant calories consumed by obese and overweight patients, some nutrients have clearly become suboptimal in their diets primarily because of the overconsumption of high calorically dense foods of poor nutritional quality; it is estimated that 27%–30% of calories consumed by American children and adults are nutritionally impoverished processed foods and that sweeteners and desserts contribute 18%–24% of those total calories.

Studies have also identified eating patterns in the obese population that need to be flagged: As a rule when nutrient-poor processed foods increase in the diet, nutrient-dense food intake proportionally declines. For instance, when fat intake is greater than 30% of total calories, there is a tendency to observe a decline in the dietary intake of vitamins A, C, and folate. It is additionally concerning that as sweetened beverages increase in the diet, milk consumption decreases, thus causing calcium and vitamin D to plummet. Fat-soluble vitamins and antioxidants tend to be unusually low in the morbidly obese, most notably vitamin A, ß-carotene and α-tocopherol (vitamin E). Baseline iron deficiency anemia has been reported in 44% of adults prior to undergoing gastric bypass surgery. Vitamin D deficiency is more widespread in the general population than previously thought and besides impairing calcium absorption, vitamin D deficiency is suspected to affect the immune system, thereby increasing the body's susceptibility to cancers, diabetes mellitus, autoimmune diseases, and cardiovascular disease (Xanthakos, 2009).

Clinicians should also question patients about their intake of nutrient supplements. Willett and colleagues identified folate as a nutrient at risk in developing countries that are westernizing and has recommended the fortification of the food supply with folate in order to decrease the incidence of neural tube defects. Fiber intake is also a concern as chronically low intakes are responsible for constipation, which greatly impacts gastrointestinal disease (Willett et al., 2006).

Environmental factors have possibly the most significant impact on the way people eat and may explain in part why obesity is a disease that afflicts the poor and immigrants with modest financial reserves. Indeed, fast food restaurants abound in low-income urban areas whereas grocery stores are fewer. One-parent families may tend to eat in cheap restaurants or fast food chains outside the home because tight schedules, financial constraints, and work obligations that make home cooking challenging.

But it is not only the poor who are becoming obese. Professionals bound to their desks for long hours are prone to significant weight gain. Accountants, financial analysts, and customer service representatives are all glued to their seats, some of them for long hours. The prospect of making a meal at home is not likely as there is simply not enough time. On the way home, having dinner at the restaurant with a client is far more likely than sitting down to a full cooked meal with the family. Eating out frequently is indeed tied to excess caloric intake because restaurant food is loaded with salt, sugar, and fat. Tie in the larger portions and alcohol consumption, and it is far more likely to exceed caloric needs than the dinner table at home.

To round out a prognosis, ask the patient about exercise. In this environment of financial stress, poverty, and tight schedules, the ability to include regular exercise is also difficult. Sedentary jobs that occupy long hours can cause employees to expend far few calories than they did in previous decades. The opportunity to exercise in a gym after work is less likely for single parents with children at home or for professionals with long work hours. Ask about the patient's exercise history. Here the clinician is attempting to uncover if the patient did sports as a child, an adolescent, and as a young adult. This is relevant because if physical activity was introduced early on in a person's life then it is far more likely that they will

more easily accommodate a physical activity prescription and feel the benefit then if they had never done sports as a youth. This is important to assess as it tempers the prognosis.

It is necessary, in the final stages of the interview, to establish a weight-loss goal and to clarify the reasons for wanting to lose weight. This helps the dietitian to ascertain the subject's readiness to make important lifestyle changes and thus to formulate a positive prognosis.

3.5. OBESITY CASE STUDY: GRADUAL WEIGHT GAIN OVER 3 YEARS IN A 27-YEAR-OLD WOMAN

3.5.1. Presentation

A 27-year-old woman on medical assistance weighing 230 lb (height: 5'10") presents with elevated LDL cholesterol, borderline hyperglycemia, high blood pressure (BP), and some anxiety. The patient's primary care physician reports that patient gained 55 lb over the last 3 years because of depression. He recommends a consultation with the clinic's registered dietitian in order to ensure a healthy weight loss diet. The goal is a minimal 10%–20% weight loss in order to positively affect blood lipids, blood sugars, and BP and ultimately avoid any BP and diabetes medication.

3.5.2. Body Composition Assessment

The clinician starts by measuring the patient's BMI (kg/m^2) to establish if the patient is overweight, obese, or morbidly obese. Taking her weight in pounds (230 lb) and multiplying it by 0.454 will provide a metric weight of 104.42 kg. Taking her height (70 in) and multiplying it by 0.0254 provides a height in meters of 1.78 m. The BMI can now be determined:

BMI = 104.24 kg/(1.78 meters)^2
BMI = 32.90

She is suffering from obesity class-1.

Next her body fat needs to be determined using one of three methods:

1. **Skinfold measurements** can be used to estimate the full body percent fat.
2. **Bioelectrical impedance assessment (BIA)** can calculate whole body percent fat using the impedance of a light electrical flow through the body. The

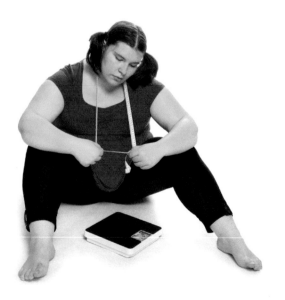

Figure 3.1. Obese and depressed woman. © Kletr/Shutterstock.com.

TABLE 3.2. Patient Chart Information.

Marla C. CHART INFORMATION	
Age: 27 Weight: 230 lb Height: 5 feet 10 inches Patient lost boyfriend and job. Has been on social assistance for 3 years and gained 55 lb.	
ACTUALS	**STANDARDS**
FPG: 120 mg/dl	80–100 mg/dl
BP: 150/110	≤140/90
BMI:	18.5–24.9
% Body fat:	20%–35%
Waist circumference:	<35 in
Kcals consumed:	2,320 kcal
A1C: <6.5%	5.9%

American Diabetes Association (2011) Standards of Medical Care in Diabetes—2012. *Diabetes Care*. Suppl. 1:S11–63. FPG: fasting plasma glucose.

greater the fat content the greater the impedance, and the lower the fat the lower the impedance.

3. **Plethysmography,** otherwise known as the BodPod measurement, can very reliably and accurately determine the total body fat through air displacement.

The clinician uses BIA to determine the patient's total body fat of 39%. The waist circumference using a measurement tape position on the top of the iliac crest equals 44 inches.

3.5.3. Dietary Assessment

The dietitian at this point assesses the patient's dietary habits using a **usual food record** and a food frequency questionnaire (FFQ). The dietician asks questions like "in the morning when you wake up, when is the first time that you consume or eat something?" From the

TABLE 3.2. Usual Food Intake Record

PATIENT NAME: **Marla C.** USUAL FOOD INTAKE

FOODS CONSUMED	QUANTITY CONSUMED	PLACE
BREAKFAST:		
Orange Tang or orange drink (beverage) Kraft white bread, toasted	2 cups 2 pieces	Kitchen
Butter (salted)	1 tablespoon	
AM SNACK		
Chocolate bar (Snickers) reg. size	52.7 g (1.9 oz wt)	Work lounge
Coca Cola (reg.)	12 fl oz (355 ml can)	
LUNCH		
Coca Cola (reg.)	12 fl oz (355 ml can)	Work lounge
Bologna sandwich	2 slices (44 g)	
Mayonnaise (Hellman's)	2 Tbsp	
Lay's Salt & Vinegar Potato Chips	1 oz bag	
PM SNACK		
Coca-Cola (reg.)	12 fl oz (355 ml can)	Work lounge
Gummy bears	19 pieces	
DINNER		
Stouffer's Lasagna Italiano	7.67 oz wt (215 g)	TV room in the house
Beer (Dos Equis)	1 bottle	
Italian bread	3 (1 oz wt)	
Butter (salted)	3 pats	
Homemade mixed green salad	2 cups	
Bottled Italian salad dressing	3 Tablespoons	
EVENING SNACK		
No snacks recorded		

TABLE 3.3. Nutrient Breakdown of Usual Food Intake vs. Recommended Intake

Nutrient	Recommended Daily Intake	Actual Daily Intake
Kcal	2,320	2,515
Carbohydrates	348 g (60% DRI kcal) (261–377 g)	385 g
Protein	87 g (15% DRI kcal) (58–203 g)	39 g
Fat	64 g (25% DRI kcal) (52–90 g)	91 g
Total sugar	<145 g (25% DRI kcal)	218 g
Total salt	<2,400 mg	3008 mg

Calories measured using the www.myfitnesspal.com website.

usual food record, the dietitian will plug foods, typically ingested on a normal day, into the diet analysis software. It will determine the total calories, grams of fat, protein, and carbohydrate usually ingested. The FFQ does not establish the quantity consumed but rather the quality of the food consumed.

3.5.4. Nutritional Interpretation of the Diet

To help interpret the ingested calories and macronutrients, the dietitian refers to the *Dietary Guidelines for Americans* reviewed in the previous chapter. She uses the preferred macronutrient ranges for carbohydrates (45%–65%), protein (10%–35%, with the usual requirement set at 15%), and fat (20%–35%, with the maximal cut-off usually set at 30%).

The patient is exceeding her daily caloric goal by 23%. She also exceeds her carbohydrate goal by 11%, and her fat intake greatly surpasses her dietary goal of 25% of DRI calories by 42%. Total sugar refers to sugars consumed through fruits, vegetables, and milk in addition to sugars added to processed foods (added sugar). The patient's total sugar intake of 218 g exceeds her maximal allowance by 50% because of the soft drinks and Tang she usually consumes. Her excessive sodium intake is not surprising given that she eats a lot of very processed food, notably the lasagna and the salad dressing.

3.5.5. Interpretation of Medical Indices. The dietician considers the key medical symptoms of blood sugars, hemoglobin (Hb) A1C, and blood pressure. In 2009, the American Diabetes Association, the International Diabetes Federation (IDF), and the European Association for the Study of Diabetes (EASD) formed an International Expert Committee that recommended the use of Hb A1C cut-off of ≥6.5% in diagnosing a patient with diabetes mellitus. Pre-diabetes could be reasonably diagnosed with an Hb A1C between 5.7% and 6.4%. This means the patient is at an elevated risk of developing diabetes in the future. Similarly the fasting plasma glucose (FPG) value falls within the range of 100–125 mg/

dl and confirms pre-diabetes. Also a random blood glucose ≥200 mg/dl signifies hyperglycemia. This patient's A1C at 5.9% and fasting plasma glucose of 120 mg/dl confirms that this patient is at a high risk of becoming diabetic. The blood pressure is above the normal range established for normotensive patients and can decidedly be interpreted as hypertension.

3.5.6. Dietary Recommendations

As is the case so often in patients who have gained weight, there are only a few dietary aberrations that need to change to significantly cut back on her calories consumed. In this case eliminating Coca-Cola and Tang from the menu would eliminate 560 kcal from her intake. Additionally, it would be a good idea to drop the chocolate bar and the gummy bears. In total, the excess calories coming from snacks and sweetened beverages at lunch and breakfast total 950 kcal in a typical day. This dietary correction would realign the patient's caloric intake to 1,896 kcal per day. It would be necessary to add 3 cups of 2% milk back to the diet, which would add 366 kcal. Her total caloric intake for weight maintenance would therefore be 2,262 kcal.

The clinician wants to ensure that the patient can maintain weight stability and refrain from further weight gain. (Once this is achieved for a period of time lasting 2 weeks to 1 month, the clinician helps the patient develop a diet for mild to moderate weight loss using both caloric restrictions and regular exercise.) To do this, she recommends some food exchanges. First, white bread should be changed to a whole wheat bread. Second, the Tang at breakfast needs to be replaced by a 4 fl oz pure orange juice and one to two fruit servings (for example, one small banana and half a grapefruit). Third, a high fiber cereal should be included such a Raisin Bran, Grape Nut Original, Bran Buds, Bran Flakes, All Bran, Fiber One, or Kashi Original. There are others but these are all considered excellent sources of fiber as they contain at least 5 g per serving. Fiber is all too often suboptimal in the diet because of the highly processed food consumed by North Americans. Unless a high fiber cereal is consumed in the morning, it is very difficult to meet fiber requirements by the end of the day. Fourth, a minimal of three vegetable servings need to be added throughout the day. Perhaps one vegetable at lunch and two at dinner could be selected such corn, green beans, broccoli, brussels sprouts, cabbage (or coleslaw), turnips, carrots, and sweet potato (yams).

3.5.7. Determining the Body Weight Goal

The clinician then sets a weight goal for the patient. Using the two compartment model of body composition, it is possible to determine the patient's fat free mass (FFM): total body weight (TBW) = body fat + fat free mass. Since the clinician knows the total body weight (230 lb) and the percent body fat (39%), it can be calculated that the FFM equals 61% of the total body weight (100% − 39% = 61%). This means that 39% fat mass equals 89.7 lb (0.39 × 230 lb) and that FFM = 140.3 lb (230 lb − 89.7 lb). The equations are written below:

$$(3.1) \quad FFM = TBW \times 0.61$$
$$(3.2) \quad FFM = 230 \text{ lb} \times 0.61 = 140.3 \text{ lb}$$

Now it is possible to more precisely to determine a weight goal with the understanding that the patient's FFM must NOT decline with weight loss, but rather the body fat must decrease with weight loss. Consequently the following equation can now be established using a healthy percent body fat of 25%. This is a healthy goal to aim for as it is within the healthy range of 20%–35% for women. It is now possible to write the following two equations:

$$(3.3) \quad (100 - 25\%) \times TBW = 140.3 \text{ lb}$$
$$(3.4) \quad TBW = 140.3/0.75 = 187 \text{ lb}$$

The healthy weight that this patient should aim for is therefore 187 lb, which would represent a 43-lb weight loss.

Next, the clinician decides upon the rate of weight loss. Traditionally, 1–2 lb per week has been advised by the frontline providers and the dietitians. This is achieved by subtracting 500–1,000 kcal from her current maintenance diet.

In practice, this approach would advocate for a daily energy intake of 1,320–1,820 kcal per day while maintaining her current sedentary lifestyle. The prognosis for this type of approach is not very good. Most patients, while capable of dropping excess weight rapidly, tend to regain significant weight within a year of achieving their goal if their energy expenditure does not increase. Therefore the clinician prescribes weekly exercise in order to offset the caloric restriction needed to achieve this rate of weight loss. By adding a brisk walk (3.5 miles per hour) of 75 minutes every day to her routine, the patient can burn an additional 496 kcal per day. In total, then, she would experience an overall daily energy deficit of 745 kcal.

It would be possible to predict the rate of weight loss knowing that a 3,500 kcal deficit causes 1 lb of weight loss. Assuming the patient could maintain this regime, she would be experiencing a weekly caloric deficit of 5,215 kcal. This can be translated in pounds lost by dividing 5,215 3,500, which equals 1.5 lb of weight loss per week. Given that her goal is to drop 43 lb, she should expect to take almost 29 weeks to achieve her final goals. The primary care physician should be satisfied with a weight loss of 23 lb, which is enough to cause a medical improvement in BP and FPG.

NOTE

1. Certain sections of this chapter have been copied from chapters 6 and 10 of the textbook: IT'S ALL ABOUT NUTRITION: Saving the Health of Americans, and blended into this chapter with the permission of the copyright holder © David Bissonnette

REFERENCES

1. American Diabetes Association. (2011). Standards of medical care in diabetes—2012. *Diabetes Care.* 35 Suppl. 1:S11–63.
2. American Dietetic Association. (2009). Position Paper on Weight Management. *J Am Diet Assoc.* 109:330–346.
3. Astrup A, et al. (2004). Atkin's and other low carbohydrate diets: hoax or an effective tool for weight loss. *The Lancet* 364(9437):897–899.
4. Bissonnette D. (2013) *It's All about Nutrition: Saving the Health of Americans.* Lanham, MD: University Press of America.
5. Bissonnette DJ. (2009). *Obesity in America: A National Crisis.* DVD. Mankato MN: St-Jude Nutrition Medical Communications. Distributed by Films for the Humanities and Sciences.
6. Bleich S, et al. (2007). Why Is the Developed World Obese? NBER Working Paper 12954. Cambridge, MA: National Bureau of Economic Research (NBER); 43.
7. Bouchard C. (1997). Genetics of human obesity: recent results from linkage studies. *J Nutr.* 127(9):1887S–1890S.
8. Bouchard C, et al. (1988). Inheritance of the amount and distribution of human body fat. *Int J Obes.* 12:205–215.

9. Bray, G (1998). Classification and Evaluation of the Overweight Patient. In: Handbook of Obesity. George A Bray, Claude Bouchard, WPT James (eds) New York: Marcel Dekker Inc: 831-854

10. Farooqi S, O'Rahilly S. (2009). Leptin: a pivotal regulator of human energy homeostasis. *Am J Clin Nutr.* 89 Suppl.:980S–984S.

11. Gallagher D, et al. (2000). Healthy percentage body fat ranges: an approach for developing guidelines based on body mass index. *Am J Clin Nutr.* 72(3):694–701.

12. Haddock CK, et al. (2002) Pharmacotherapy for obesity: a quantitative analysis of four decades of published randomized clinical trials. *Int J Obes.* 26(2):262–273.

13. Harvard School of Public Health. (2012). The obesity prevention Source: Globalization. Available at http://www.hsph.harvard.edu/obesity-prevention-source/obesity-causes/globalization-and-obesity/.

14. Kelly T, Yang W, Chen CS, Reynolds K, He J. (2008) Global burden of obesity in 2005 and projections to 2030. *Inter J Obesity (Lond).* 32:1431–1437.

15. Ma Y, et al. (2007) A dietary comparison of popular weight loss plans. *JADA* 107(10):1786–1791.

16. Mann T, et al. (2007) Medicare's search for effective obesity treatments. *American Psychologists.* 62(3):220–233.

17. National Institute of Diabetes and Digestive and Kidney Disease (2014). Weight Control Information Network. Available at http://www.win.niddk.nih.gov/publications/low_calorie.htm#lcd.

18. National Institutes of Health/National Heart Lung and Blood Institute/North American Association for the Study of Obesity (NHLB). (2000). Obesity Education Initiative. The Practical Guide Identification, Evaluation, and Treatment of Overweight and Obesity in Adults. NIH Publication Number 00-4084. Available at http://www.nhlbi.nih.gov/guidelines/obesity/prctgd_c.pdf.

19. Ogden CL, et al. (2006). Prevalence of overweight and obesity in the United States, 1999–2004. *JAMA.* 295:1549–1555.

20. Perry B, Wang Y. (2012). Appetite regulation and weight control: the role of gut hormones. *Nutrition and Diabetes.* 2, e26; doi: 10.1038. Available at http://www.nature.com/nutd/journal/v2/n1/full/nutd201121a.html.

21. Popkin BM (2007). The world is fat. *Scientific American,* September; 88–95.

22. Roger VL, et al. (2012). AHA Statistical Update: Heart Disease and Stroke Statistics 2012. *Circulation* 125:e2–e220.

23. Schoeller DA, Shay K, Kushner RF. (1997) How much physical activity is needed to minimize weight gain in previously obese women? *Am J Clin Nutr.* 66:551–556.

24. Sturm R, Hattori A. (2013). Morbid obesity rates continue to rise rapidly in the United States *Int J Obes (Lond).* 37(6):889–891. Available at http://www.ncbi.nlm.nih.gov/pmc/articles/PMC3527647/.

25. Sturm R. (2007). Increases in morbid obesity in the USA: 2000–2005. *Public Health.* 121:492–496.

26. U.S. Army. Army Regulation 600-9 (revised June 28, 2013). The Army Body Composition Program. Available at http://www.apd.army.mil/jw2/xmldemo/r600_9/main.asp.

27. Willett WC, et al. (2006) Prevention of chronic disease by means of diet and lifestyle changes. In: Jamison DT, ed. *Disease Control Priorities in Developing Countries.* 2nd ed. Washington, DC: World Bank.

27. Xanthakos SA. (2009). Nutritional deficiencies in obesity and after bariatric surgery. *Pediat Clin North Amer.* 58(5):1105–1121. Available at http://www.ncbi.nlm.nih.gov/pmc/articles/PMC2784422/.

28. Yarnell S, et al. (2013). Pharmacotherapies for overeating and obesity. *J Genet Syndrome and Gene Therapy.* 4(3):131. Available at http://www.ncbi.nlm.nih.gov/pmc/articles/PMC3697760/.

CHAPTER 4

THE PROBLEM OF CARDIOVASCULAR DISEASE

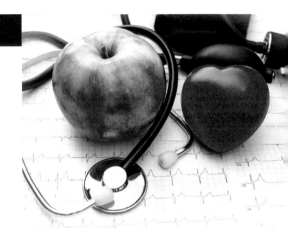

4.1 THE PREVALENCE OF CARDIOVASCULAR DISEASE (CVD)

The obesity epidemic carries serious long term health implication because of the increased morbidity associated with being overweight and obese. There is a tendency towards heightened risk factors and a greater incidence of diabetes mellitus, cardiovascular disease (CVD) endpoints such as coronary heart disease, stroke and heart failure. In addition, degenerative joint disease, asthma and cancer are intimately tied to obesity. Cardiovascular disease refers to people suffering from hypertension, heart disease (HD), stroke, peripheral artery disease (PAD), and diseases of the veins. It is the most prevalent medical disorder in the U.S. with a total of 82.6 million Americans who have one or more types of CVD, representing about 24% of the U.S. population. It is not surprising then that as many as 76.4 million suffer from hypertension. As of 2008 both CVD and stroke alone carried a price tag of $297.7 billion in direct and indirect costs. By contrast cancers and benign neoplasms cost $228 billion in direct and indirect medical expenses (Roger et al AHA 2012). It is also responsible for the greatest mortality in the U.S., representing 810,810 deaths in 2008 or 32.8% of all reported deaths in the U.S. that year. Although death rates from CVD have declined 30.6% between 1998 and 2008, CVD still remains a significant health burden. This is especially true when specific metrics of good cardiovascular health are measured in the population. It is estimated that 63% of adult whites, and 71% of adult African and Mexican Americans have only 3 or fewer ideal metrics of good health out of 7 (Roger et al AHA 2012).

4.2 THE CAUSES OF CARDIOVASCULAR DISEASE

4.2.1 Poor Diet & Lifestyle Habits

There 4 basic behaviors that are considered healthy and conducive to keeping CVD in check in the population. First, moderate to high levels of physical activity need to be included on a daily basis; daily commitments of 60 minutes or 420 minutes per week greatly contribute to managing stable body weights in addition to increasing the HDL cholesterol, known as the good cholesterol. It is concerning that only 61% of teenagers and adults consider themselves as physically active. Second, the decision not to smoke sizably decreases a person's risk of developing heart disease. Approximately 84% of teenagers and 73% of adults are non-smokers in the U.S.;

45

third, maintaining a BMI<25 has been clearly associated with lower risks of CVD; however, as many as 38% of teenagers and 68% of adults fail to meet that weight standard; fourth, meeting 5 healthy dietary practices can substantially decrease CVD risks. The American Heart Association affirms the importance of 1- consuming ≥4.5 cups/day of fruits and vegetables; 2-serving ≥2-3.5oz-wt of oily fish/week; 3-maintaining sodium intake to <1500 mg/day; 4-keeping sugar-sweetened beverages to weekly intakes that are ≤450Kcal; 5-ensuring the consumption of 3oz-wt/day of whole grains containing 1.1g of fiber per 10g carbohydrates; 6-nuts, legumes and seeds should be consumed in excess of 4 servings/week; 7-processed meats need to be ≤ 2 servings/week; and 8-staturated fat intake should be kept at <7% of total calories.

The NHANES 2007-2008 survey data measured a number of cardiovascular health risks in the U.S. population, and the findings are setting off alarms at the national level. In the 12-19 year old age group there are a number of dietary and lifestyle practices that heighten this age group's risk of developing CVD early on in their lives (**Figure 4.1**). At a most fundamental level, impoverished eating habits are now forcibly making this crisis alarmingly dangerous. An imposing 92% of teenagers fail to consume more than 4.5 cups of vegetables/day, whereas 88% of those older than 20 years do not meet this basic healthy nutrition goal.

And it is the quality of the fats that are consumed specifically that impact the vascular system. Atherosclerosis is defined as a chronic inflammatory disease that generally culminates in athero-thrombotic complications, after several decades of silent development. A gradual thickening of the arterial walls by an atheroma causes a slowed circulation because of a narrowing of the artery leading gradually to obstruction. The end point is acute coronary syndromes, which often occur as a heart attack or stroke. Indeed, arterial obstruction prevents the oxygen-rich blood from reaching specific tissues. A heart attack occurs when a specific region of the heart muscle receives inadequate oxygen; a stroke is when regions of the brain are deprived of blood because of a vascular obstruction (**Figure 4.1**). It is specifically cardiovascular risk factors such as hypercholesterolemia, hypertension, smoking or diabetes that are often at the source of the inflammation. There are other circumstances however, when inflammation precedes atherosclerotic alterations. One of the theories behind atheroma formation begins with an arterial wall injury resulting from elevated BP. Damage to the inner wall of the artery called the endothelium, initiates an inflammatory response which causes a convergence of free and esterified cholesterol, monocytes and macrophage which form a foam like substances that attempts to heal the injury through fibrosis and calcification. It is precisely at the location of arterial lesions that platelets begin to aggregate and stick to the injury site, leading often times to the formation of blood clots and to an eventual obstruction to blood flow, resulting in a heart attack (Balanescu et al 2010; Grundy, 2006). The diet can protect against the formation of an atheroma and heart attack most notably through the consumption of omega-3 fatty acids, abundantly found in oily fish. These fish are particularly rich in EPA and DHA, which are known fatty acids that protect against strokes and cardiovascular events. Sadly, only 9.2% of teenagers and 18.3% of adults over 20 years of age consume ≥ 2-3.5oz-wt of oily fish servings/week. Sodium intake in foods tends to be very elevated the more processed the food. The ingestion of sodium needs to be controlled because of its tie to hypertension. Here again there are concerns at the population as less than 1% of teenagers and adults maintain their sodium intake < 1500mg/day. The NHANES 2005-2006 survey revealed that 90.4% of adult Americans do in fact exceed their maximal daily allowance of 2400 mg.

Sugary beverages are being ingested in larger volumes at an earlier age. In fact, 68% of teenagers fail to drink ≤450 kcal/week, and as many as 48% of adults fail to keep soft drinks and other sugary beverages in check. When a composite of 4-5 healthy eating behaviors were monitored in the NHANES 2007-2008 survey, none of the teenagers and a mere 0.3% of the adults met 4-5 out of the 8 recommended healthy eating practices. Is there any wonder that CVD risk factors still remain elevated?

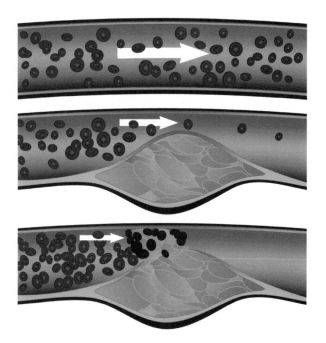

Figure 4.1 Atherosclerosis in the arteries Credit Line © Monkey Business /Shutterstock.com

4.2.2 Abnormal Lipid Metabolism

The lipid profile of patients with heart disease reveals high LDL cholesterol, low HDL cholesterol, elevated triglycerides (TG) and often times there is hyperglycemia. Understanding how lipoproteins are formed and work within the scheme of lipid metabolism is critical for understand the diagnosis of heart disease risks as well as the treatments. It begins with fat ingestion in our diet and the absorption of that fat from the lumen of the intestine into the blood and then to the various tissues either for deposition or energy production. The ideal model would be that all the fat ingested at a meal would be taken up by the individual cells and oxidized in the Tricarboxilic acid (TCA) cycle to ATP. In this way there would be no surplus fat to deposit in any of the adipocytes. Obesity would not be a problem in this context. Unfortunately, obesity and heart disease are two of the main epidemics currently afflicting American society. The main dietary deviances that are causing these problems are the excess total and saturated fats consumed regularly by the population.

Once fat is ingested, the bile, secreted from the gallbladder, emulsifies the fat into dispersed droplets, called micelles, which are then easily hydrolyzed principally by the "lipase" enzyme secreted by the pancreas. Pancreatic lipase is considered the most important fat digestive enzyme. It cleaves the fatty acids from the glycerol backbone thus resulting in free fatty acids. The latter are absorbed into the enterocytes—the cells lining the small intestine—where they are encapsulated into a large lipoprotein called "**chylomicron.**" Inside this lipoproteins are found long and some medium chain fatty acids, glycerol, phospholipids, proteins and cholesterol. These chylomicrons are released into the circulation first via the **lymphatic system,** which eventually connects with the subclavian vein (superior vena cava), and onwards to the liver (**Figure 4.1**). As the chylomicron circulates in the blood leading to the liver, it deposits its main cargo of triglycerides into muscle cells, where the fatty acids are eventually oxidized, and into the adipocytes for storage. Afterwards, having lost most of the triglycerides, the chylomicron becomes a **chylomicron remnant (CR)**, containing significantly less triglycerides and proportionally more cholesterol which it deposits in the liver. From there, very light-density lipoproteins (VLDLs) are released into circulation with the objective of redistributing the triglycerides into lean tissue and adipose tissue (Hegele, 2009).

As this lipoprotein makes its deposits, it becomes first an intermediary density lipoprotein (IDL) and finally a light-density lipoprotein (LDL) containing mostly cholesterol. It is this lipoprotein that accumulates in the blood of patients with high cholesterol. The high density lipoproteins (HDLs), by contrast, are considered cholesterol scavengers; they are generated from peripheral tissues like the intestines, and from the liver (Figure 4.1). They scavenge the cholesterol from the vascular epithelium and return it to the liver to be repackaged again as VLDLs and recirculated in the blood or utilized for the synthesis of bile by the liver. The clinician, looking over a patient's lipid profile, wants to see elevated HDLs, low LDLs and triglycerides (TG) (See Table-4.2 for lipid standards). The primary targets of lipid-lowering therapy are the LDLs according to the National Cholesterol Education Program (NCEP).

4.3 ASSESSMENT OF CARDIOVASCULAR DISEASE

An important and valuable tool used in the assessment of CVD is **metabolic syndrome**. The NHANES 2003-2006 survey data confirmed that 34% of adult Americans suffer from metabolic syndrome. A cluster of risk factors for CVD and diabetes are used by the frontline clinicians to screen for patients with metabolic syndrome. These are patients with 3 or more of 5 risk factors:

Fasting blood glucose > 100 mg/dl

HDL cholesterol < 40 mg/dl in men and < 50 mg/dl in women, or who are receiving pharmacotherapy for low HDLs

Serum triglycerides ≥ 150mg/dl or receiving medication for hypertriglyceridemia

Waist circumference ≥102 cm in men, and ≥88 cm in women

BP with a systolic value ≥130 mm Hg and a diastolic ≥85mm Hg or a patient treated with antihypertensive drugs who has a history of hypertension.

While most patients with diabetes have metabolic syndrome, some prefer to stratify these patients into a distinct risk category because of the diabetes. Nevertheless, the criteria used to screen patients with metabolic syndrome is consistently used in the healthcare field and so must be well known by dietitians, nurses and other health care professionals.

4.4 STRATEGIES TO CONTROL CVD

The American Heart Association's (AHA) 2020 goal is to improve cardiovascular health by 20% in the U.S population by the year 2020. The AHA defines "Ideal cardiovascular health" as the absence of any of the clinical symptoms of CVD, and of the presence of 7 health behaviors such as increased lean body mass—this intimates a low but healthy % body fat,—avoidance of smoking, heightened and regular physical activity [PA], and healthy dietary intake practices that are consistent with the standards of the **Dietary Approaches to Stop Hypertension [DASH] (Table 4.1)**. In addition the AHA recommends reaching and maintaining these blood markers: i-untreated total cholesterol <200 mg/dl; ii-untreated BP <120/<80 mm Hg; and, iii- fasting blood glucose <100 mg/dl. Achieving these health behaviors may prove to be more challenging than most people think.

Strategies for complying with the DASH Diet—The DASH diet encompasses strict dietary guidelines that are healthy but stringent enough to reduce the risks of heart disease in the population if followed closely. The guidelines overlap with the U.S. Food Guide and the Healthy Eating Guidelines for Americans. In many ways the DASH diet is more stringent and therapeutic in decreasing BP. The DASH diet is generated from extensively studying the dietary factors that are most protective against hypertension. Historically, sodium and salt were thought to be the most influential factors in the etiology of hypertension. The DASH diet still encourages a target sodium intake of no more than 1500mg per day, but now recognizes the importance of calcium, magnesium, potassium, and fiber in maintaining BP in a healthy zone. The goal is to achieve the nutrient intakes recommended in Table 4.1.

Dietary Recommendations of the DASH Diet—Respecting the DASH diet guidelines means eating 4-5 serving of vegetables / day, an amount most of the

American public is not likely to consume. Nevertheless, the standard DASH diet recommends vegetables that are rich in magnesium and potassium such as tomatoes, carrots, broccoli, sweet potatoes, and include greens of various types like spinach, kale, and cabbage, all good sources of fiber. One serving of leafy greens is 1 cup and so is ½ cup of cooked or raw vegetables. The idea is to creatively decrease meat portions by increasing the proportion of vegetables in a dish, for instance.

Fruits servings need to increase to 4-5 servings/day. One serving is understood to be 1 medium size fruit, ½ cup of fresh, frozen or canned (with no syrup or added sugar), or ½ cup of juice. Fruits need very little preparation, and so can be eaten on the run, as a dessert or as a flavorful snack any time of the day. The snacking industry in the U.S. is controlled by large multinational corporations that flood the grocery stores with cheap non-nutritious snack foods; their goal is not to feed the population but to make a lot of money. Hence massive snacking publicity campaigns flood the media and the market place, whether on billboards, TV, internet commercials or magazines. The ads encouraging the consumption of soft drinks, candies, cakes, pastries and chips are everywhere. The catastrophic consequences of these expensive campaigns, is that the desire to eat fruit instead has gone down considerably since the 1980s.

Dairy intake needs to represent 2-3 servings a day as this is a major source of calcium, vitamin D and protein. Indeed, three servings of milk contain 24g of high quality protein, 900 to 1100 mg of calcium, and 120 to 300 IU of vitamin D. Vitamin D is fortified in the U.S. following the standard of 40-100 IU/100 Kcals. One serving of dairy equates to 1 cup of milk (skim or 1%) and 1.5oz-wt of cheese. Plain yogurt can be incorporated in the diet with much greater ease than sweetened yogurts. For desserts, it is a good idea to mix frozen unsweetened berry blend fruit mixes into plain yogurt; this strategy maximizes dairy and fruit consumption without including any added sugar.

Grains need to be included to the tune of 6-8 servings/day. One serving consists of ½ cup of cooked cereal, pasta or rice; it will also include 1oz-wt of dry cereal, or 1oz-wt of bread. The goal is to select whole grain products that are elevated in fiber. For instance, brown rice, whole grain pasta and a high fiber cereal containing at least 5g/serving are excellent choices for reaching the fiber intake goal of 30g/day.

Lean meats, poultry and oily fish are encouraged. The goal is to consume 6 or less servings / day. One serving has been defined as 1oz-wt of meat or 1 egg. Eating enough protein in the diet has not been a problem for the American public in recent years because of the abundant meat consumed in the U.S. However, the quality of that

TABLE 4.1 Daily Nutrient Goals Achieved by following the DASH Diet

Total Fat	≤27% of calories
Saturated Fat	≤6% calories
Cholesterol	<150 mg/day
Protein	18% of calories
Carbohydrate	55% of calories
Std. Na DASH Limit	<2300 mg/day
Low Na DASH diet	1500 mg/day
Potassium	4700 mg/day
Magnesium	500 mg
Calcium	1,250 mg/day
Fiber	30 g/day

Source: NHLBI's Guidelines retrieved from: https://www.nhlbi.nih.gov/health/health-topics/topics/dash/

protein needs to be scrutinized more closely. As a rule the U.S. is not a great consumer of fish and seafood, but yet, history and research informs us that the omega-3 fats found in salmon, herring and tuna, are highly protective against heart disease. Otherwise, leaner cuts of poultry and red meats need to be purchased more frequently. The goal here is to decrease saturated fat to ≤6% of calories (DASH diet standard).

Nuts, seeds and legumes should be consumed more frequently and in greater abundance. The goal is to reach 4 to 5 servings /week. One serving is characteristically ⅓ cup of nuts, 2 tablespoons of seeds, or ½ cup of cooked legumes like lentils, Romano beans, kidney beans, navy beans or soy beans. These are excellent sources of vegetable protein which when complemented with grains in the diet, form complete proteins. These foods are rich in healthy oils that contain omega-3 and monounsaturated fatty acids. Legumes are also rich in magnesium and potassium, not to mention soluble fibers that help regulate serum cholesterol and decrease the risk of some cancers (Mayo Clinic).

Fats and oils are valuable in regulating cardiovascular risks. The vilification of fats in recent years has led to the adoption of low fat weight loss diets by many individuals, and to a significant decline in healthy fat intakes. The DASH diet encourages consuming no more than 27% of calories as fat, and giving preference to monounsaturated fats. In order to maintain saturated fats to <6% of calories, it is imperative that individuals limit their intakes of meat, butter, cheese, whole milk, cream and eggs, in addition to lard, solid shortenings, palm and coconut oils. There is also intent to restrict the trans-fats by avoiding baked goods, crackers and fried foods made from shortenings and hard margarines.

To help the patient maintain a healthy weight, the recommendation is to consume 5 or fewer servings of sweets/week. This includes limiting the ingestion of regular soft drinks, candies and pastries of various types.

Therapeutic Lifestyle Change (TLC)—The Third Report of the Expert Panel on Detection, Evaluation, and Treatment of High Blood Cholesterol in Adults (Adult Treatment Panel III or ATPIII) has updated a set of guidelines for interpreting blood cholesterol values (Table 4.2). These parameters have been adopted by the National Cholesterol Education Program's (NCEP) clinical guidelines that can help clinicians understand the severity of the hypercholesterolemia and better interpret the dietary and lifestyle guidelines the patients might have to follow in order to significantly alter the clinical risks.

The TLC has specific dietary therapeutic recommendations that can assist the patient in significantly reducing blood lipid values without medications. A minimal 10% weight reduction in combination with regular

TABLE 4.2 ATP III Classification of Blood Cholesterol

Bio measures	Goals mg/dl	Interpretation
LDL Cholesterol (mg/dl)	<100	Optimal
	100-129	Near optimal
	130-159	Borderline High
	160-189	High
	≥190	Very high
TTL Cholesterol (mg/dl)	<200	Desirable
	200-239	Borderline High
	≥240	High
HDL Cholesterol (mg/dl)	<40	Low
	≥60	High

Source: Shils, M.E (2006), p: 1896

physical activity will benefit a patient if minimal dietary adjustments are made: saturated fat should be kept <7% of total kcals, total dietary cholesterol <200 mg/day, 2g/day of plant stanols/sterols can be taken in combination with viscous soluble fibers (10-25g/day). The recommendations in Table 4.3 are the complete TLC dietary guidelines.

TABLE 4.3 Nutrient Composition of the TLC Diet

Nutrients	Recommended Intake
Saturated Fat	<7% calories
Polyunsaturated fat	Up to 10% calories
Monounsaturated fat	Up to 20% calories
Total fat	25-35% calories
Carbohydrates	50-60 % calories
Fiber	20-30g/day
Protein	~15% calories
Cholesterol	<200mg/day

Shils, M.E. et. al. (2006) p: 1898

4.5 CVD CASE STUDY-4.1: A 54 YEAR OLD MALE WITH HYPERLIPIDEMIA

4.5.1 Presentation

John B. is a 54 year old male business executive who came for his yearly checkup. He presented with no specific complaints and has maintained a clean bill of health for all of his life. The yearly review documented early hypertension, and hypercholesterolemia. His current weight: 183lbs, his height: 5 feet 9inches. Patient admits

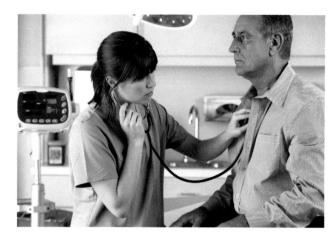

Figure 4.2 A 54 Year Old Male Being Treated for Hyperlipidemia—Credit Line © Monkey Business Images /Shutterstock.com

TABLE 4.4 Results of Medical Tests

Tests	Actual	Goal
Glucose (mg/dl)	85	≤100
LDL Cholesterol (mg/dl)	135	<100
HDL Cholesterol (mg/dl)	48	≥60
BP mmHg	138/87	<120/80
Triglycerides (TG) (mg/dl)	179	<150
Total Cholesterol (mg/dl)	223	<200

Source: NCEP 2001 report JAMA 16 (285): 2486- 97

gaining 20lbs over the last year because of excessive work-related travel. Consequently he has not been able to maintain his normal YMCA exercise commitment of 3 times a week for 1hr and 30 minutes.

4.5.2 Diet Assessment

His dietary habits changed slightly in that he has been eating out more because of traveling and business meetings. He is also drinking more beer and wine at meals compared to previous years. Otherwise his meals are balanced according to the MyPlate food guide.

4.5.3 Body Composition Assessment

Patient's BMI of 24 has been maintained stable for many years, which is within the healthy range of 18.5 to 25. His current 20lb weight gain in the last year now results in a BMI=27 which places him in the overweight category as he is situated within the range of 25 to 29.9. His weight circumference equals 41 inches. Because the circumference measure is >40 inches, he is at risk.

4.5.4 Medical Assessment

His blood biochemistry and general medical exam results are displayed in the table below.

The profile indicates than John B has hypertension, that blood sugars are normal, but that LDL cholesterol is borderline elevated in addition to total cholesterol; HDL is too low, and triglycerides are borderline elevated. This

is an ideal candidate for diet therapy and lifestyle modification to help bring risk factors down.

4.5.5 Recommendations

Exercise Prescription: First, weight-loss is the primary goal to aim for; losing 20lbs over the next 40 weeks should bring his BP down. Aiming for slow but regular weight loss is possibly the ideal way to lose weight as it decreases the chances of weight regain after dieting. In addition, including an exercise schedule could possibly accomplish two things: first, accelerate the weight loss from heightened energy expenditure; second, exercise is known to increase HDL cholesterol in the blood. According to the **2008 Physical Activity Guidelines for Americans**, adults should complete 150 minutes/week of moderate intensity aerobic exercise (2hrs 30 minutes). Spread over 5 days that works out to be 30 minutes/day. The patient should additionally dedicate 2 days or more of muscle strengthening exercises at a rate of at least 30 minutes per day. This would help the patient lose the weight or at the very least prevent further weight gain (Health & Human Services, 2008). Physical activity can be increased to 300 minutes/week and split between vigorous and moderate aerobic activity in addition 2 days of muscle strengthening exercise.

Diet Prescription: A restrictive diet would not be recommended as the patient only recently gained weight because of excess alcohol intake and more meals eaten in restaurants while traveling. Patient should simply be advised to drink only one alcoholic beverage with meals, and to consistently eat only 50-75% of the plate served at a restaurant; this will decrease total fat, saturated and sodium in amounts sufficient to bring down LDLs and TGs. The rationale here is simply that larger portions are generally served in restaurants, and often the entrées are cooked in oil and salt to enhance the taste. It is a successful approach used to increase sales and repeat food acquisition behaviors. Otherwise, recommend that the patient continue to eat normally.

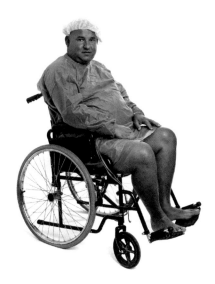

Figure 4.3 A 38 Year Old Heart Attack Victim—Credit Line © Luis Louro /Shutterstock.com

4.6 CVD CASE STUDY-4.2: A 38 YEAR OLD MALE WHO SUFFERED A HEART ATTACK

4.6.1 Presentation

Ryan V. is a 38 year old pharmaceutical sales representative with a family history of heart disease. He suffered a heart attack about 5 weekends ago while doing home repairs. He underwent bypass surgery 2 weeks ago and is now stable.

4.6.2 Medical Assessment

The BMI reveals that Ryan is obese. There is a family history of heart disease and obesity; both his father and mother are obese. Prior to the heart attack his weight was 305lbs; since the surgery he has lost 49lbs resulting from a loss of appetite. Since the heart attack he stopped eating snacks, drinking beer and barely eats his regular meals. He admits experiencing a fear of eating as he perceived most of his dietary selections as being responsible for his heart attack. His chart information is described in Table 4.5.

This patient has serious hypertension that will require medication. His LDL cholesterol is high and will need to be managed by diet and statins (Stone et al 2013). His total cholesterol is also high. The low levels of HDLs represent a second risk factor that can be related to smoking, elevated trans-fatty acid intake, low exercise, excessive weight or consuming a lot of refined foods. The patient should be questioned about these possibilities

TABLE 4.5 Patient Chart Information

Ryan V... CHART INFORMATION		
Age: 38 Current Weight: 256lbs Usual Weight: 305lbs Height: 5 feet 11 inches Patient lost 49lbs since suffering a heart attack and going through bypass surgery		
Tests	**Actual**	**Goal**
*Glucose (mg/dl)	178	≤100
LDL Cholesterol (mg/dl)	165	<100
HDL Cholesterol (mg/dl)	36	≥60
BP mmHg	162/92	<120/80
Triglycerides (mg/dl)	221	<150
Total Cholesterol (mg/dl)	309	<200

Source: NCEP 2001 report JAMA 16 (285): 2486- 97; American Diabetes Association (2011) Standards of Medical Care in Diabetes—2012 *Diabetes Care.* Suppl. 1:S11-63. * Fasting plasma glucose

(Harvard Publications, 2010). Mildly elevated triglycerides usually indicate abundant sugar consumption in the form of sucrose or fructose. Being overweight, smoking and alcohol consumption can also contribute to rising serum triglycerides (Malloy, 2007). Very elevated triglycerides tend to be the result of diabetes. The patient's TG levels are in the high risk range of 200 to 499mg/dl. Considering his elevated fasting glucose (178gm/dl) it would be reasonable to suspect type-2 diabetes mellitus. Weight loss will still be recommended in order to avoid having to prescribe oral hypoglycemic agents to control the blood sugars.

4.6.3 Body Composition Assessment

The dietitian used skinfold calipers to determine the percent body fat using a four site approach: Biceps, triceps, subscapular and supra-iliac. Using specific tables a total fat of 47% was established

Waist circumference= 56 inches

His weight: 256lbs; height 5feet 11 inches; BMI= $(256lbs \times 0.454lbs/Kg)/(71 \text{ inches} \times 0.0254 meters/inch)^2$

The BMI= 116.22 Kg/ (1.803 meters)^2 = 35.75 He is therefore classified as "obese Class-2."

This assessment indicates that the patient is over fat, and has an overabundance of highly atherogenic visceral fat, as indicated by the waist circumference greater than 40 inches.

4.6.4 Lifestyle Assessment

A review of the patient's chart reveals that the patient works long hours and is often traveling nationally. He covers a large territory and so admits to being in motels and hotels most of the time. He refers to his lifestyle as stressful as he is unable to partake in leisurely exercise except on weekends when he is home with his wife and two children. He reports going out to eat in the restaurant to give his wife a break when he is home on weekends. He rates his activity level as low.

Dietary Assessment—The dietitian sat down with the patient and questioned him about his regular eating habits prior to the heart attack. She used a Usual Food Intake assessment in order to evaluate his usual caloric consumption (Table 4.6), and a Food Frequency Questionnaire (FFQ) to ascertain the quality of his diet. The dietitian also assessed the patient's caloric requirements based on his initial reported weight prior to the heart attack (305lbs). She used the following equation for total energy expenditure:

For men:

TEE = [864 − (9.72 × Age-$_{years}$)]+[PA × ((14.2 x wt.$_{kg}$) + (503 × ht. $_{meters}$))]

TEE= [864-(9.72x38)]+[1.12x(14.2 x 138.47Kg) +(503 x 1.803 meters).

TEE= [494.64 + 3218] = 3713 Kcal/day

The usual food intake record (Table 4.6) reveals that prior to the heart attack the patient usually consumed 6700 Kcal/day, an amount that could justifiably cause significant weight gain for it was 80.4% in excess of his caloric needs.

Of particular interest was the alarming amount of fat regularly consumed, representing 44.3% of his caloric intake, and amount that far exceeded the recommended macronutrient range of 20 to 35%, proposed by the DASH and TLC diets. Also carbohydrate intake far

exceeded his recommended healthy range of 418-603g. His protein intake was acceptable, but his total sugar intake—most of which was added sugar—exceeded his maximal allowance of 232g/day. Since maximal added sugar is <10% of calories, or 93g, his actual intake can therefore be considered alarmingly elevated. This elevated sucrose intake can, in part, explain the elevated triglycerides (Mallow, 2007). Fiber intake was 45g/day which on the surface appears to meet the daily requirement of 30g. However, when broken down per 1000 kcals to be consistent with ADA guidelines, the patient is actually consuming 6.92g/1000 Kcals, which is far less than the recommended 14g/1000 Kcals. It can be concluded therefore, that the patient's diet is poor in fiber content.

4.6.5 Diet Prescription

He has been referred to a dietitian who is a member of cardiac rehabilitation services; she will be reviewing his usual diet and teaching him the DASH diet. The first step consists of prescribing a weight maintenance diet that will first stabilize his weight at his current weight of 256lbs, while taking into account his low activity factor. Since the heart attack the patient has lost a lot of weight through a fear of eating and poor appetite. It is important at this point to introduce him to healthy eating, reassuring him that it is safe to eat. Once his weight has stabilized, then a more thoughtful plan for slow and gradual weight reduction in combination with increased physical activity may be introduced. Again, the dietitian used the previous TEE equation to assess his daily caloric needs:

For men:

TEE = [864 − (9.72 × Age-$_{years}$)]+[PA × ((14.2 x wt.$_{kg}$) + (503 × ht. $_{meters}$))]

TEE=[864-(9.72x38)]+[1.12x(14.2 x 116.22Kg) +(503x1.803 meters) = 494.64+[2556.91]=3052 Kcals/day.

So then, the total daily calories necessary to maintain this patient's weight at 256lbs for a short transition period and assuming a low activity factor is: 3052 Kcals/day. The goal is to prescribe a low fat and a high carbohydrate intake rich in complex starches that are high in fiber and consistent with DASH dietary standards.

Using the recommended macronutrient ranges of the Healthy Eating Guidelines for Americans as a guidepost, the dietitian prescribed 55% of calories as carbohydrates, 18% as protein and 27% as fat. Her intent was to

TABLE 4.6 Usual Food Intake Record

PATIENT NAME: **Ryan V**	USUAL FOOD INTAKE	
FOODS CONSUMED	**QUANTITY CONSUMED**	**PLACE**
BREAKFAST: TIME		
Never consumes breakfast Coffee (Starbucks Grande + cream)	3 cups (900 ml) or 30fl-oz	Kitchen & car
AM SNACKS TIME:		
Chocolate bar (snickers) Reg. size Pepsi Cola(Reg.) Donut (Dunkin donut jelly-filled)	105.4g (3.76 oz-wt) 12fl-oz (355 ml can) 3	Office/car
LUNCH TIME:		
Pepsi Cola (Reg.) French Fries (McDonald's) Lay's plain Potato Chips (bag)	12fl-oz (355 ml can) Large 5oz bag	restaurants
PM SNACK TIME:		
Pepsi Cola (Reg.) Big Mac	12fl-oz (355 ml can) 1(7.6oz-wt)	McDonald's
DINNER TIME:		
Sirloin Steak (Logan's Roadhouse) Beer—Indian Pale Ale (IPA) Baked Potato (Logan's Roadhouse) Butter (salted) Pasta salad	16oz-wt (448g) 20fl-oz 1 whole 4 pats 2 cups	restaurant
ENEVING SNACK TIME:		
Orville Reddenbacher…butter popcorn Pepsi Cola (Reg)	9 cups popped 20fl-oz (591 ml)	

NUTRIENT BREAKDOWN OF USUAL FOOD INTAKE	
Kcals recommended: 3713 kcal/day (3342-4084 Kcals/day) Carbohydrates recommended: 557g/day (60% DRI Kcals) (418-603g) Protein recommended: 139g/day (15% DRI Kcals) (93g-325g) Fat recommended: 103g (25% DRI Kcals) (83-144g) Total Maximal Sugar: <232g (25% DRI Kcals) Total Maximal Sodium: <2400 mg/day	Kcals eaten: **6700 kcals** Carbohydrates eaten: **770g** Protein eaten: **185g** Fat eaten: **320g** Total Sugar eaten: **272g** Sodium eaten: **5505 mg**

Calories measured using the www.myfitnesspal.com website

maintain saturated fat < 6% of calories and dietary cholesterol <150 mg/day. Taking into account the elevated BP, the dietitian recommended keeping sodium intake to < 1500 mg/day. Consistent with the full rationale governing the DASH diet, the dietitian also recommends a diet rich in foods abundant in fiber, magnesium (Mg), potassium (K) and calcium (Ca) as they are helpful in controlling BP.

The dietitian's diet prescription for weight maintenance is found in Table 4.7.

There are a number of foods that will need to disappear from his usual menu while he is on the maintenance diet. This means that the food items are non-negotiable; he needs to eliminate them from his normal fare in order to break away from the addictive nature of these foods: soft drinks (regular and diet), fast food, and unhealthy snack foods (chips, donuts, chocolate bars). These foods are important contributors of total and saturated fats, and therefore need to be removed from the menu, and replaced by a broad variety of fruits. Here, innovative

TABLE 4.7 Diet Prescription for Weight Maintenance

Macronutrients	Diet prescribed	Goal
Carbohydrates	420g (1680Kcal)	55%
Protein	137g (548Kcals)	18%
Fat	92g (828Kcals)	27%
Total Calories	3056 kcals	3052 Kcals
Saturated fat	<20g	<20g
cholesterol	<150mg	<150mg
Sodium	<2300 mg	<2300 mg

approaches will need to be taken into to get these fruits consumed. This will be rather difficult in the beginning because of the patient's taste preference for foods high in sugar, salt and fat. Innovative strategies involve the use of plain yogurt, high fiber breakfast cereals and food carvings. Here are some suggestions:

Plain yogurt added to frozen berry blend fruits which have no added sugar. Spoon out ⅓ cup of berry blend fruit into a small plastic container, top with ½ cup of plain yogurt, sprinkle 1 Tablespoon of granola, and then seal the lid and store in the refrigerator. These are quick snacks that can be easily accessed. This will increase the patient's calcium and antioxidant intake (Figure 4.4).

For breakfast, 1 cup of high fiber cereal consisting of ⅓ cup of Kellogg's bran buds, ⅓ cup of old fashioned whole oats, ⅓ cup of dried fruits (raisins, dates, cranberries and apricots). Serve with skim milk or yogurt

A smoothie can also be a creative method of consuming vitamin and mineral-rich foods. Mix together in a blender, ½ cup of yogurt (low fat), 1 medium banana, and ½ cup of thawed frozen berry fruits (blackberry, strawberry and cherry mix). Blenderize until smooth, pour in a container that can be sealed and refrigerated.

4-Carve out the center of a watermelon, and fill with pineapple chunks, apples, grapefruit pieces, orange quarters, cantaloupe, strawberries and blueberries. Mix in about ½ cup of pure orange juice. Serve at meal time so that the whole family can learn to love fruits. This is especially attractive to children (Figure 4.5).

After it becomes clear that the patient's appetite is good and his weight stabilized, a slow weight loss diet can be introduced. Rapid weight loss should be discouraged as the evidence appears to indicate that weight regain is almost inevitable (Mann et al. 2007). The only non-surgical approaches, that seem to work so far, are mild calorie restrictions in combination with regular exercise. The dietitian aimed for about ½lbs weight loss/week from diet restriction alone. Given that a 3500 kcal deficit in a week equates to a 1lbs weight loss, and that this can be achieved with a 500 kcal deficit/day, it is therefore correct to advance that a 250 kcal restriction

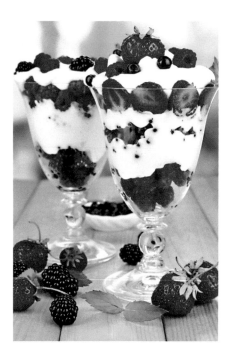

Figure 4.4 Fresh & frozen fruits mixed with yogurt— shutterstock_145095274. Credit Line © Africa Studio / Shutterstock.com

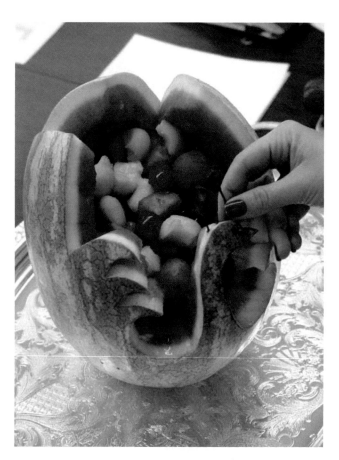

Figure 4.5 Carved Melon Swan with Fresh Fruit

would result in a ½lbs weight loss per week. Hence the diet prescription for slow weight loss, would amount to a 2806 Kcal/day diet.

The exercise prescription should not involve rigorous high intensity workouts, but should be of long duration but mild in intensity. The patient does not have an extensive history of exercise.

Walking 3 mi/hr at moderate pace for 2hrs/day for a total of 3 days/week will cause an expenditure of 0.025Kcal/ lb/min. This 256 pound man will therefore be able to expend 768 Kcals/2hrs of walking. In combination with his dietary restriction of 250kcals/ day, this patient will be able to afford 1.16lbs of weight loss/week. Below, I outlined the calculations.

A caloric restriction of 250 Kcals/day equates to 1750 Kcals/week (250 kcal x 7 days). Energy expenditure from walking= 768 Kcals/2hrs of waking. If patient walks three times per week the total energy expenditure from walking = 2304 Kcals (3 days x 768 Kcals). The total energy deficit arising from both caloric restriction and exercise equates to 4054 Kcals (1750Kcals + 2304 Kcals). Since a 3500 kcals deficit equals 1lb of weight loss, then a 4054 kcal deficit/week will equal a loss of 1.16lbs/ week (4054/3500Kcals).

As the patient loses weight the risk indicators of heart disease such as waist circumference, hyperglycemia, hyperlipidemia and BP should greatly diminish. In addition, regular exercise should allow HDLs to rise.

REFERENCES

1. Balanescu, S. et al. (2010) Systemic inflammation and early atheroma formation. Are they related? Maedica (Buchar). 5(4): 292–301.
2. Bissonnette, D.J. (2014) It's All About Nutrition: Saving the Health of Americans. Lanham, MD: University Press of America 232pp
3. Grundy, S. Nutrition in the Management of Disorders of Serum Lipids and Lipoproteins. In: Modern Nutrition in Health and Disease 10th edition. New York: Lippincott, Williams and Wilkins. p:1076-1094
4. Harvard Health Publication (March 2010: HDL: The good but complex cholesterol. Retrieved April 9, 2014 from:
5. http://www.health.harvard.edu/newsletters/Harvard_Heart_Letter/2010/March/hdl-the-good-but-complex-cholesterol
6. Hegele, R.E. (2009) Overview of Lipoprotein Metabolism *Nature Reviews Genetics* **10**, 109-121
7. Malloy, M.J. and Kane, J.P. (2007) Disorders of lipoproteins metabolism in: D.G. Gardner and D. Shoback, eds Greenspan's Basic and Clinical Endocrinology (New York: McGraw-Hill/Lang pp: 770-795
8. Mann, T. et al. (2007). Medicare's Search for Effective Obesity Treatments: Diets are not the Answer. Am Psychol. 62(3):220-33
9. Mayo Clinic. Nutrition & Healthy Living—DASH Diet: Healthy Eating to Lower your BP. Retrieved April 4, 2014 from:
10. http://www.mayoclinic.org/healthy-living/nutrition-and-healthy-eating/in-depth/dash-diet/art-20048456?pg=1
11. National Cholesterol Education Program (NCEP) (2001) Expert Panel on Detection 3rd Report on The Evaluation and Treatment of High Blood Cholesterol in Adults. JAMA 16 (285):2486-97
12. National Heart, Lung and Blood Institute (NHLBI). NIH. What is the DASH Eating Plan? Retrieved April 4, 2014 from:
13. https://www.nhlbi.nih.gov/health/health-topics/topics/dash/
14. National Heart, Lung and Blood Institute (NHLBI), NIH, What is atherosclerosis. Retrieved April 4, 2014 from:
15. https://www.nhlbi.nih.gov/health/health-topics/topics/atherosclerosis/
16. Roger, V.L et al. (2012) AHA Statistical Update: Heart Disease and Stroke Statistics 2012. Circulation 125: e2-e220. Retrieved April 7, 2014 from: http://circ.ahajournals.org/content/125/1/e2.full
17. Shils, M.E. et al. (2006). Part VIII Appendix Table A-9-b-1-a ATP-III Classification of LDL, Total and HDL Cholesterol. In: Modern Nutrition in Health and Disease 10th edition. New York: Lippincott, Williams and Wilkins. p: 1896
18. Shils, M.E. et al. (2006). Part VIII Appendix Table A-9-b-6-a Nutrient Composition of the TLC Diet In: Modern Nutrition in Health and Disease 10th edition. New York: Lippincott, Williams and Wilkins. p: 1898
19. Stone, N.J. et al. (2014) 2013 ACC/AHA Guideline on the Treatment of Blood Cholesterol to Reduce Atherosclerotic Cardiovascular Risk in Adults. Journal of the American College of Cardiology
20. doi:10.1016/j.jacc.2013.11.002 Retrieved April 10, 2014 from: https://circ.ahajournals.org/content/early/2013/11/11/01.cir.0000437738.63853.7a.full.pdf
21. U.S Department of Health & Human Services. The 2008 Physical Activity Guidelines for Americans, chapter 4: Active Adults. Retrieved April 9, 2014 from: http://www.health.gov/paguidelines/guidelines/chapter4.aspx

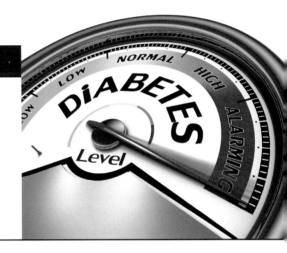

CHAPTER 5

THE PROBLEM OF DIABETES MELLITUS

5.1 THE PREVALENCE OF DIABETES

Health care in the United States is changing dramatically as the number of young obese and type-2 diabetic patients is exploding. The consequences are terrifying as the medical system is now under siege by patients who are more complicated and more time-consuming to manage. There has been an exponential growth of the diabetic population in the U.S. in recent decades, going from 5.6 million cases in 1980 to 17.4 million cases in 2007, and more recently jumping to an astounding 26 million American adults in 2010 according to the Center for Disease Control's 2011 report. This represents a 364% increase in the overall diabetic population in the last thirty years. But most surprisingly, there are an additional 79 million American adults or 35% of the adult population who are classified as pre-diabetic. In total, then, there are 105 million adult Americans who are either suffering from diabetes or are at risk of developing diabetes. Epidemiologists have identified the top 10 states forming the diabetes belt with an adult diabetes prevalence that varies between 10-12%; the highest prevalence is exclusively found in the southern states, except for Ohio. Notably, Alabama and West Virginia have the honors of being the two states with the highest prevalence of adult diabetes in the nation.

While it is understood that 90 to 95 percent of all diabetes mellitus cases are type-2, it is important to note that the prevalence of type-2 diabetes is still rare in less than 10 year old children (0.4 per 100,000 cases). The most numerous cases in the youth, nevertheless, have been observed in the 10-19 year olds (8.5 cases per 100,000).

Type-2 diabetes, a disease that was historically documented in adults over the age of 40 is now, in fact, growing in prominence among children and adolescents. A study by Pinhas-Hamiel and co-workers (1996) reported that the incidence of newly diagnosed type-2 diabetics in children jumped from 2-4% in 1982 to 16% by 1994 which when stratified represented 33% of the 10-19 year-olds. In the U.S. the prevalence of type-2 diabetes becomes more accentuated if cases are stratified by ethnicity. Indeed, increases of between 8% and 45% have been observed among recently diagnosed diabetic children and adolescence, depending on their ethnic heritage (American Diabetes Association, 2000). The American Indian children ages 10-14 are particularly vulnerable; the prevalence of type-2 diabetes among Pima Indians for instance, rose 200% between the decades 1967-1976 and 1987-1996, and 150% in the ages 15-19. Also, the Asian Pacific Islanders, Hispanics and the Non-Hispanic blacks ages 10-19, residing in the U.S. between 2002-2005, are also specifically at risk, as close to 50%

or more of the newly diagnosed diabetics in these groups tend to suffer from type-2 diabetes (CDC, 2011).

In the UK the story is most notable because researchers found that the risk of type 2 diabetes is 13.5 times greater among Asian than white children (Ehtisham et al. 2000; Drake et al. 2002). They also found that girls are 1.7 times more likely than boys to have type-2 diabetes. Worldwide the prevalence of diabetes has more than tripled since 1985. Dr Zachary Bloomgarden (2004), an endocrinologist affiliated with Mount Sinai School of Medicine in New York, writes in the April 2004 issue of Diabetes Care: "*The topic has become a clinical and health economic priority, with important implications for an increasing health care burden throughout the world.* "

Looking ahead, the Centers for Disease Control and Prevention predicts that by the year 2034 there will likely be an estimated 44.1 million diabetics, representing over a 24 year period, a 69.61% prevalence increase, which is projected to be accompanied by a shocking 197.34% increase in direct medical expenses. There is no doubt that the financial burden on the system will be difficult to bear and could ultimately cripple the American Health Care system (Pinhas-Hamiel, 1996 O. and Zeitler, P et al. 2001). The alarming medical costs only make sense, if one considers the treatment costs for many chronic diseases that are attached to diabetes. Indeed, a much bleaker picture gets drawn over the American landscape. Consider that the 2011 National Diabetes Fact Sheet published by The Center for Disease Control and Prevention, reveals that the total costs associated with diagnosed diabetes in 2007 amounted to $174 billion, consisting in $116 billion in direct medical costs and $58 billion in indirect costs involving disabilities, work loss and premature mortality. These kinds of medical problems become costly but also time consuming to manage since the life course of diabetes is plagued with crippling secondary conditions and diseases.

The increased prevalence of diabetes in the US and worldwide is so alarming that it has health care providers struggling with this epidemic as so many of the young appear to be suffering from chronic illnesses at younger ages thereby increasing their risk of developing long term health problems by middles age (Wilde, 2004).

Type-2 diabetes has risen concurrently in prevalence with obesity which has been steadily increasing since the mid-1970s. Close to 70% of American adults are either overweight or obese, and approximately 34% of adults are obese (Ogden, et al., 2006). Internationally, the problem is also becoming quite concerning as Scotland reported 25-26% obesity among adults in 2008, and Greece exhibited 26-28% obesity in 2001-2003 (International Obesity Task force).   The consequences of a nation becoming significantly overweight and obese are numerous and profound. This growth is unrelenting, sweeping adults and children into inescapable lives of chronic and debilitating diseases, and unspeakable suffering. Can a nation support this level of illness? What can we do to halt its progress? One thing is certain, and that is we must intervene in haste less we end up ruining the health of our youth and the very fabric of our society.

5.2 TYPE-1 DIABETES

A broader look at diabetes may be necessary at this stage in order to fully appreciate the complexity of this devastating disease. Historically, the most prevalent form of diabetes among children and young adults has always been type-1 or juvenile-onset diabetes, however, type-1 diabetes only represents 5% of the people who have diabetes according to the American Diabetes Association. It is rather type-2 diabetes that is gaining prominence, representing between 90 to 95 percent of all diabetic cases.

Type-1 diabetes occurs when the beta cells of the pancreas can no longer produce sufficient insulin, a hormone that is secreted in the blood, and which allows serum glucose to enter the cells where it is converted to energy (**Figure 5.1**). Without insulin, the sugar remains high in the blood after a person consumes complex starches or simple sugars. In type-1 and type-2 diabetics, blood sugars remain elevated for extended periods of time after carbohydrate intakes, a phenomenon known as **hyperglycemia**.

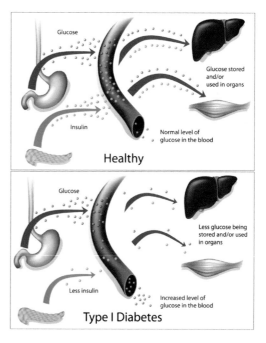

Figure 5.1 Causes of Type-1 Diabetes. Credit line © Alila Medical Media /shutterstock.com

The diagnosis of either type-1 or type-2 diabetes is based on the detection of hyperglycemia using accepted blood sugar concentration standards in various settings:

1. When random blood sugar concentrations are 200 mg/dl or greater
2. When blood sugar levels are 126 mg/dl or greater after an 8 hour fast
3. When blood sugar concentrations following a 75 g glucose challenge are 200 mg/dl or greater two hours after the challenge (Anderson, 2006).

There are usually 6 classic symptoms found concurrently with hyperglycemia in patients with diabetes Mellitus:

1. Polyuria: frequent urination
2. Weight loss: because sugar is not converted to calories
3. Polydipsia: Increase in excessive thirst
4. Ketoacidosis: acidosis produced by excessive ketone body production
5. Ketonuria: When ketone bodies in the blood reach dangerously elevated levels and spill over into the urine.
6. Glycosuria: when glucose concentrations in the blood surpass the renal threshold of 200 mg/dl and begin to spill into the urine.

Of equal importance, at the clinical level, is the detection a sub-clinical form of diabetes Mellitus called pre-diabetes or Impaired Glucose tolerance using blood screening among patients who are at risk:

Screening for pre-diabetes allows health practitioners to begin early prevention strategies such as weight loss and controlling sugar intake. The criteria for establishing pre-diabetes are featured here and were established in 1979 by the World Health Organization and the National Diabetes Data Group (Ramlo-Halsted, and Edelman, 2000).

1. A normal fasting blood glucose of < 126 mg/dl
2. Post-prandial plasma glucose of ≥140 mg/dl but < 200mg/dl 2 hrs after drinking a 75 g glucose solution

The importance of detecting and controlling elevated blood sugars is paramount in getting the upper hand on the long term devastating effects on the vascular systems, the eyes, and the kidneys. The problem with chronically elevated blood glucose levels is the eventual cell and tissue damage that takes place through **glycosylation**. This process is characterized by glucose non-enzymatically attaching to proteins and producing advanced glycation

end products (AGEs). When these compounds accumulate they can damage the integrity of cells and blood vessels thereby leading to macro and microvascular complications in addition to diabetic neuropathies. These problems invariably lead to poor circulation which slows the healing of injuries such as foot wounds for instance. The neuropathies translate into poor sensitivity thus preventing the recognition of pain as a key signal that injury has occurred. This usually means an important delay in treating these injuries which lead to infections and ultimately to foot injuries becoming gangrenous, and thus requiring amputation. It is estimated that between 15-20% of diabetics require hospitalization because of foot complications.

It becomes clear that the financial implications that are tied to the secondary effects of type-2 diabetes such as heart disease, retinopathies, neuropathies, nephropathies and amputations are likely to be financially cumbersome to a health care system that is already overburdened by a populace plagued by chronic disease.

Indeed the 2011 CDC report indicates that of those individuals with diabetes about 60% to 70% have mild to severe forms of nervous system damage and that 60% of non-traumatic lower-limb amputations occur in people with diabetes. In addition, diabetes also accounted for 44% of new cases of kidney disease in 2008.

Though hyperglycemia is the primary disordered outcome of both types of diabetes, each type remains nevertheless distinct in terms of the etiology of these elevated blood sugars. The main physiological impairment in type-1 diabetes is the necrosis or destruction of the pancreatic beta cells which can no longer produce insulin. The only medical treatment available, to counter this problem, is the subcutaneous injections of insulin along with a well-controlled diet. The reason behind the death of these cells is not clear, but scientists believe that it may be caused by an autoimmune disorder, environmental toxins or an infection of some sort. The question is: what makes certain individuals more susceptible than others to such viral attacks?

There appears to be some inherited risk factors which can heighten the chance of a person developing type-1 diabetes, but overall, the genetic influence remains relatively weak. In fact, even if both parents have type-1 diabetes the child has between a 1 in 4 and a 1 in 10 chance of also developing the disease (American Diabetes Association). By contrast, in type-2 diabetes the primary defect is **insulin resistance** which also leads to hyperglycemia because of a loss of balance between insulin sensitivity and secretion (Bloomgarden, et al. 2004). The important difference with type-1 is that in type-2 diabetes, even though insulin can still be produced by the pancreas, it is not very effective in allowing sugar to move into the cells because there are insufficient insulin-receptors imbedded within the muscles. In that sense, insulin becomes insensitive. In type-2 diabetes there can even be hypersecretion of insulin resulting in hyperinsulinemia in response to high sugar intakes, as seen with frequent soda intake and insulin resistance. Over time, a high demand for insulin can exhaust the beta cells thus leading to the possibility of insufficient insulin production. This type of diabetes, in contrast to type-1, is more heavily associated with genetics in that it is more intricately tied to family lineage and history. In fact, if both parents have type-2 diabetes the child has a 1 in 2 chance of also developing diabetes—a genetic association that is much stronger than in type-1 diabetes. This blood sugar disorder has been historically referred to as adult onset diabetes because it was most often diagnosed in adults over the age of 45.

5.3 TYPE-2 DIABETES

The cause of type-2 diabetes is currently unknown, but body fat appears to be an important determinant in causing insulin resistance. Indeed, between 80 to 90 percent of people with type-2 diabetes, are obese, and it appears that it is specifically the visceral fat accumulation or the android-type of obesity that can promote atherogenesis or the buildup of atheromas in the vascular lining, thus leading to atherosclerosis.

The impact of excessive weight in the form of fat is even more worrisome among American Indian children among whom, 40% of the less than 10 year old children are classified as overweight or obese (Styne, 2010). In addition, Styne (2001) describes a glucose metabolism that is 40% slower in obese children compared to normal weight children. This is the pre-clinical manifestation of insulin resistance, also called pre-diabetic which occurs when the tissues of the body begin to lose their sensitivity to the action of insulin, thus preventing the blood glucose from entering the cells and producing energy (**Figure 5.2**). This culminates in a rise in the blood levels of glucose, which is referred to as hyperglycemia, and it is this kind of diabetes that is called type-2 diabetes.

The mechanism was previously reported by Professor Yuji Matsuzawa from Osaka University in Japan. His team showed that accumulated abdominal fat causes impaired glucose metabolism, lipid disorders and hypertension (Matsuzawa, et al. 2008). They report, in their review, that the visceral adipocytes may link directly to the liver via the portal circulation. This fat mass is readily prone to lipolysis causing abundant free fatty acids (FFA) to flood the portal circulation leading to the liver and thus producing abundant release of VLDLs from the liver into the blood circulation. This lipoprotein circulates to muscles, vascular

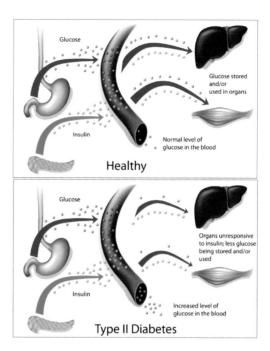

Figure 5.2 Causes of Type-2 Diabetes. Credit line © Alila Medical Media /shutterstock.com

endothelium and adipocytes where it deposits it fatty cargo and eventually becomes the more atherogenic lipoprotein called LDL or light density lipoprotein (Kuriyama, 1998). This is likely the mechanism that enhances atherogenesis in obese patients with visceral fat accumulation. However, Dr Matsuzawa completes the story further, by demonstrating that visceral adipose tissue tends to abundantly secrete bioactive compounds called adipocytokines, which have been tied to thrombogenic vascular disease. Importantly, they identified an adipocytokine produced mostly by peripheral adipocytes called adiponectin that has been found to be protective against heart disease and diabetes. This is because it appears to induce the production of anti-inflammatory cytokines and thus protect the body against disease. Interestingly, adiponectin is abundantly found in the circulation, when visceral fat reserves are low and suboptimal when there is an accumulation of visceral fat in obesity. They proposed that visceral fat accumulation may prevent the release of adiponectin from subcutaneous adipocytes because of the inhibitory effect that comes from abundant secretion of tumor necrosis factor alpha, a nefarious cytokine secreted from visceral adipocytes (Matsuzawa, et al. 2008).

5.4 CAUSES OF TYPE 2 DIABETES

Dr. Lucy Candib, a professor of family medicine and community health at the University of Massachusetts'

Medical School, explains the multiple factors that come into play in the etiology of type-2 diabetes.

The factors that are the most influential in promoting diabetes to such important degrees that it is likely to afflict entire populations and nations are outlined here:

1. Fetal and maternal explanations
2. The thrifty genotype
3. The nutritional transition
4. The health impact of urbanization and immigration
5. Social attributions and cultural perceptions of increased weight
6. The impact of globalization (Candib, 2007)

The prominent use of high fructose corn syrups in sodas is now being considered as an important source of the obesity and diabetes crisis. In the 1900s fructose coming essentially from fruits represented only 15g/day or 4% of total calories. Before World War II, fructose consumption had jumped to 24g/day and then to 37g/day by 1977. However, with the introduction of high fructose corn syrup into sodas by 1994, fructose consumption sharply rose to 55g/day. Currently, when stratified by age, it is estimated that adolescents consume 73g/day. The consumption of fructose has in fact increased 5-fold since the early 1900s and doubled since the 1980s. If one considers high fruit juice intake in addition to sodas, the total fructose consumption per capita can be adjusted upwards to 194 g/ day or a total of 156 Lbs per year (Lustig 2010).

The initial interest in fructose was fuelled by the understanding that intakes of fructose do not increase blood glucose levels. So it seemed like the ideal sweetener for diabetics. However, elevated fructose consumption can drive denovo hepatic lipogenesis or in other words new synthesis of fat from fructose. In a sense the overabundance of fructose consumed through sodas can metabolically overwhelm the mitochondrial TCA cycle, resulting in the abundant deposits of fat in the liver thus producing steatosis and inflammation. In fact, when carbohydrate intakes exceed the energy expenditure of the body, hepatic fat synthesis increases 10-fold (Aarsland, et al., 1996). Most importantly, both fructose and ethanol metabolically produce reactive oxygen species (ROS) which increases the risk of hepatocellular damage. In response to this overabundance of sugar being consumed by the US, the American Heart Association recommends cutting sugar consumption by more than 50%. Health practitioners and dietitians needs to revise current sugar intake standards as it is clear that things are getting out of hand. Indeed, high fructose corn syrup doesn't act like other sweeteners. There is now evidence emerging that, chronic intakes of fructose may actually prevent dopamine clearance from the brain, thereby stimulating

continued caloric intake despite regenerated energy stores (Anderzhanova, et al. 2007).

5.5 THE TREATMENT OF TYPE-2 DIABETES

The increasing numbers of overweight and obese patients are mostly immigrants, and low income and colored populations who consult doctors more frequently for weight problems, but who also have undiagnosed hypertension, diabetes, metabolic syndrome with significant dyslipidemia (Candid, 2007). These patients become medical train wrecks, tying up much of the medical practitioners' time with complicated issues such as high blood pressure and heart disease in addition to all of the medication management issues associated with these diseases.

We are dealing with an insulin-resistant diabetic epidemic that is resulting from obesity and lack of exercise (Bloomgarden, 2004). Logically then, it comes as no surprise that one of the most important goals in the treatment of type-2 diabetes is to lose weight and significantly decrease abdominal fat, as it will greatly assist in diminishing the risks of heart disease and insulin resistance. In fact, increased physical activity will heighten insulin sensitivity thus decreasing fasting blood sugars in children (Schmitz, et al., 2002).

An effective treatment to reduce the size of visceral fat is frequent exercise. This is based on the notion that caloric expenditure through aerobic exercise requires fat as the main fuel to support activities such as brisk walking, swimming, running and hiking. The goal is to engage in exercise routines that occupy significant time commitments such as 3 hours, and to expend significant calories. A study by Schoeller and colleagues (1997), published in the American Journal of Clinical Nutrition (Schoeller, et al. 1997) established, using doubly-labeled water, that sizable daily caloric expenditures needed to be attained that equated to 11-12 kcal/Kg/day in order to better manage body weight. The National Weight Control Registry estimates that members, who have successfully lost weight and kept if off, regularly engage, on average, in exercises that expend 2682 Kcal/week (ADA, 2009). Also, the Federal Physical Activity Guidelines for Americans 2008 recommend that, in order to achieve significant health benefits, people should engage in 300 minutes per week of exercise of moderate intensity. This represents a 5 hour weekly commitments to disciplined exercise in order to burn sufficient calories and lose significant weight.

Schoeller's recommendations represent a demanding expenditure that many would have trouble meeting on a daily basis. For instance, a man weighing between

155-210 lbs would need to expend between 1050 to 1144 kcal/day in order to successfully lose weight; this is the equivalent of 5400 to 8000 kcal/week, depending on body weight. This demanding recommendation is nevertheless relatively consistent with the guidelines provided by **the Federal Physical Activity Guidelines for Americans 2008** which advocates for moderately intense exercise occupying 300 minutes per week. In this setting, a man weighing 189 lbs who runs at a speed of 6 mi/hr—this equates to burning 0.072 kcal/lb/ min—for one hour five times per week would in fact expend 4082 kcal/week. Likewise, for individuals who are older and / or compromised by physical disabilities, who cannot engage in rigorous forms of activities, walking becomes a gentler alternative. Hence regular walking at a speed of 3 miles/hr (0.0249 kcal/lb/min), a man weighing 189 lbs would have to walk 3 hours/day or 9 miles per day in order to expend 5929 kcal/week, a total caloric expenditure that becomes meaningful. This is also consistent with the 2005 dietary guidelines for American which encouraged 60 to 90 minutes/day or between 420 to 630 minutes/ week of exercise of moderate intensity in order to prevent weight regain.

A more recent recommendation to increase physical activity may not be strictly tied to losing body fat, but also to augmenting lean body mass or muscle mass. An observational study by UCLA medical researcher, Preethi Stikanthan, published in the September 2011 issue of the Journal of Clinical Endocrinology and Metabolism, concluded that higher muscle mass was associated with a lower risk of diabetes. This is an important study that detracts from the single-minded focus of weight reduction, through dietary caloric restrictions alone, and emphasizes the notion of improved fitness as well. The therapeutic strategy of caloric restriction has not, historically been shown, to be effective in causing obesity prevalence to decline (Fagot-Campagna, 2001; Mann et al 2007) and consequently does not appear to be effective in diminishing the prevalence of diabetes.

A more realistic goal in managing overweight and obese children is to aim for weight maintenance or even delaying weight gain (Bloomgarden, 2004) while focusing at guiding the children and parents towards healthier food choices over the long term, in addition to increasing physical activity.

The main conclusions drawn from the 90% weight loss success stories filed with The National Weight Control Registry, is that individuals with weight problems need to embrace low fat and high carbohydrates diets; they need to regularly eat breakfast, become physically active and frequently monitor their weight. To be part of the Registry, the more than 3000 subjects had to have lost and maintained 30 lbs of weight loss for more than one year. Their commitment to weekly exercise is anything but small. On average, they report expending 2682 Kcal/week which involved daily walking schedules of 4 miles/day seven days per week. This level of exercise tends to be too taxing for most adults who have professional and family responsibilities (ADA, 2009). Bloomgarden (2004) points out several limiting factors in diet management that prevent more positive and measurable outcomes such as weight loss. First, he describes a clear decrease in fitness level among obese and overweight children, thus making physical activity more difficult and continued weight gain more likely. Second, the mean 0.6 kg weight gain that tends to occur prior to and during holidays, that affects both children and adults, is described as a phenomenon that is not offset by the mean 0.1 kg in weight loss that follows after the holidays. Third, physicians tend to consider obese patients as non-compliant to medical directives, leading them to not address weight problems during patient visits (Hiddink et al. 1999).

5.5.1 Public Health Strategies

However, let there be no mistake, obesity is the most significant driver of the diabetes epidemic in the US and around the world, and there needs to be a long focus on resolving the obesity epidemic according to Dr. Lucy Candib, a researcher in the Department of Family Medicine and Community Health at the University of Massachusetts. Her work suggests that neither enhanced clinical management of diabetes nor improved screening strategies for pre-diabetics will impact death rates from diabetic complication or the enormity of this epidemic (Candid, 2007). Dr. Candib advances that for successful outcomes in battling the obesity and diabetic epidemics, *"clinicians need to be involved at a broader level"* implying that physicians should be involved in community collaborations that establish relationships, for instance, between health clinics and local fitness centers, thereby fostering safer and easier patient access to exercise programs. It's a strategy that helps front line health care providers assess the sociological and economic factors that define the realities that limit patients' abilities to comply with medical directives. In doing so, physicians are adopting more of a syndemic orientation that sees human affliction intertwined with living conditions and public strength. This approach essentially advocates for a strong public health initiate in combatting obesity and diabetes. As such, physicians need to communicate with community groups and foster ties between their patients and meaningful organizations such as churches, neighborhood associations and radio stations. In this setting the clinicians become the instruments for change and education at the community level, teaching, as it were, along with the dietitian, about healthy nutrition, spearheading efforts to rid junk food from local vending machines, schools, community centers, and replace them with healthy choices. They can, along with the dietitian, organize community gardens, farmer markets and activity programs for children (Candib, 2007).

Public health strategies for combatting the rise of type-2 diabetes are, nevertheless, plagued with difficulties, as multifactorial causes, associated with the disease, make it a difficult to manage. Indeed, weight loss and increased physical activity are difficult outcomes to reach given the complexity of causes tied to overeating and sedentary lifestyles. The **Bienestar School-based Diabetes Prevention Program**, aimed at implementing a total of 93 educational sessions at 27 elementary schools in Texas, is one such effort that intended to implement changes in health behavior among a network of social support personnel that affected 1,420 Mexican kids. The sessions involved nutrition education in the home, classroom, school cafeteria, friends and classmates. Attempts were made to educate cafeteria staff and parents in order to decrease saturated fat levels in food in addition to increasing fruits and vegetables in the diet of the children. The study consisted of separating the students into control and intervention groups. The study found, after one year, that the intervention group experienced greater physical activity, and an increase in caloric intake, that was consistent with increased exercise, in addition to a higher BMI. The study also showed a significant decrease in fasting blood sugars in the intervention group but virtually no clinically significant change in body fat (Travino et al. 2003). Other studies, attempting to change school foodservices and introduce healthy lifestyles to the students, failed to show significant changes in the body weight and blood sugar levels, despite some declines in soft drink consumption. However, exercise-based intervention studies such as the **Trim and Fit program** implemented in Singapore between 1992 and 2000, reported that the prevalence of obesity in primary and secondary schools fell from 16 to 14% (Toh and Cutter, 2002). A Japanese exercise intervention study caused the prevalence of overweight in junior high school students to decline 3% in boys and 8% in girls (Kida et al. 2000). These were important studies that magnify the difficulties with changing eating habits, especially in children. They have acquired taste preferences which are conditioned by the high fructose content of the North American diet and that result from habituation and dependence on certain foods. (Lustig, 2010).

5.5.2 Prenatal Nutrition

In the US, it is the blacks, Hispanics, Native Americans, and the poor or immigrants that represent the groups most vulnerable to the epidemics of obesity and type-2 diabetes. In fact, obesity and diabetes are regarded as markers of inequalities in health, in the US and in other developed nations. These are the very groups that struggle to change dietary habits and exercise more regularly, and who do not consistently take prescribed medications, thus leading to worsening medical problems. From the clinical view point, the difficulties in getting these groups to slim down have been assigned to behavioral decisions or individual characteristics, but recently, there is mounting evidence that compliance to medical directives could be more difficult than initially thought because of a constellation of factors. In a review paper by doctor Lucy Candid (2007) she writes: *"Nevertheless, the epidemic increase in obesity and diabetes around the world suggests that factors far beyond individual behaviors must be at work to explain this recent global process"*.

Indeed, one of the most meaningful findings in recent years, is the key observation that low birth weight babies, resulting from adverse intrauterine environments, can predispose these small infants to obesity and metabolic syndrome later in life (Yajnik, 2004). The explanation for this paradox resides with the **thrifty gene phenotype** hypothesis, formulated by the geneticist Dr James Neel in 1962 from his interest in Diabetes Mellitus. It was a novel concept that introduced that idea that the phenotype of a fetus could be altered in utero in order to accommodate impoverished conditions during pregnancy such as undernutrition. Hence, infants born underweight may likely have a thrifty gene that would permit a rapid and abundant synthesis of fat, once food becomes available, in order to compensate for the low body weight and a possible environment of food scarcity. This gene, however, tends to backfire in a world of abundant and unrestricted calories as we currently see in the North American context. In this environment, the body becomes an efficient synthesizer of fat and eventually produces excessive amounts of body fat thus resulting in obesity, type-2 diabetes and metabolic syndrome in adulthood (Caballero, 2005). It is common, then, to see premature or underweight babies becoming skinny-like kids or adolescents, but developing insulin resistance in late adolescents, when weight begins to get packed on—the result of rapid fat synthesis from the thrifty genotype. In early adulthood, further weight gain becomes apparent as activity levels drop with more academic and professional responsibilities concurrently with unabated food and alcohol intake, and a worsening of dietary practices. In this context, insulin resistance worsens and transitions into type-2 diabetes by early adulthood. In other family environments, low birth weights translate into early fat deposition and obesity in childhood, as poor nutrition and lack of physical activity dominate households. Presently, there are now more numerous cases of insulin resistance being reported by clinician among children older than age 10, a worrisome scenario, as this invariably can lead to an adult population prone to obesity and diabetes (Candib, 2007).

A viable solution that needs to be seriously considered is the implementation of programs that influence prenatal nutrition practices at a public health level by using both healthy concepts of nutrition and socioeconomic status of the families. Strategic efforts also need to be placed on promoting breast feeding programs, as it currently understood that lower rates of obesity are found among breastfed children. According to the CDC 2010 report, only 13.3% of US mothers breastfeed through 6 months.

Internationally, the story appears to be different, since it is not necessarily the poor who are becoming obese, but rather those individuals who have access to cheap food and inexpensive vegetable oils. It is in fact mostly the immigrants, the low income and minority communities that are disproportionately struggling with obesity and diabetes. The primary reason that developing and emerging nations like Mexico, are struggling with diabetes and obesity, is related to global trade policies that lead to the production of cheap cash crops such as corn and soy from which are derived cheap vegetable oils and sugar. These cash crops tend to be produced by large corporate farms, a practice which has invariably led to the closure of the smaller farms as they can no longer compete.

Moreover, the industrialization and mechanization of nations influenced by the mass media complex creates urbanization and immigration. Indeed, these become economic driving forces which attract workers from all around the world seeking opportunity and prosperity. However, this trend also create large urban centers that become **obesogenic environments** that foster poverty, decreased physical activity, and an explosion of fast food restaurants that essentially prey on the poor. These urban environments foster abundant and easy access to high calorie foods within a social environment that offers limited access to nutritious foods but easy embracement of sedentary forms of entertainment. In this context, parents, more concerned about the safety issues in playgrounds, prefer to see their kids playing X-box, in the safety of the home, rather than playing in the unsafe parks and neighborhoods. This has a significant impact on the overall energy expenditure of the kids on a daily basis.

The time is short and so we must act in haste to reverse these epidemics. It does appear that government support for community health interventions is needed, if we are, as a society, going to get the upper hand. In the end, the prevention rather than the treatment of disease appears to be a more affordable and beneficial alternative. But how can we begin to the process? The notion that the genetics load the gun, but that the environment pulls the trigger describes fairly accurately how poor dietary and exercise habits can set up genetically-predisposed individuals to developing obesity and type-2 diabetes. By exposing our children to a toxic food environment, early on, we trap them into developing a sort of habituation to food, based on heightened taste sensations that create food preferences based on addiction and which clearly competes with the much milder tastes found in fruits and vegetables. Is there any wonder that most of our young in the US fail to meet minimum requirements for fruits and vegetables. For nutritionists and epidemiologists, this translates into something of a nightmare since these food habits are, in fact, almost impossible to reverse in the young. Programs focused on prenatal nutrition and teaching mothers how to purchase food and feed their children remain possibly the strategies which may carry the greatest impact.

5.6 TYPE-2 DIABETES CASE STUDY-5.1: A 32 YEAR OLD WOMAN WITH HYPERGLYCEMIA

5.4.1 Presentation

Female patient is a 33 year old secretary who presents with a recent increase in fatigue, hirsutism, frequent urination (polyuria), very thirsty (polydipsia), and numbness in her feet and hands. Her weight is 333lbs, her height: 5 feet 5 inches. She complains of sleep apnea, and of pain in her joints and lower back.

5.4.2 Medical Assessment

Patient's BP is very high and will require antihypertensive medication. Patient complains of extreme fatigue concurrently with polyuria, polydipsia, hyperglycemia and hypertriglyceridemia, all of which suggest diabetes mellitus. Type-2 diabetes has been ruled in based on the extreme form of obesity she appears to suffer from, the hyperinsulinemia and the very noticeable hirsutism on her face and back. Her lipid panel, body weight and BP indicate Metabolic Syndrome.

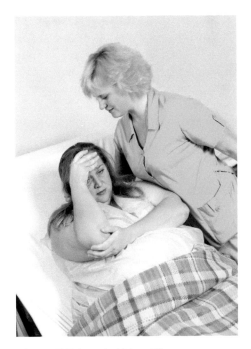

Figure 5.3 Angela K is a 32 year old secretary diagnosed with hyperglycemia—credit line © Nata-lunata/shutterstock.com

5.4.3 Body Composition Assessment

The patient's BMI suggests extreme obesity also called morbid obesity or super-obesity.

$$BMI = Weight (Kg)/[Height (meters)]^2$$

$$BMI = 151.19Kg/ (1.65 meters)^2 = 55.5$$

Waist circumference measurement = 65 inches

Percent body fat measured by bioelectrical impedance assessment (BIA) = 57% fat.

5.4.4 Lifestyle and Diet Assessment

Patient has a long history of obesity that began around 10 years of age. Both parents are classified at least as class-2 obesity. She has one brother who is obese and one sister of 23 who does not have a weight problem. The patient leads a sedentary life with no real physical activity, except the habitual movements of standing and sitting typically associated with office work. Her total energy expenditure (TEE) is calculated using equation-1:

TABLE 5.1 Patient Chart Information

Angela K... CHART INFORMATION		
Female Age: 32; Current Weight: 333lbs Usual Weight: 357lbs; Height: 5 feet 5 inches Patient lost 24lbs trying to diet in the last year. She has a long history of chronic dieting; she has lost and regain weight frequently		
Tests	**Actual**	**Goal**
*Glucose (mg/dl)	304	≤100
Insulin (μIU/ml)	9.1	<5.0
LDL Cholesterol (mg/dl)	230	<100
HDL Cholesterol (mg/dl)	27	≥60
BP mmHg	189/98	<120/80
Triglycerides (mg/dl)	475	<150
Total Cholesterol (mg/dl)	380	<200

Source: NCEP 2001 report JAMA 16 (285): 2486- 97; American Diabetes Association (2011) Standards of Medical Care in Diabetes—2012 *Diabetes Care.* Suppl. 1:S11-63. * Fasting plasma glucose

1- TEE **For women:**

$$TEE = [387 - (7.31 \times Age_{years})] + [PA \times ((10.9 \times wt._{kg}) + (660.7 \times ht._{meters}))]$$

$$TEE=[387-(7.31\times32]+ [1\times(10.9\times151.18Kg)+ (660.7\times1.65 meters)]$$

$$TEE= [150.08] + [2738 Kcal]= 2888 Kcals$$

$$TEE=2888Kcal/day$$

Her usual food intake (Table 5.2) reveals an excessive amount of calories (5241 Kcals/day) which represents a 81.5% calorie excess. Because of the excessive soft drink consumption, she consumes a little over 1lbs of sugar/day. Her fat intake (181g) can be looked at from two perspectives: first, as a percent of her actual caloric intake of 5241 kcal/day. From the outset, it appears that she is only consuming 31.08% of her actual caloric intake as fat, which is within the accepted macronutrient fat range of 20-35%. However, when it is expressed as a percent of her daily caloric need (DRI), it jumps to 56.4% of her body's requirement for calories. This is indeed a substantive fat load for her body size and caloric expenditure, and does support her abnormal blood lipid profile. Indeed, LDL and total cholesterol are reported as high. Moreover, her blood glucose, insulin and triglycerides are consistent with the high sugar intake recorded in her usual food intake. Hyperinsulinemia and hyperglycemia are typically found in cases of type-2 diabetes since it is more of a problem of insulin resistance, rather than insulin insufficiency.

5.4.5 Recommendations

This patient will require first, a weight stabilizing diet that will prevent further weight gain. The purpose of this diet, it to get the patient acquainted to healthy eating without the added stress of caloric deprivation. The focus here is to negotiate the elimination of a few critical foods that are greatly affecting her diabetes and lipid profile. The restriction should include: soft drinks, donuts and cakes. Rather than strictly focus on eliminating food, it is psychologically helpful to speak about introducing foods as well, albeit healthy foods. Here more vegetables and fruits will need to be slowly introduced. The dietitian needs to recognize that there is quite a high likelihood of these new foods being rejected by the patient. Patience and creativity is called for in this case. Using recipes that are healthy and tasty is essential to the success of this approach. Remember that the dietitian's role is to reeducate the patient and re-sensitize the taste buds to a new standard, which is a task that will take time.

Caloric Recommendation—The patient's new caloric intake should be consistent with her sedentary need of 2888 kcal/day. Because the patient has metabolic syndrome, the diet will need to be broken up in accordance with the DASH diet and TLC guidelines:

1. Fat: 27% of calories/day
2. Protein: 18% of calories/day
3. Carbohydrates: 55% of calories/day
4. Saturated fat<6% of calories/day
5. Monounsaturated fats (MUFAs): up to 20% of calories/day
6. Polyunsaturated fats (PUFAs): 5-10% of calories
7. Sodium:<1500 mg/day

The patient should follow this diet for a period of 4 to 8 weeks. During this time, body weight should not increase significantly; there may be a noticeable loss of weight in the first 2 to 3 weeks, the consequence of no longer eating the junk foods and not being able to fully comply with the new dietary directives—the tendency is to eat less than what is prescribed.

The second step is to establish a new caloric prescription that will favor slow weight loss (0.5 -1.0Lbs/week). The calculations pertinent to this new objective are below:

Since 1lbs weight loss arises from a 3500 kcal deficit, then a ½lbs loss would equal a 1750 kcal deficit (3500Kcal/2). Since the goal is to achieve this rate of weight loss over one week, then the daily caloric deficit would equal 250 Kcal/day (1750 kcal/7 days). Similarly, a 1 lb weight loss would require a 500 Kcal/day deficit (3500 Kcal/7 days). The diet prescription for weight loss could vary between: **2388-2638 Kcal/day**.

The third step should involve setting a healthy goal weight while taking into account the percent body fat. This is important because the patient should not lose any lean body mass while following the diet. The body composition assessment, conducted by BIA calculated a 57% body fat or fat mass (FM). Using the two compartment model (Total Body Weight = FFM (Fat Free Mass) + FM (Fat Mass)) it is possible to determine the FFM otherwise known as the lean body mass. It is the latter that should not decrease in size during dieting. The calculations are outlined here:

TBW (Total Body Weight)= FFM + FM

FFM= TBW-FM

Since the percent body fat= 57% then the FM is equal to: 0.57 x 333Lbs= 189.81lbs.

This means then that the FFM would equal:

FFM = 333lbs- 189.81lbs.

Remember that this mass must remain constant throughout the weight loss process. The objective at this stage is to aim for a percent body fat that is considered healthy (See the obesity chapter for acceptable percent body fat ranges for women). It is best for this patient to aim for the upper healthy range for percent body fat; that would be 35% body fat. The equation then to determine a healthy body weight goal for this patient is written out below:

Weight goal x (% FFM) = 189.81lbs
Weight Goal x (100-35%) = 189.81lbs

The premise of this equation is that even once the patient reaches that new body weight, the amount of FFM will not be different than the original obese body weight, which is 189.81 lbs. So then, the new weight goal is calculated as follows:

Weight goal = 189.81lbs/65%
Weight goal = 189.81lbs/0.65
Weight goal = 292lbs

The plan is to allow the patient to lose a total of 41lbs over an undetermined amount of time. If the diet prescription is for ½lbs of weight loss/week, then it will take 82 weeks to lose this weight or 1.58 years (19 months). Aiming for a 1lb weight loss/week would require 41 weeks or a little over ¾ of a year. Although these calculations are mathematically correct, the reality is that weight loss does normally take place following this kind of linear model. The general rule is that while a 500 kcal/day deficit should afford 26lbs over a 6 month period, only 20lbs of weight loss actually occurs. Similarly, while a 1000 kcal/day deficit should permit 2lbs of weight loss/week and 52lbs of lost weight after 6 months, the reality is that only 25lbs is normally recorded (Williamson et al., 1992). The same kind of proportional adjustment can also be made for 1 year of weight loss.

TABLE 5.2 Usual Food Intake Record

PATIENT NAME: **Angela K**	USUAL FOOD INTAKE	
FOODS CONSUMED	**QUANTITY CONSUMED**	**PLACE**
BREAKFAST: TIME		
Never consumes breakfast		
AM SNACKS TIME: 10:00 am		
Pepsi Cola(Reg.) Little Debbie Coco cream mini cakes	30fl-oz (900 ml bottle) 8 individual mini cakes	Office/car At work
LUNCH TIME:		
Pepsi Cola (Reg.) Fish & Chips Medium –Jack in the Box	20fl-oz (600 ml can) 2 Medium servings	Cafeteria Restaurant
PM SNACK TIME:		
Pepsi Cola (Reg.) Dunkin Donut Muffin-Banana chocolate chips	20fl-oz (600 ml can) 1 complete muffin	Dunkin Donuts
DINNER TIME:		
Domino's meat lover pizza Pepsi Cola (Reg)	8 medium slices 20fl-oz (600ml)	Order out
ENEVING SNACK TIME:		
Pepsi Cola (Reg)	20fl-oz (600 ml)	Home
NUTRIENT BREAKDOWN OF USUAL FOOD INTAKE		
Kcals recommended: 2888 kcal/day (2599-3177 Kcals/day) Carbohydrates recommended: 433g/day (60% DRI Kcals) (325-469g) Protein recommended: 108g/day (15% DRI Kcals) (72g-253g) Fat recommended: 80g (25% DRI Kcals) (64-112g) Total Maximal Sugar: <181g (25% DRI Kcals) Total Maximal Sodium: <2400 mg/day	Kcals eaten: **5241 kcals** Carbohydrates eaten: **823g** Protein eaten: **80g** Fat eaten: **181g** Total Sugar eaten: **504g** Sodium eaten: **5911 mg**	

Calories measured using the www.myfitnesspal.com website

REFERENCES

1. Aarsland, A et al. (1996) J. Clin. Invest 98:2008-2017
2. American Diabetes Association (2000). Diabetes Care. 23: 381-9
3. American Dietetic Association (ADA) 2009. Position Paper on Weight Loss Diets. J. Amer. Diet. Assoc. 109(2): 330-346)
4. Anderson. J.W. (2006). Diabetes Mellitus: Medical Nutrition Therapy. In: Modern Nutrition in Health and Disease 10th edition, (Shils, ME et al Eds) Baltimore MD: Lippincott, Williams & Wilkins p: 271-285
5. Anderzhanova, E. et al. (2007) Am. J Physiol. Regul. Integr. Comp Physiol. 293; R603-R611
6. Bloomgarden, Z et al. (2004). Diabetes Care 27(4): 998-1010.
7. Caballero, B. (2005) N.Engl.Med. 352 (15):1514-1516
8. Candib, L.M. (2007). Annals of Family Medicine 5(6): 547-556
9. Center for Disease Control and Prevention (CDC, 2011). The 2011 National Diabetes Fact Sheet
10. Drake AJ, Smith A, Betts PR, Crowne EC, Shield JP (2002): *Arch Dis Child* 86:207–208
11. Ehtisham S, Barrett TG, Shaw NJ (2000): *Diabet Med* 17:867–871
12. Fagot-Campagna, A. (2001). BMJ 322:377-8
13. Hiddink GJ et al. (1999). Eur. J Clin Nutr. 53:S35-S43
14. Kida K et al (2000); Deckelbaum RJ Eds Humana Press: 435-446
15. Kuriyama, H. (1998) Hepatology. 2: 557–562
16. Lustig, RH. (2010) JADA.110:1307-1321
17. Matsuzawa, Y. (2008) International journal of obesity 32 Suppl 7:S83-S92
18. NIH/NHLBI/NAASO (2000) The Practical Guide Identification, Evaluation, and Treatment of Overweight and Obese Adults. Retrieved April 17, 2014 from: http://www.nhlbi.nih.gov/guidelines/obesity/prctgd_c.pdf
19. Ogden, C.L. et al. (2006). JAMA. 295: 1549-1555
20. Pinhas-Hamiel, O. et al (1996) Increased Incidence of Non-Insulin Dependent Diabetes Mellitus among Adolescents. J. Pediatrics 128:608-615
21. Romalo-Halsted, B and Elelman, S.V.(2000) Clinical Diabetes 18(2)
22. Rosenbloom AL, Joe JR, Young RS, Winter WE (1999): *Diabetes Care* 22:345–354
23. Schmitz, KH et al (2002) Int. J. Obes Relat Metab Disord 26; 1310-1316
24. Schoeller, DA et al. (1997) Am J Clin Nutr 66: 551-556
25. Styne, D.M. (2010). JPHMP. 16(5):381-387
26. Styne, D. M. (2001). Childhood and Adolescent Obesity: Prevalence and Significance. Pediatric Clinics of North America, 48(4): 823-854
27. Toh CM and Cutter, J.(2002) BMJ 324: 427
28. Travino RP et al. (2003) Diabetes 52 (suppl. 1): A404
29. Wilde S. et al. (2004) Diabetes Care 27: 1047–1053
30. Williamson DF, Serdula MK, Anada,RF, Levy A, Byers T. Weight loss attempts in adults: goals, duration, and rate of weight loss. Am J Pub Health. 1992;82:1251-1257
31. Yajnik, CS. (2004) J. Nutr. 134(1):205-210
32. Zeitler, P et al.,(2001) Lancet *36 (9575),* 1823-1831

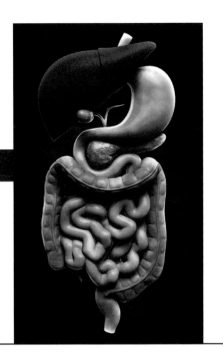

CHAPTER 6

THE PROBLEM OF GI DISEASES

6.1. THE PREVALENCE OF GASTROINTESTINAL (GI) DISEASES

The U.S. is greatly afflicted by gastrointestinal (GI) diseases of various types, which affect 60 to 70 million people and caused as many as 245,921 deaths in 2009. These diseases are of such a serious nature that they were responsible for the hospitalization of an estimated 21.7 million Americans in 2010. GI diseases encompass a wide variety of disorders such as abdominal wall hernias, constipation, diverticular disease, gallstones, gastroesophageal reflux disease (GERD), GI infections, liver disease, pancreatitis, peptic ulcer disease, hemorrhoids, viral hepatitis, and inflammatory bowel diseases (U.S. Department of Health and Human Services [DHHS], 2013a). Of the GI disorders, GERD affects 70 million people, constipation about 63 million, diverticular disease about 2.2 million, and irritable bowel syndrome (IBS) about 15.3 million. These disorders are significantly associated with diet and lifestyle and can be prevented by eating diets high in fiber and low in fat and by implementing good stress management strategies such as regular exercise.

6.2. THE PROBLEM OF CONSTIPATION

Constipation affects 10%–15% of the general population in the U.S. and Canada, but it is particularly in those over 65 years of age that the prevalence rises to 30–40%. Interestingly, women are three times more likely to suffer from constipation than men (Dennison et al., 2005). Criteria for diagnosing functional constipation follow the ROME system of objective diagnosis. The top three standards frequently used by physicians are first, fewer than three defecations/week; second, straining for >25% of defecations because of the hardness of the stool; and third, a sensation of incomplete evacuation for >25% of defecations (Dennison et al. 2005). The symptoms of abdominal pain—usually in the lower left quadrant— and bloating result from the buildup of stool and gas in the descending colon and in the rectum (Figure 6.1), causing an expansion of the colonic wall.

While short-term constipation can be easily treated with laxatives, chronic constipation represents a greater challenge as it can lead to long-term abdominal discomfort. In rare cases, it can trigger fecal impaction and ultimately bowel perforation, thus requiring hospitalization. In the U.S. in 2009, there were 4 million ambulatory care visits tied to constipations, 1.1 million hospitalizations in 2010, and 5 million laxative prescriptions in 2004 (DHHS, 2013a). These represent a needless cost burden on our health care system that would normally be preventable through lifestyle changes at the population level. Chronic constipation is usually the consequence of insufficient dietary fiber (<25 g per day) and fluid intakes. It also arises from extensive immobility or lack

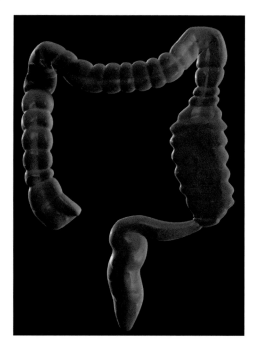

Figure 6.1. Constipation in the descending Colon and rectum. shutterstock_2578426 credit line © Sebastian Kaulitzski/shutterstock.com

of exercise, the aftereffect of an inactive lifestyle, typified by individuals glued to their desks at work or fastened to their sofas at home, either looking at TV, playing video games, or surfing the Internet.

Also medications such as analgesics, antacids, antihistamines, antidepressants, antihypertensive drugs, and iron supplements can cause constipation. A study conducted in the UK, for instance, found that up to 40% of hospitalized women over the age of 65—frequently prescribed multiple medications—suffer from fecal impaction (Dennison et al., 2005). This is the result of stool that is so tightly compacted in the large intestine that it offers a very small likelihood of natural evacuation and also increases the risk of perforation. A tear or puncture of the colon leads to stool seeping into the peritoneum, causing peritonitis and ultimately sepsis if prompt intervention is not forthcoming. Interestingly, chronic constipation in hospitalized elderly has also been tied to mental confusion, although the actual mechanism is not clearly understood. Individuals who suffer from anxiety and depression have a tendency to exaggerate the severity of their constipation thus consulting physicians more frequently for remedies (Dennison et al., 2005). This impacts the health care system by way of expensive resource mobilization, for indeed, doctors, PAs, and nurse practitioners frequently encounter patients suffering from abdominal pain caused by chronic constipation. This requires a bit of an expensive workup before other causes can be ruled out and translates into sizable dollars.

The standard recommendations for people suffering from chronic constipation is to increase dietary fiber to between 25 and 38 g per day (American Dietetic Association [ADA], 2008). This can be easily achieved by regularly consuming a high fiber cereal in the morning with dried fruit. For instance, a half cup of Kellogg's Bran Buds has 13 g of fiber. Mixed with 1 cup of Total Raisin Bran cereal, containing 5 g of fiber, the total fiber intake for breakfast approximates 18 g of fiber, or 72% of a minimal fiber recommendation (Bissonnette, 2014). If the patient opts for whole wheat bread instead of white, in addition to a minimum of 5 servings of fruit and vegetables, the patient will likely meet fiber requirements by the end of the day. Combined with good fluid intake and regular exercise, high fiber intake will resolve chronic constipation within a week to a month for most individuals; this makes sense given that Americans, on average, only consume 15 g of fiber per day (ADA, 2008).

6.3. THE GI DISEASES: GER AND GERD

Gastroesophageal reflux disease (GERD) is a condition that caused as many as 8.9 million ambulatory care visits in 2009. The prevalence of the problem is difficult to estimate, but based on pharmaceutical sales, about 1 in 10 Americans purchase antacids at least once a month to relieve the discomfort of GERD, representing in 2010 about $1.2 billion in sales. When the sales of the top four antacids are broken down—Protonix with $690 million in sales, Prilosec OTC racking up $288.5 million, Zantac 150 posting $72.7 million, and Pepcid Complete with $53.9 million in sales—it is relatively easy to grasp the full scale of the problem of overeating in the U.S. (Hunsinger Benbow, 2011). Indeed, the use of antacids is intimately tied to overeating, eating abundant fatty foods, or both. It is an indictment of the cultural eating habits of a nation and represents an urgent cry to intervene in haste before overeating compromises the population. This is no exaggeration, as the medical expenses in 2004 tied to GI diseases was estimated at $141.8 billion, with $97.8 billion in direct medical costs and $44 billion in indirect costs related to disabilities and mortality.

Another way to look at the importance of GERD in the U.S. is to consider where antacid sales figure from the perspective of pharmaceutical sales overall. Among the top patented drugs in 2011, an antacid—Pfizer's Protonix—took fifth place in sales. Interestingly, the top position belonged to Lipitor—a cholesterol-lowering drug—which is another Pfizer product; the second position went to an antipsychotic drug—Ili Lily's Zyprexa (Alazraki, 2011). This may not be a coincidence, as obesity is intimately tied to hypercholesterolemia and to overeating, and not surprisingly, obesity is also associated with depression and anxiety. There is a connection here that is worth paying attention to for health care providers. Greater numbers of patients are now coming to outpatient clinics with a broad assortment of diseases and conditions that are secondary to obesity and morbid obesity. It is no longer uncommon for a frontline health care provider to encounter a 375 lb, 5 feet 5 inch female who presents with hypercholesterolemia treated with Lipitor, who takes Zantac for acid reflux, and takes a selective serotonin reuptake inhibitor (SSRI) to manage depression.

The problem of gastroesophageal reflux (GER) results from a regurgitation of acid from the stomach into the esophagus. Individuals experience what is medically described as acid indigestion or heartburn. It is a widespread digestive problem that can be treated with antacids (DHHS, 2013b).

This problem of GER can be alleviated through strategic lifestyle and dietary changes. The first is a dietary change that involves consuming fewer fatty foods in the diet. This can generally be achieved by eliminating junk or fried foods and unhealthy snack foods. The second meaningful change would be to avoid overeating, a common problem in obesity. The third strategy consists of controlling the ingestion of coffee, alcoholic beverages, and spicy foods. There are also lifestyle changes that would be beneficial such as losing weight if the patient is either overweight or obese, not smoking, and not eating 2–3 hours before retiring for the night (DHHS, 2013b).

GERD is a more chronic condition of heartburn caused by a laxed lower esophageal sphincter (Figure 6.2) taking longer to shut or not forming a complete seal after the passage of food into the stomach. The consequence is stomach acid—consisting of hydrochloric acid

(HCL)—chronically refluxing through the sphincter opening and back into the esophagus, therefore causing a burning sensation in the chest area. Patients suffering from GERD do not consistently experience heartburn. Other symptoms tied to this condition include dry cough, sore throat, nausea, pain in the chest or upper abdomen, bad breath, and difficulty swallowing. These symptoms could be the consequence of a secondary condition called Schatzki's ring. This is a membranous ring structure that partially obstructs the lumen of the esophagus, thus leading to dysphagia or a difficulty swallowing (Smith, 2010). GERD is a condition often associated with obesity, pregnancy, the use of certain medications such as antihistamines, sedatives, antidepressants, analgesics (pain killers), and smoking. If left untreated, GERD can lead to chronic esophagitis, which can evolve into an erosive esophagitis. This signifies an injury to the esophageal lining caused by chronic gastric acid irritation, sometimes leading to bleeding and ulceration. The damage that can ensue over many years of gastric acid reflux may culminate in precancerous changes in the esophageal lining. One form of esophageal anomaly is called Barrett's esophagus, characterized by the lining of the esophagus adopting cells similar to those of the intestine. Sometimes it has been known to lead to a rare but deadly form of esophageal cancer (Figure 6.3) (DHHS, 2013b).

The treatment strategies for GERD are to lose body weight, avoid smoking, consume small but frequent meals as opposed to fewer large meals, and keep the head in the upright position for at least 3 hours after a meal. Finally, raising the head of the bed an additional 6–8 inches could help control symptoms. Otherwise, antacids such as Alka-Seltzer or Maalox are regularly prescribed. Alternatives to antacids are Tagamet and Zantac, which are proton pump inhibitors (PPIs). Metoclopramide is

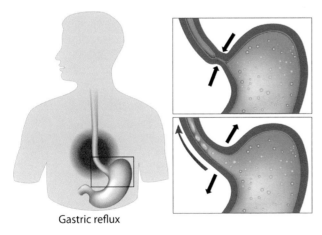

Gastric reflux

Figure 6.2. Gastroesophageal reflux disease (GERD). shutterstock_74586250. Credit line © Alila Medical Media/ shutterstock.com.

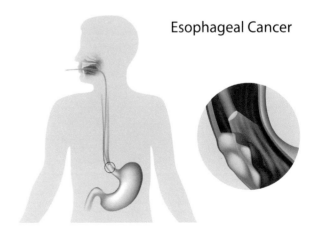

Esophageal Cancer

Figure 6.3. Esophageal cancer arising from chronic esophagitis. shutterstock_128826997. Credit line © Alila Medical Media/ shutterstock.com.

a class of prokinetic drug that can also be used, but it has many unwelcomed side effects such as nausea, diarrhea, tiredness, depression, anxiety, and problems with physical movement. Antibiotics, such as erythromycin, work just as well a prokinetics but with fewer side effects (DHHS, 2013a).

6.4. PEPTIC ULCER DISEASE

Ulcerations or sores along the inner lining of the esophagus, stomach, or duodenum affect about one half million people every year in the U.S. and are referred to as peptic ulcers. They create a great deal of abdominal discomfort often experienced as a dull burning pain that is accentuated especially when the stomach is empty. Patients with ulcers also experience nausea, bloating, vomiting, and weight loss *(DHHS, 2010)*.

Originally, it had been thought that spicy foods, stress, and excessive alcohol consumption caused ulcers. Consequently the long-term management of ulcers consisted of prescribing bland and tasteless diets with very little spices or alcohol allowed. Over time, the diet prescription evolved to "an as-tolerated diet," because the practice of over-restricting foods sometimes compromised the nutritional status of patients. The consumption of milk was encouraged as it relieved symptoms of discomfort fairly rapidly, but it is now known that milk elicits acid secretion and therefore may actually even

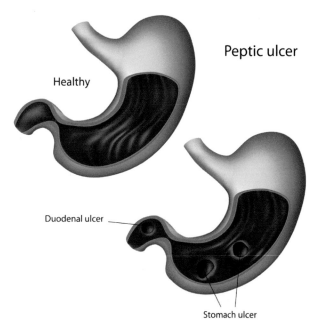

Figure 6.4. Peptic ulcer disease of the stomach/ duodenum. shutterstock_75515089. Credit line © Alila Medical Media/shutterstock.com.

worsen the ulcers or prevent them from healing. However, back in the 1980s, a bacterium called *Helicobacter pylori (H. pylori) was identified* by Australian scientists Barry Marshall and Robin Warren and found to be *responsible for the majority of gastric and duodenal ulcers (Yamaoka, 2008). The therapeutic goals are to kill the bacterium using the antibiotic amoxicillin, reduce acid production, using proton-pump inhibitors (PPIs) or histamine receptor blockers (H2 blockers), and protect the lining of the stomach and duodenum, through the use of bismuth subsalicylates like Pepto-Bismol. However, in recent years antibiotic-resistant bacteria have become more prominent throughout the world, making it more difficult to kill H. pylori. Therefore doctors now verify the efficacy of antibiotic therapy by using breath and stool tests and often implement several rounds of therapy in order to successfully kill the bacterium (DHHS, 2010). Nevertheless, resistance to amoxicillin specifically is still relatively rare.*

6.5. DIVERTICULAR DISEASE

Diverticulosis is a condition characterized by the formation of out-pouches, most often found along the transverse and descending colon, created through an increased intraluminal pressure on the colonic wall. It arises from chronic constipation in most cases. This intraluminal pressure, resulting from the hard and voluminous stool compacted inside the colon, pushes along the colonic wall and creates out pouches called *diverticula* over 10 to 20 years. When pieces of fecal material get caught in the out-pouches they become infected, thereby creating an inflammatory condition called *diverticulitis*, characterized by inflammation of and around the infected area, abdominal pain, nausea and fever. Sometimes there can be numerous diverticula that begin to bleed and become infected. These advanced forms of diverticulitis will often require surgery. The surgical intervention, most often executed in these advanced cases, is the partial colectomy or surgical resection of the infected segments of the colon.

Figure 6.5. Diverticular disease of the colon. shutterstock_75923548. Credit line © Alila Medical Media/shutterstock.com.

The disease begins normally to appear in people over the age of 40, but the prevalence increases significantly every 10 years afterwards; between the ages of 60 and 80, about 50% of people suffer from diverticular disease, but almost every individual over the age of 80 has diverticulosis (DHHS, 2007). In 2009 there were 2.7 million ambulatory care visits linked to diverticular disease in the

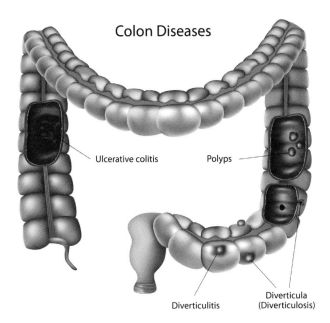

Colon Diseases

Ulcerative colitis

Polyps

Diverticulitis

Diverticula
(Diverticulosis)

Figure 6.4. Peptic ulcer disease of the stomach/ duodenum. shutterstock_75515089. Credit line © Alila Medical Media/shutterstock.com.

U.S. which only represents those individuals acutely affected (DHHS, 2013). The physician will use a **barium enema** in order to observe through X-ray the extent to which the out-pouches or *diverticula* are spread throughout the colonic wall. A **colonoscopy** can be used by a gastroenterologist to visually observe the colonic wall using a miniature camera attached to a tube that moves along the colon after it enters through the anus.

The causes of diverticular disease, from an epidemiological perspective, are tied to the low-fiber westernized diet. Fiber's role in maintaining a healthy GI tract tends to be greatly underestimated. Food processing has been responsible for the most significant loss of fiber in the U.S. diet. This has mostly taken place in the processing of wheat used for bread making and breakfast cereals. Also the shift from a fruit- and vegetable-based diet to more animal-based and calorically dense food choices has had inevitable consequences on the health of the American population.

6.5.1 Recommend a High Fiber Diet

The low-fiber content of the U.S. diet translates into harder stools and longer transit times through the GI tract. The soluble fibers, found mostly in fruits and vegetables, are colloidal in structure and richly found in the pectin of fruits for instance. This means that the colloids attract and trap water within the structure. This feature is responsible for softening the stool; the pay-off is less

intraluminal pressure against the intestinal wall. The insoluble fibers, by contrast, are mostly located in cereals and tend to not capture and bind water. Instead, the insoluble fibers draw water into the GI tract without binding it. Hence, its role is less for softening the stool but more for flushing the stool down the GI tract. In other words, insoluble fibers provide a shorter transit time or a faster flow of stool down the colon and into the rectum.

The notion of disease prevention applies to this condition very well, because once the disease sets in, there is no escaping it afterward. The out-pouches become permanent features of the colon and susceptible to infections. The prevention strategy most suitable to averting this condition is to begin early on to consume a diet that is rich in fruits such as apples, pears, peaches, nectarines, prunes, dates, figs, raisins, and dried apricots. It is also pertinent to include vegetables of all sorts, such as broccoli, squash, carrots, turnips, cauliflower, spinach, and cabbage. Most forgotten in the North American diet are legumes, like navy, lima, kidney, and romano beans, soybeans, and lentils. These need to find their way back into the diet as source of vegetable protein and soluble fiber. This should ideally decrease the reliance on animal protein from beef and pork.

The added benefit from frequently ingesting soluble fibers is that it decreases the risk of cardiovascular disease. In addition, soluble fibers tend to be fermented by gut bacteria that line the GI tract. Fermentation produces short and medium chain fatty acids that play an important role in managing an ideal pH that favors the colonization of a friendly microflora, considered instrumental in minimizing GI diseases and some cancers. The insoluble fibers, found in whole wheat bread, brown rice, bran flake, and bran bud cereals are important in minimizing chronic problems of constipation. Soluble and insoluble fibers consumed regularly can work together preventing diverticular disease in many people.

6.6. HEMORRHOIDS, ANAL FISSURES, AND FISTULAS

About 75% of the U.S. population will develop hemorrhoids at some point during their lives. Hemorrhoids affect mostly adults between the ages of 45 to 65 and are diagnosed when there is inflammation of the veins surrounding the lower rectum or the anus. Hemorrhoids can bleed, leaving bright red blood in the toilet bowel after defecating or on toilet paper. Hemorrhoids can be *internal* (located in the lower end of the rectum) and can prolapse or fall through the anus (Figure 6.6). Prolapsed hemorrhoids tend to be painful, uncomfortable, and associated with itching but will tend to recede on

Anal Disorders

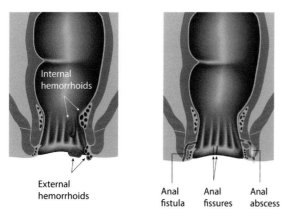

Figure 6.6. Hemorrhoids, anal fistulas and fissures resulting from constipation. shutterstock_125891603 Credit line © Alila Medical Media/shutterstock.com.

their own. However, sometimes prolapsed hemorrhoids permanently protrude and may require treatment or surgery. Non-prolapsed hemorrhoids tend to not be painful or uncomfortable. Hemorrhoids are also classified as *external*, situated under the skin in proximity to the anus. Hemorrhoids occur from chronic straining resulting from constipation and from the increase pressure on the abdominal wall during pregnancy and from pushing during delivery. Pregnancy-derived hemorrhoids tend to disappear after parturition (DHHS, 2013c).

Anal fissures are really only slight linear cracks or tears of the mucosa lining the anus. These fissures are often observed in young infants more than in children and will generally heal on their own if the anal area is kept clean; otherwise anal abscesses can arise. A perianal abscess is an infected area surrounding the anus that fills up with white blood cells and debris in a process of a pus pocket formation. This can occur from blocked anal glands, sexually transmitted infections, or an infected anal fissure (National Institutes of Health [NIH], National Library of Medicine [NLM], 2012). Anal fissures are prevalent as well in young adults—both men and women are equally susceptible—and are less prevalent in older adults.

Fissures can occur in adults who tend to strain when defecating large hard stools or who experience frequent bouts of diarrhea, but in about 90% of cases these fissures spontaneously heal over time with constipation management (Jonas and Scholefield, 2001). The solution is the ingestion of a diet containing 25–38 g of fiber per day (ADA, 2008). This can be achieved by ingesting a high-fiber, bran-based cereal such as Raisin Bran, Bran Flakes, Bran Buds, or regular cereals with added natural bran. Adding dried fruits like raisin, apricots, figs, and

dates will provide soluble fibers and some natural laxative agents that assist with stool softening and shorten the transit time of the stool. If dietary changes are not implemented, then fissures can evolve to abscesses (Figure 6.6), which most often pierce through into the anal canal and spontaneously heal; however, occasionally the abscesses can undergo a submucosal spread that produces a transphincteric route or track that pierces through the buttocks called a *fistula* (Figure 6.6). In these circumstances, the area surrounding the fistula exit site becomes tender and sore and will tend to have purulent drainage and thus must be surgically treated with a fistulotomy (Mappes and Farthmann, 2001).

6.7. INFLAMMATORY BOWEL DISEASE (IBD)

The onset of inflammatory bowel disease is more frequently seen in 15- to 30-year-olds of Caucasian and Ashkenazic Jewish origin with about 10% of cases occurring under the age of 18. This condition, because it is chronic, involves a lifetime of medical care and currently carries a price tag of $1.7 billion a year in health care costs; it is, in fact, the most prevalent form of gastrointestinal disease in the U.S. IBD generally refers to Crohn's disease and ulcerative colitis, which is primarily an immune response characterized by chronic inflammation of the gastrointestinal (GI) tract (CDC, 2014). Recent studies have been able to show that the incidence of IBD is more frequent in developed countries, particularly in urban centers. It has been advanced that the westernized lifestyle may be a significant contributor to the disease. It has also been hypothesized but not proven that the western diet, oral contraceptives, perianal and childhood infections, and atypical myocardial infections may be playing a role in the onset of the disease (CDC, 2014).

6.7.1. Crohn's Disease

This is a type of inflammatory bowel disease that characteristically causes deep fissures through all the layers of the intestinal wall, potentially affecting both the small and large intestine (Figure 6.7). The symptoms of abdominal pain and diarrhea are, however, common with other types of inflammatory bowel disease such as ulcerative colitis and irritable bowel syndrome (IBS); this makes it difficult to diagnose unless confirmed by sigmoidoscopy, colonoscopy, a computerized tomography (CT) scan, or an upper or lower GI series using barium (DHHS, 2011a). However, it is mostly the end of the small intestine (ileum) in 35% of cases, the ileum and

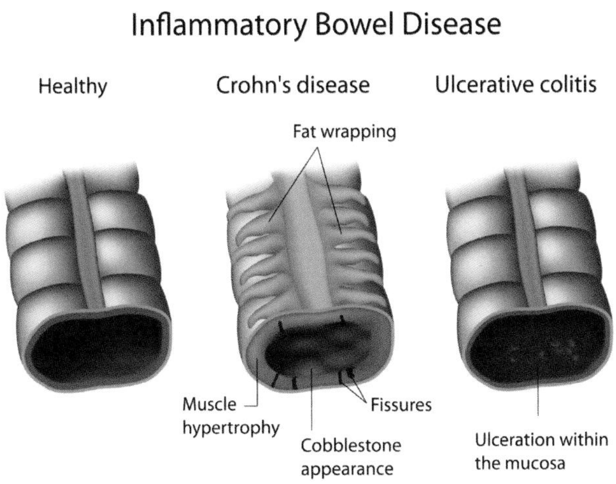

Inflammatory Bowel Disease

Figure 6.7. Crohn's disease and ulcerative colitis. shutterstock_147789395. Credit line © Alila Medical Media/shutterstock.com.

the beginning of the colon in 45% of individuals, and only the colon in 20% of patients (CDC, 2014; Merck, 2012a). Consequently Crohn's disease, if not well managed, causes a great deal of malabsorption and weight loss; many nutrients such as vitamins D and B12, in particular, and iron in children, are of concerns as they cannot be completely absorbed in the inflamed areas thereby causing anemia and growth retardation (Merck, 2012a). Moreover, there are significant protein losses resulting from the fissure damage of the intestinal wall and villi. Low dietary intake of calories and protein, secondary to the anorexia that accompanies the disease, further contributes in a significant way to the weight loss (DHHS, 2011a). Not helping matters, fistulas are reported in about 30% of patients with Crohn's disease, which exacerbates patient discomfort and heighten the fear of eating (CDC, 2014).

The Vienna Classification of Crohn's and its recent Montreal modification identify three clinical presentations of Crohn's that provide a broad perspective to the disease: First, it presents primarily as an inflammation that persists over several years; second, it evolves into a stenotic or narrowing of the GI tract leading to obstruction; and third, it becomes penetrating in the way it affects the mucosa, submucosa, and muscularis layers of the intestinal tract. It is also fistulizing in that fistulas become more prevalent in about 30% of patients.

As a means of monitoring patients with Crohn's it is advisable to conduct lab tests for anemia, hypoalbuminemia, and electrolyte imbalances. Every 1 to 2 years, patients need have their serum hydroxy-25 (OH-25) vitamin D and B12 status checked. Other vitamins such a niacin and folic acid in addition to the minerals, zinc, selenium, and copper can be monitored as well. No

matter the patients' ages, bone density measurements using DEXA (Duel Energy X-Ray Absorptiometry) should be conducted periodically (Merck, 2012a). Those individuals prone to Crohn's disease are people of Jewish heritage and smokers, and those less likely to contract this disease are African Americans (DHHS, 2011). The causes of this condition are still being studied, but presently it is believed to be the result of an interaction between inherited genes, a compromised autoimmune system, and some elements in the environment (DHHS, 2011a). One credible hypothesis suggests that the immune system attacks friendly bacteria and foods located in the GI tract, causing white blood cells to migrate to specific sites along the lumen of the intestine. This sets into motion an inflammatory response which, over time, results in inflammation, followed by ulcerations and sores that chronically injure the intestinal wall (DHHS, 2011a). Crohn's patients are at risk of cancer. Symptoms experienced by patients tend to be frequent watery stools, abdominal cramps, fever and rectal bleeding (CDC, 2014).

Historically, it had been theorized that feelings of guilt, stress, and anxiety were associated with the onset of the disease; this has since been shown to be false. However, emotions have most certainly been tied to the worsening of the problem particularly as they relate to chronic stress, which has been shown to heighten abdominal pain and cause frequent diarrhea (Crohn's and Colitis Foundation of America [CCFA], 2014).

6.7.1.1. Treatments of Crohn's Disease

This condition can be managed by a combination of medications, surgery, and nutritional supplementation to ensure the patient is adequately fed. This kind of disease can often times go into remission for many years before reappearing. There is really no cure for this condition, but rather long-term management strategies that involve the use of anti-inflammatory medications like Sulfasalazine—the most popular in use—or, as alternatives, Asacol, Dipentum, or Pentasa—all mesalamine-based medications classified as 5-aminosalicylic acid (5-ASA) agents, which are reported to have side effects such as nausea, diarrhea, vomiting and headaches (DHHS, 2011a).

In order to manage inflammatory flare-ups of the disease, especially in the early periods of the disease when inflammation is prominent and symptoms difficult to manage, steroids such as prednisone and budesonide frequently prescribed in large doses. About 67% of patients suffering from Crohn's will require surgery to deal with intestinal blockages, perforations, bleeding, or abscesses. Intestinal resections are time performed because of extensive and irreparable damage to the intestine or colon (DHHS, 2011a).

During periods of inflammation, doctors will prescribe intravenous nutrition in the form of total parenteral nutrition (TPN). Bypassing the GI tract for a brief period is a strategy aimed at providing bowel rest so that lesions, inflammation, or abscesses can heal, often with a combination of antibiotics and prednisone (DHHS, 2011a). Although it is clear that foods do not cause Crohn's disease, certain foods like bulky grains, hot spices, alcohol, and milk products are known to cause diarrhea and cramps in some patients; these foods tend to be on a cautionary list. Otherwise, patients are encouraged to eat a liberal diet as tolerated.

6.7.2. Ulcerative Colitis

This is also an inflammatory bowel disease that is more prevalent than Crohn's disease. It usually begins in the rectum and slowly progresses to involve part of the colon, but rarely the entire large intestine. Unlike Crohn's disease, ulcerative colitis (UC) is strictly limited to the large bowel or colon and does not affect all the layers of the intestine (Figure 6.7), but rather the inflammation remains in the mucosa and the submucosa with a complete absence of abscesses or fistulas (Merck, 2012b). In severe cases of the disease, there are mucosal ulcers formed with purulent exudates. Consequently, patients experience abdominal cramps followed by frequent bowel movements, often in the form of diarrhea containing blood and mucus. Because only the mucosa is affected, malabsorption is less of a problem compared with Crohn's disease. The implication is that there are fewer nutrients at risk of becoming deficient. Nevertheless, iron deficiency anemia is likely and should be monitored closely in these patients because of the blood loss in the stool. Hence, it is appropriate for physicians to measure hemoglobin levels to ensure proper iron status. Also, a loss of appetite with weight loss is commonly observed in patients with ulcerative colitis, and can lead to poor growth in children (CDC, 2014).

About half of the individuals with UC only experience mild symptoms and have long periods of months or even years between flare-ups that are asymptomatic. Therefore, far fewer patients with UC—only 25 percent—require surgical interventions (CDC, 2014).

6.8. IRRITABLE BOWEL SYNDROME (IBS)

This is not an inflammatory bowel disease, but a functional GI disorder with symptoms of abdominal pain and diarrhea that resemble what would be observed in IBD (DHHS, 2013d).The onset of the disease usually takes place in the early twenties and tends not to occur after 45 years of age (FDA, 2014). Historically this disorder was given different medical terms such as colitis, mucous colitis, spastic colon, nervous colon, and spastic bowel. The expression *irritable bowel syndrome* was finally adopted to enforce the notion that the condition had both a mental and physical dimension. Although the GI tract has no physical damage to it when viewed by colonoscopy, the symptoms of abdominal discomfort, distension, constipation, and diarrhea are still real and affect the patient's quality of life (DHHS, 2013d). IBS is diagnosed in individuals that experience abdominal pain or discomfort at least three times a month for at least 3 months in the absence of diseases or injuries that could explain the pain.

While there is no physical sign that is diagnosable, the functional disorder impacts normal motility or movement of the GI tract that moves the chyme down the small intestine towards the colon and onward to the rectum. Instances of slow motility translate into constipation, whereas fast motility produces diarrhea. Spasms that contract the GI muscles can generate mild to acute cramps that are very uncomfortable. The reasons for the erratic and unpredictable motility irregularities are not very well understood. The research is unanimous however, in identifying a strong mental health component that appears based in anxiety, depression, panic disorder, and post-traumatic stress disorder. Some have also found an inexplicable link between bacterial gastroenteritis and IBS. However, the mechanism remains elusive (DHHS, 2013d). Certain foods like carbohydrates, spicy or fatty foods, coffee, and alcohol do appear to trigger symptoms. The mechanism may be tied to suboptimal bile secretion for fat emulsification that leads to poor fat digestion and intestinal discomfort. Additionally, it has been proposed that large amounts of fructose, mannitol, and sorbitol may be poorly absorbed, thereby leading to cramps and osmotic diarrhea (DHHS, 2013d; Merck, 2013).

6.8.1. Therapeutic Strategies for IBS

The treatments for IBS are based on making important dietary modifications. The general rule is to follow a liberal but healthy diet as tolerated. If discomfort is experienced it is best to follow these four basic steps: First, eat small frequent meals at a slow pace or small portions at mealtime; second, consume foods low in fat; third, include foods high in complex carbohydrates such as pastas, rice, and whole grain breads and cereals; and fourth, consume many varieties of fruits and vegetables, but avoid those that are gas-producing like cabbage and legumes. The goal behind steps three and four is to heighten the total fiber intake, which appears to alleviate most of the symptoms of IBS. One tablespoon of raw bran can be added to some foods at meals in order to boost fiber. Fiber supplements have also been recommended with some success, but it is important to keep total daily fiber intake below 40 g to avoid gas and abdominal distention; individual tolerance must be considered. The frequent consumption of probiotics has had significant benefits in patients with IBS. Probiotic foods like yogurt with *Bifidobacteria* help recolonize the microflora of the GI tract. The idea here is that the gut of IBS patients may not have a healthy microflora possibly because of previously poor dietary habits involving a lot of junk and processed foods that caused more nefarious bacteria to dominate the lumen of the GI tract (DHHS, 2013d).

The possibility of lactase deficiency can be addressed by restricting milk. Antispasmodic drugs such as hyoscine, cimetropium, and pinaverium have been used with some success, in addition to antidepressant medications (DHHS, 2013d). A more natural approach using aromatic oils such as peppermint are popularly used and effective in relaxing the GI muscles and minimizing cramps (Merck, 2013). Regular exercise has also been documented as an effective approach to manage both stress and the symptoms of IBS (Asare et al., 2012)

6.9. SHORT BOWEL SYNDROME

Also called malabsorption syndrome, short bowel syndrome arises from the surgical resection of more than two-thirds of the small intestine—overall less than 2 m of bowel (6.6 feet) remaining—usually because of damaged gut from Crohn's disease, cancer, or congenital anomalies (Merck, 2012c; Nightingale & Woodward, 2006).

Resection of the distal small intestine, which includes more than 100 cm of the ileum, almost always invariably leads to diarrhea and malabsorption, which are the typical symptoms of short bowel syndrome. By contrast, when the jejunum is partially resected with >100 cm of remaining jejunum, there is a moderate but temporary malabsorption of many nutrients that takes place. However, the ileum will tend to adapt and compensate for this loss by increasing the size and absorptive capabilities of its villi (Merck, 2012c). The removal of a significant section of the ileum—more than 100 cm—is, however, critical, as it will tend to compromise absorption of bile and vitamin B12. This has serious consequences because normally most of the bile is reabsorbed in the ileum via the enterohepatic pathway (Figure 6.8), which brings bile acids back to the liver for the regeneration of new bile, and the conversion of **cholic acid**—main compound of bile—to cholesterol. In short bowel syndrome, large

amounts of bile therefore move into the colon and causes a secretory diarrhea to occur. If <100 cm of the jejunum is left after resection and the ileum is completely resected, then the GI tract loses its ability to absorb fat and many micronutrients, which normally occurs in the jejunum. In addition, vitamin B12 absorption which exclusively takes place in the ileum, with the help of **intrinsic factor** (IF), is compromised, justifying the need for intramuscular injections of vitamin B12 (Merck, 2012a).

The loss of such a large segment of the jejunum necessitates a lifetime of total parenteral nutrition (TPN). Surgeons tend to want to preserve at least 100 cm of jejunum, as it is the minimal length needed to ensure an adequate absorption of protein and fat. Carbohydrates, by contrast, especially simple carbohydrates, contribute such a significant osmotic load to the GI tract that it exacerbates short bowel syndrome. The goal is to recommend a diet consisting of 40% fat—steatorrhea must not be observed—15% protein and 45% carbohydrates consumed as small but frequent meals. The carbohydrates should be mostly in the form of complex starches such as potatoes, rice, pastas of all types, couscous, and cereals like oats, rye, and bulgur. It important to minimize the intake of simple sugars like table sugar (sucrose), drinks with high fructose corn syrup, corn syrup, and maple syrups, as they will precipitate diarrhea in many circumstances (Merck, 2012a).

There are three standard medications commonly used in managing short bowel syndrome. The first is an anti-diarrheal medication, Loperamide, taken about one hour before a meal. It acts via the enterohepatic

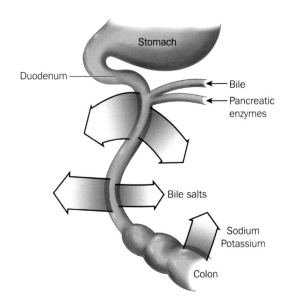

Figure 6.8. The enterohepatic circulation. shutterstock_103901657. Credit line © Blamb/ shutterstock.com.

(EH) circulation by reducing GI motility. A higher than usual dose may be needed as the EH circulation is compromised in short bowel, resulting in a short transit time through the intestine. The second strategy is to prescribe cholestyramine at meal time as it will bind the bile salt pool in the gut and diminish the availability of the salt that serve as a vector for secretory diarrhea (Nightingale and Woodward, 2006). The third involves taking proton (H2) pump inhibitors to mitigate the larger than usual gastric acid secretions and ensuing diarrhea (Merck, 2012a). The acid, in this instance, leaks into the proximal end of the duodenum and deactivates the pancreatic enzymes, lipase, and amylase, therefore causing poor digestion of sugars and fats (Nightingale andWoodward, 2006).

Preserving the integrity of the colon is essential in preventing the excessive loss of fluids—water is reabsorbed back into the body through the colonic wall—and electrolytes such as sodium (Na^+), potassium (K^+), calcium (Ca^{2+}), magnesium (Mg^{2+}), chloride (Cl^-), hydrogen phosphate (HPO_4^{2-}), and hydrogen carbonate (HCO_3^-). Should the terminal ileum and ileocecal valve be resected in surgery, the risk of bacterial overgrowth then becomes elevated. Colonic bacteria, in this instance, can move into the intestine and populate the anastomotic area linking the intestine and the colon (Merck, 2012a).

6.10. BOWEL DISEASE CASE STUDY: A 55-YEAR-OLD MALE WITH ABDOMINAL PAIN

Background. A 45-year-old male presents to urgent care with a complaint of (c/o) a gradually worsening lower left quadrant (LLQ) abdominal (ABD) pain, duration previous 3 days. His pain is described as aching, at times sharp. Associated symptoms include low grade fever 100.2F°, fatigue, and nausea, without vomiting and malaise. Past medical history (PMH) is significant for chronic constipation but no history of inflammatory bowel disease or irritable bowel syndrome. Otherwise the patient is in good health, with no daily medications taken.

Pertinent Negatives: No diarrhea, rectal bleeding, melena, chest pain, shortness of breath (SOB) or anorexia.

Exam. The patient appears mildly ill and in no distress. Exam is normal except for moderate tenderness with palpation of LLQ, no guarding or rebound tenderness.

Summary of Biochemistry.
Complete blood count (CBC): normal except white blood count (WBC) elevated 13.1
Comprehensive metabolic panel (CMP): normal

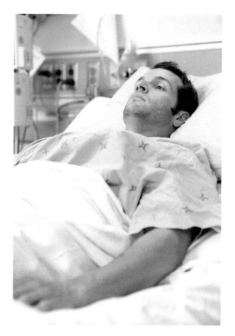

Figure 6.9. Robert B. is a 45-year-old construction worker with abdominal pain. shutterstock_158643689 credit line © Tyler Olson/shutterstock.com.

Erythrocyte sedimentation rate (ESR): normal
C-reactive protein (CRP): normal
Urine analysis (UA): normal

Imaging Assessment.
Flat and UR ABD XR unremarkable gas pattern
CT ABD with contrast: left-sided colonic diverticulitis.

Treatment.
Stool softeners, cipro 500mg BID 14 days, Flagyl 500mg TID 14 days.
Constipation prevention strategy of high fiber diet recommended.
Referral to dietitian was made.

6.11. INFLAMMATORY BOWEL DISEASE CASE STUDY: A 23-YEAR-OLD FEMALE WITH INFLAMMATORY BOWEL DISEASE (IBD)

Background. A 23-year-old female presents to family practice with 2 weeks history gradually worsening ABD pain and diarrhea. At illness onset, loose stools occurred three to four times per day but have gradually progressed to frequent liquid stools eight to nine per day and sometimes bloody. Pain location right upper and lower ABD. Pain described as aching and at times burning, initially mild but gradually worsening to severe. Patient states she

Robert B. CHART INFORMATION		

Male Age: 45
Current Weight: 220 lb (has poor dietary habits)
Usual Weight: 230 lb
Height: 5 feet 11 in.
Patient lost 10 lb in last 3 months from ABD pain. He has a long Hx of chronic constipation; he has frequently dieted for weight loss. Regular BP: 110/79

TESTS	ACTUAL	GOAL
*Glucose (mg/dl)	98	≤100
Albumin (g/dl)	4.7	3.9–5.0
Creatinine (mg/dl)	0.92	0.8–1.4
BUN (blood urea nitrogen) (mg/dl)	8	7–20
Sodium (Na) (mEq/L)	138	136–144
Hemoglobin (mg/dl)	10.8	
Alkaline phosphatase (IU/L)	48	44–147
ALT (alanine aminotransferase) IU/L	12	8–37
AST (aspartate aminotransferase) IU/L	15	10–34

Source: NCEP. (2001). Report. *JAMA.* 16(285):2486–2497; American Diabetes Association. (2011). Standards of Medical Care in Diabetes—2012. *Diabetes Care.* Suppl. 1:S11–63.

*Fasting plasma glucose.

MedlinePlus: comprehensive metabolic panel: http://www.nlm.nih.gov/medlineplus/ency/article/003468.htm

is now so ill she cannot work, is weak and has noticed clothes are loose due to weight loss. Her boyfriend says she looks pale and miserable. Pain becomes worse 2 hours after a meal and is milder with food intake avoidance.

Associated Symptoms. nearly complete loss of appetite, fevers up to 102 that do not reduce entirely with ibuprofen, debilitating fatigue, malaise, pallor, bloody stools.

Pertinent Negatives. N/V, melena, body aches, chills.

Past Medical History. Negative, patient has been in excellent health until this illness, no chronic health problems, no daily medications.

Social History. College senior, works part time at a grocery store.

Family History. Mother has rheumatoid arthritis, otherwise negative.

Exam. Young adult female who appears stated age, ill and tired appearing but in no distress. Thin body habitus but no cachexia. Skin: pale, slightly diaphoretic but no cyanosis, Turgor normal. Heart: tachycardic 120, rate regular, no murmur. Lungs: clear to auscultation, no cough or dyspnea. ENT: mucous membranes moist, no urinary tract infection (URI).

Abdomen (ABD): Soft, non-distended, pain with palpation over right upper and lower ABD. No palpable masses or enlarged organs. Rectal: hemoccult positive.

Biochemistry.
CBC: normal except low hemoglobin 8.2
CMP: normal except low potassium 3.3
UA: normal except moderate proteinuria
ESR: elevated 12.1
CRP: elevated 7.1

Imaging Assessment.
Flat and UR ABD XR: normal
CT ABD with contrast: transmural colonic inflammation at ileocecal valve consistent with active Crohn's disease.

Course of Action: Patient is hospitalized and transfused with 2 units PRBCs, IV rehydration. NPO is prescribed for bowel rest. Colonoscopy findings were significant for inflammation and constriction at the ileocecal valve. Colitis is consistent with Crohn's disease. Biopsy results also consistent inflammation associated with Crohn's.

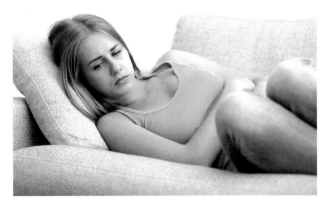

Figure 6.10. Sally C. is a 23-year-old female college student with abdominal pain. shutterstock_163286378 credit line © Alexander Raths/shutterstock.com.

Treatment. Patient stabilized initially with prednisone then changed to immune modulator therapy to affect remission. Patient will need lifetime monitoring of this condition with up to twice yearly colonoscopy and monitoring of serum inflammatory markers.

REFERENCES

1. Alazraki M. (2011). The 10 biggest-selling drugs that are about to lose their patents. *Daily Finance*, February 27. Available at http://www.dailyfinance.com/2011/02/27/top-selling-drugs-are-about-to-lose-patent-protection-ready/.
2. American Dietetic Association (ADA). (2008). Position of the ADA: Health Implications of Dietary Fiber. *J Am Diet Assoc.*108:1716–1731.
3. Asare F, et al. (2012). Meditation over medication for irritable bowel syndrome? On exercise and alternative treatments for irritable bowel syndrome. *Curr Gastroenterol Rep.* 14(4):283–289. Available at http://www.ncbi.nlm.nih.gov/pubmed/22661301.
4. Bissonnette D. (2013). *It's All about Nutrition: Saving the Health of Americans.* Lanham, MD: University Press of America.
5. Centers for Disease Control. (2014). Inflammatory Bowel Disease (IBD). Available at http://www.cdc.gov/ibd/.
6. Crohn's and Colitis Foundation of America (CCFA). (2014). Crohn's Disease and Ulcerative Colitis: Emotional Factors. Available at www.CCFA.org.
7. Dennison C, et al. (2005). The health-related quality of life and economic burden of constipation. *Pharmacoeconomics.* 23(5):461–476.
8. U.S. Food and Drug Administration (FDA). (2014). Irritable Bowel Syndrome Treatments Aren't One Size Fits All. FDA's Consumer Update. Available at http://www.fda.gov/ForConsumers/ConsumerUpdates/ucm392396.htm.
9. Hunsinger Benbow D. (2011) Recalls are making antacids harder to find. *Indianapolis Star*, March 6. Available at http://usatoday30.usatoday.com/money/industries/health/2011-03-01-antacid-shortage_N.htm.
10. Jonas M, Scholefield JH. (2001) Anal fissures. In: Holzheimer RG, Mannick JA, eds. *Surgical Treatments: Evidence-based and Problem-Oriented.* Munich: Zuckschwerdt. Available at http://www.ncbi.nlm.nih.gov/books/NBK6878/.
11. Mappes HJ, Farthmann EH. (2001) Anal abscess and fistula. In: Holzheimer RG, Mannick JA, eds. *Surgical Treatments: Evidence-based and Problem-Oriented.* Munich: Zuckschwerdt. Available at http://www.ncbi.nlm.nih.gov/books/NBK6943/.
12. Merck Manual for Healthcare Professionals. (2012a). Inflammatory Bowel Disease: Crohn's Disease. Available at http://www.merckmanuals.com/professional/gastrointestinal_disorders/inflammatory_bowel_disease_ibd/crohn_disease.html?/.
13. Merck Manual for Healthcare Professionals. (2012b). Inflammatory Bowel Disease: Ulcerative Colitis. Available at http://www.merckmanuals.com/professional/gastrointestinal_disorders/inflammatory_bowel_disease_ibd/ulcerative_colitis.html.
14. Merck Manual for Healthcare Professionals. (2012c). Gastrointestinal Disorders: Short Bowel Syndrome. Available at http://www.merckmanuals.com/professional/gastrointestinal_disorders/malabsorption_syndromes/short_bowel_syndrome.html.
15. Merck Manual for Healthcare Professionals. (2013). Inflammatory Bowel Disease: Irritable Bowels Syndrome. Available at http://www.merckmanuals.com/professional/gastrointestinal_disorders/irritable_bowel_syndrome_ibs/irritable_bowel_syndrome_ibs.html?qt=IBS&alt=sh#v896655.
16. National Institutes of Health (NIH), National Library of Medicine (NLM). (2012). Abscesses. Available at http://www.nlm.nih.gov/medlineplus/ency/article/001519.htm.
17. Nightingale J, Woodard JM. (2006). Guidelines for the management of patients with a short bowel. *Gut.* 55(5): iv1–iv12. Available at http://www.ncbi.nlm.nih.gov/pmc/articles/PMC2806687/.
18. Smith MS. (2010) Diagnosis and management of esophageal rings and webs. *Gastroenterol Hepatol (NY).* 6(11):701–704. Available at http://www.ncbi.nlm.nih.gov/pmc/articles/PMC3033540/.
19. Stevenson WF. (2006). The esophagus and stomach. In: Shils ME, Shike M, Ross AC, Caballero B, Cousins RJ, eds. *Modern Nutrition in Health and Disease.* 10th ed. Philadelphia: Lippincott Williams & Wilkins; 1179–1188.
20. U.S. Department of Health and Human Services (DHHS), National Digestive Diseases Information Clearinghouse (NDDIC). (2013a). Digestive Disease Statistics for the United States NIH Publication No. 13-3873. Available at http://digestive.niddk.nih.gov/statistics/statistics.aspx.
21. U.S. Department of Health and Human Services (DHHS), National Digestive Diseases Information Clearinghouse (NDDIC). (2013b). Gastroesophageal Reflux (GER) and Gastroesophageal Reflux Disease (GERD) in Adults. NIH Publication No. 13-0882. Available at http://digestive.niddk.nih.gov/DDISEASES/pubs/gerd/.
22. U.S. Department of Health and Human Services (DHHS), National Digestive Diseases Information Clearinghouse (NDDIC). (2013c). Hemorrhoids. NIH Publication No. 11-3021. Available at http://digestive.niddk.nih.gov/ddiseases/pubs/hemorrhoids/index.aspx#what.
23. U.S. Department of Health and Human Services (DHHS), National Digestive Diseases Information Clearinghouse (NDDIC). (2013d). Irritable Bowel Syndrome (IBS). NIH Publication No. 13-693. Available at http://digestive.niddk.nih.gov/ddiseases/pubs/ibs/index.aspx#what.

24. U.S. Department of Health and Human Services (DHHS), National Digestive Diseases Information Clearinghouse (NDDIC). (2011a). Crohn's Disease. NIH Publication No. 12-3410. Available at http://digestive.niddk.nih.gov/ddiseases/pubs/crohns/.

25. U.S. Department of Health and Human Services (DHHS), National Digestive Diseases Information Clearinghouse (NDDIC). (2011b). H Pylori and Peptic Ulcers. NIH Publication No. 12-1597. Available at http://digestive.niddk.nih.gov/ddiseases/pubs/colitis/index.aspx#what.

26. U.S. Department of Health and Human Services (DHHS), National Digestive Diseases Information Clearinghouse (NDDIC). (2010). H Pylori and Peptic Ulcers. NIH Publication No. 10-4225. Available at http://digestive.niddk.nih.gov/ddiseases/pubs/hpylori/#1.

27. U.S. Department of Health and Human Services (DHHS), National Digestive Diseases Information Clearinghouse (NDDIC). (2007). What I Need to Know about Diverticular Disease. NIH Publication No. 07-5535. Available at http://digestive.niddk.nih.gov/ddiseases/pubs/diverticular/#cause.

28. Yamaoka Y. (2008). Helicobacter pylori. In: *Molecular Genetics and Cellular Biology*. Caister Academic Pr. ISBN 1-904455-31-X.

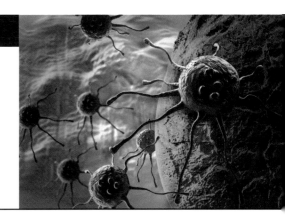

CHAPTER 7

THE PROBLEM OF CANCER

7.1 PREVALENCE OF CANCER

The prevalence of cancer is widespread throughout the U.S. with total cancer deaths increasing between 1971 and 2004 for lung, colorectal, prostate and pancreatic cancers (Sporn, 2006). Cancer carries financial and human costs that are troubling. Even though death rates from overall cancers have been recently declining in the United States (NCI, 2014), the lifetime risk of contracting cancer at some point, for a U.S. male, is still 1 in 2 or 43.92%, and it is 1 in 3 or 22.94% for a female (ACS, 2014B). According to the NIH, cancer takes the second position after heart disease, for the greatest number of deaths in the U.S., and the future does not look any better, as current forecasts rank cancer as the leading cause of death by 2015. The economic burden to this country is alarming because of the direct long term treatment costs that tax the healthcare system. In 2010 alone, cancer cost an estimated $263.8 billion in both direct and the indirect costs associated with mortality, losses to the labor force and sick time (ACS, 2010). The human cost is dreadfully high as well, as it affects the physical, emotional and spiritual dimensions of the person; it changes people's lives and the lives of their families in a

significant manner (CDC, 2013). A total of 1.45 million people reportedly had a cancer diagnosis in 2010, and there were roughly 575,000 people who died from the disease that same year (CDC, 2013). After cardiovascular disease, cancer is the most significant cause of death in the U.S. and in most westernized nations (Willett & Giovannucci, 2006). The highest risk of cancer in men is prostate cancer (CDC, 2014) (**Figure 7.1**) whereas in women it is breast cancer (CDC, 2013B). The second most prevalent form of cancer, in both men and women, is bronchial and lung cancer, and in third position, is the prevalence of colorectal cancer in both genders (CDC, 2014; 2013B). It is reassuring that the three most prevalent forms of cancer, currently in the U.S., are directly associated with lifestyle. Indeed, if Americans would quit smoking, start to exercise regularly and consume a diet rich in fruits and vegetables, cancer rates would begin to dramatically decline over the following 10 to 20 years. Worldwide, the prevalence of cancer is on the rise. The WHO estimates that between 2001 and 2020, cancer will grow at a rate of 20 million cases per year (Bissonnette, 2013). The incidence of new cancers is shocking and motivates a fear-driven population to find a remedy or a prevention strategy that works.

Top 10 Cancer Sites: 2010, Male, United States—All Races

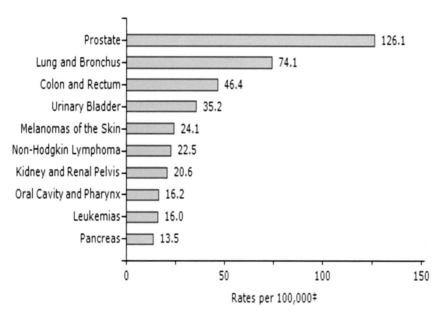

Figure 7.1 Prevalence of Male Cancers in the U.S in 2010 in all Races. Source: CDC 2014: http://apps.nccd .cdc.gov/uscs/toptencancers.aspx

7.2. PREVENTION OF CANCER

It is clear that many cancers are preventable by modifying dietary practices and lifestyles. Overall, epidemiologists have linked 45% of cancer deaths in men and 59% in women to diet and lifestyle (Anand, 2008). For instance, making a firm decision not to smoke would greatly decrease the risk of lung, bronchial and bladder cancers. Incidence rates of melanomas of the skin would also fall with use of sunscreen and limited use of tanning beds. Likewise, colon and rectal cancers would decline concomitantly with the ingestion of more fruits and vegetables in addition to maintaining a healthy weight (CDC, 2014; ACS. 2012). High physical activity levels were also tied to lower incidence of cancer at the population level (Willett and Giovannucci, 2006).

Screening is another tactic used in public health to detect a disease early in its beginning before it becomes too invasive and compromises the health of the individual. The CDC has many cancer prevention programs that are used to screen and tract the population for cancer. There is the **National Breast and Cervical Cancer Early Detection Program** (NBCCEDP), the **National Comprehensive Cancer Control Program** (NCCCP), the **National Program of Cancer Registries** (NPCR) and the **Colorectal Cancer Control Program** (CRCCP). They have all successfully coordinated either the screening or monitoring of tens of millions of Americans every year (CDC, 2013).

The most powerful incentive, however, is to study preventative ways to avoid developing cancer in the first place. Epidemiological research has also focused on the

prevention strategies built in our lifestyles and eating habits that can contain and possibly eliminate the scourge.

As far back as the early 1940s, studies on rats showed that **caloric restrictions** could hinder mammary tumor development. Much later on, in the mid-1980s, researchers demonstrated that a 30% energy restriction, in rats, diminished mammary rat tumors by as much as 90% (Willett & Giovannucci, 2006). The results were fascinating and had significant implication in human epidemiological cancer research. This was especially true for an overweight and obese population plagued with numerous secondary diseases. The growing onslaught of obese and overweight patients—the obese most typically carry a morass of costly and debilitating medical problems—began to clog the efficient delivery of medical services in the U.S as far back as the 1990s, and were becoming very expensive to manage. Indeed, by 2008, the total direct cost to manage overweight and obese U.S. adults rose to $170 billion per year according to research funded by the National Institutes of Health. It's not just that we are getting bigger, but also sicker; medically, an obese individual is at high risk of cancers of the breast, endometrium, prostate and colon. In addition to these devastating conditions, an obese person will tend to have chronic problems with their gallbladder; they will suffer from osteoarthritis, sleep apnea, asthma and possibly depression, in addition to hypertension, atherosclerosis and diabetes. All these conditions come with a hefty price tag because they are serious and complicated chronic diseases that require a constant management by medical practitioners.

At a societal level, the goal of a public health preventative program is to increase longevity and quality of life.

There is no point in living longer if it means extending lives plagues with chronic disease and suffering; the idea is to live long and healthy.

The Okinawa study, which began in 1976, is a clear example of how temperate living in an isolated Japanese sub-culture, resistant to modernization, appears to translate into health and longevity. Here is a society with a mean life expectancy of 81.2 years—much longer than the U.S.'s 76.8 years (Figure 7.2)—and an astounding 2.5 to 5 times greater number of centenarians in the population (Figure 7.3) than found in most industrialized countries (Suzuki, 2001; Willcox et al. 2006).

These are decisive statistics that greatly suggest there is an interaction between genetics and the environment. Research in the field of heritability concludes that between 10-50% of longevity is inherited with most agreeing that 33% of our lifespan is likely determined by genes. This translates into 67% of our longevity possibly being greatly influenced by factors in our environment. So then what is it in the Okinawan environment that increases longevity?

The Okinawans tend to consume only 80% of their caloric needs, or in other words, they follow a style of eating known as "*hara hachi bu.*" In this form of eating, the person is encouraged to consume low glycemic foods such as legumes and vegetables. In concrete terms, this means Okinawans rise from the table without being fully satisfied at that moment. Does this mean they remain in a state of hunger? Not likely, since that slight hungry feeling dissipates a little later on as the food settles in the stomach.

The Okinawa diet, so it appears, slows the aging process and prevents disease. In fact, the prevalence of breast and prostate cancers is 80% lower than in Western societies; also, the rates of colon and ovarian cancers are less than 50% of the rates reported in industrialized nations. One of the accepted aging theories is that free radical production can overwhelm the concentrations of antioxidants in the body and therefore overcome cellular integrity and cause cell damage and even death (apoptosis). It is this cell damage that plays into the aging process and the etiology of disease. Consistent with this theory, a population that consumes abundant antioxidants in its diet, can keep the free radicals in check, and slow down the aging process, and prevent coronary artery disease and some cancers (Suzuki et al 2001). In Okinawa, the centenarians tend to consume almost ten times (10 x) the amount of isoflavones—an antioxidant—found in the diet of Japanese Canadians.

The isoflavones—genistein and daidzein—are protective against hormone-based cancers such as breast, prostate and endometriosis, and are found in soy-based foods such as soybeans, tofu and tempeh. Researchers have also measured elevated lignans in foods like flaxseeds and grain products. Combined together, the diet content of antioxidants is elevated enough that, compared to Westerners, Okinawans have an 80% risk reduction in cardiovascular disease (Willcox 2006, 2006B).

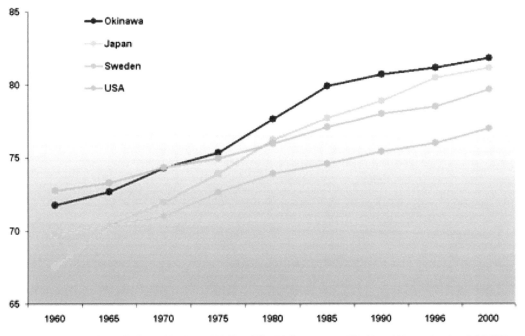

Life Expectancy in Long-lived Populations and the US

Source: W.H.O. 1996; Japan Ministry of Health and Welfare 2004; US Department of Health and Human Services/CDC 2005

Figure 7.2 Source: WHO 1996 and Japan Ministry of Health and Welfare 2004, U.S. Department of Health & Human Services/ CDC 2005

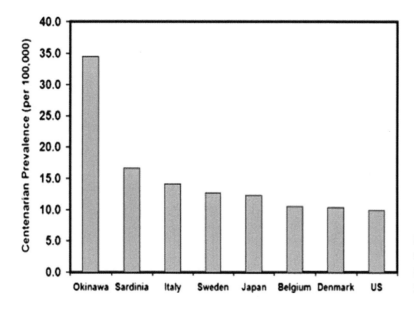

Figure 7.3 Prevalence of Centenarians in Okinawa versus US in 2002.
Source: Wilcox, DC et al AGE 2006; 28(4):313-332

Okinawa residents manage to maintain a consistent Body Mass Index (BMI) that varies between 18 and 22. This rather lean physical consistency is achieved through a combination of calorie-controlled intakes and regular physical exercise. From a very young age, the martial arts like karate and judo are taught to their children. Judo, in particular, is Japan's national sport and one of the most effective self defence systems around. The warm ups alone are intense and can cause even the most adept aerobics instructor to run for the vomit bag before the end of the 20 minute warm up; the intense Judo training then lasts an additional 1hr 10 minutes.

Agility, resistance and flexibility are the main physical attributes that are developed by a judoka. Often, this sport/martial art is practiced from anywhere between 30—70 years; it is not uncommon to see a seventy year old Okinawan still practicing judo or karate regularly. Over time, joints tend to be more flexible, physical resistance and endurance significantly greater than westerners. It would not be surprising to see a 70 year old Okinawan demonstrate greater flexibility and agility than a typical young man in the West. The schedule followed by most of the youth, is a 90 minute judo practice three to five times per week. In this setting, a Japanese teenager weighing 150 lbs. would expend 0.075 kcal/lb/minute or at total of 844 kcal per practice, and a total of 2531 kcal per week if practiced three times (3x) per week.

Maintaining energy balance appears to be the strategy that works. Other epidemiological studies appear to reaffirm the position that body fat accumulation in humans, invariably lead to the development of several cancers in humans (Nightingale & Giovannucci, 2006).

The important point that comes out of the Okinawa studies is that a diet high in antioxidants does appear to protect the body against cancer and aging. Suzuki and colleagues (2001) report that with high antioxidant intakes from the diet, there are lower levels of plasma lipid peroxides (LPO) compared to controls. Numerous animal studies also confirmed that exogenous antioxidants given to rats help decrease free radical levels and damage to cells and tissue (NCI, 2014B). The relevant question right now is whether antioxidant supplements can prevent cancer? There are nine randomized clinical trials that have tested the efficacy of antioxidant supplements in cancer prevention (NCI, 2014B), and they mostly show no decrease in cancer incidence rates, or increased risk of cancer with supplementation. Two of the studies had to be stopped early. One study—**Alpha-Tocopherol/ Beta-Carotene Cancer Prevention Study**—reported in 1994 that those subjects receiving beta-carotene supplements were developing lung cancer at rates greater than controls. The other study—**Carotene and Retinol Efficacy Trial**—was a U.S.-based investigation that found in 1996 that smokers on beta-carotene were developing lung cancer at a faster rate than non-smokers, and that the cause of death from all studied sources was also more elevated. More surprising and troubling was that cancer risk persisted up to 6 years after ending the intake of supplements. Interestingly, another study during the late nineties as well—**Physicians' Health Study I (PHS I)**—found that a 50mg beta-carotene supplement, taken over the long term, had no effect on either mortality or cancer incidence rates in smokers and non-smokers. In 2001, a U.S. trial—**The Selenium and Vitamin E Cancer Prevention Trial**—was stopped in 2008 because it showed that daily vitamin E supplements taken alone over a 5.5 year period had no effect in reducing the incidence of prostate or other forms of cancers in men 50 years of age and older. However, a 2011 follow up on subjects reported that subjects who took only vitamin E supplements had a 17% greater risk of developing prostate cancer than those on a placebo. Finally the Physicians' Health Study II (PHS II) showed that daily supplementation of two popular antioxidants (400 IU vitamin E every other day, 500 mg vitamin C) over a median 7.6 years had no impact on a wide variety of cancers notably, prostate, melanomas, leukemia and colorectal (NCI, 2014B). The impact of supplementation on cancer prevention is certainly not convincing at this time, and should cause some degree of alarm.

The idea of preventing cancer appears now to centrically revolve around the issue of good and wholesome nutrition. It is not enough to take a supplement while continuing to eat poorly, and expect to be protected from the long term devastation of chronic diseases like cancer. The Dietary Guidelines for Americans 2010 recommend the daily consumption of varied vegetables, notably dark green vegetables of the cruciferous type (Brassica genus). These include vegetables such as broccoli, Brussels sprouts, cabbage, cauliflower, turnips, rutabaga, collard greens, radishes and kale, which are rich in biologically active compounds called phytochemicals. For instance, they contain indols, isothiocyanates, and thiocyanates, that have been shown in-vitro and in rat studies to be protective against cancer (NCI, 2012). However, human prospective studies have not convincingly shown that abundant and regular intake of cruciferous vegetables imparts strong protection against varied types of cancers (NCI, 2012). Clearly more research is needed to elucidate this vegetable controversy. The challenge is to begin these long term prospective studies early enough—that is before the promotional phase of cancer is advanced—in order to truly measure the protective effect of these vegetables against cancer (Giovannucci et al. 2003). The more persuasive findings regarding dietary components that increase the risk of cancer are from those studies measuring the impact of meat consumption on cancer incidence.

Rat studies and in vitro tests have shown that heterocyclic amines (HCA) and polycistic aromatic hydrocarbons (PACs), formed from the high temperature treatment of beef, pork, chicken and fish have mutagenic effects on DNA with the potential of leading to development of cancer cells. High doses of PACs and HCAs, fed to monkeys and rats, caused mutagenic changes in their cells, and cancer. Using large epidemiological human studies, the association between the consumption of well done, fried or barbecued meats, and colorectal, pancreatic and prostate cancers in humans were significant (NCI, 2010). However, the link between HCAs and PACs, and cancer has not been decisively established in humans. And while several prospective studies have shown a 13-17% increase in the risk of cancer for every 100g (~3oz-wt) of red meat consumed,

it was the incremental risks tied to processed meat that was alarming. Prospective studies and a meta-analysis demonstrated a 49% jump in cancer risks for every 25g (~1oz-wt) of processed meat consumed (Willett & Giovannucci, 2006). Another set of 21 studies found between 30 and 40% risk of developing prostate cancer, with increased red meat consumption. Most notable, was a study by Pan et al (2012) that looked at data from two very large prospective studies—Health Professionals Follow-up Study (HPFS) and Nurses' Health Study (NHS)—that followed 51, 529 men and 121, 700 women respectively. Researchers are uncertain whether the cancers are caused by the fats from the meats or something else in the meat. One thing remains, and that is that frequent red meat consumption should not be encouraged, especially processed meats according to American Cancer Society Guidelines on Nutrition and Physical Activity (Willett & Giovannucci, 2006; ACS, 2012).

7.3. PATHOPHYSIOLOGY OF CANCER

Cancer, rather than being a static state, is now seen more as a dynamic process or an evolving cellular process, and thus is referred to as carcinogenesis. This is consistent with the medical community's understanding that there is a 20 year or greater latency period that spans the point of cancer initiation, in which there is DNA mutation that occurs, to the promotional phase in which cancer becomes invasive and metastatic (Sporn, 2006).

The size, structure, function, and growth rate of malignant cancer cells are very different than what is observed in normal cells. The problem begins when a cell's ability to differentiate becomes altered because of DNA mutations, taking place in the nucleus of the cell, that alter the normal functions, cell division, growth, and appearance of the cell (NCI, 2014). The consequence is an important change in the way the tissue works, ultimately leading to pain, cachexia, lowered immunity, anemia, leukopenia, and thrombocytopenia (NCHPAD, 2014). The mutated cells begin to divide, producing numerous anomalous cells that grow at irregular rates that are sometimes fast other times slow (Figure 7.4) (ACS, 2014).

They can metastasize or in other words proliferate in distant organs and tissues via the complex and far reaching lymphatic and cardiovascular circulatory systems (NCI, 2014). Most malignant cells form tumors (Figure 7.5), however leukemia does not form tumors, but rather leukemic cancer cells invade blood and bone marrow cells. In 2014, the National Cancer Institute estimateed that there will be 52,380 cases of leukemia diagnosed in the U.S., and about 24,090 deaths due to leukemia (NCI, 2014C).

The rapid development of cancer in the west coincides remarkably well with the growth of obesity in adults and the earlier onset of menarche in young girls which has been attributed to rapid growth rates prior to puberty. Whereas in China the onset of menstruations begins around 17years of age, in the U.S. the age of menarche starts at 12 or 13 years of age. What is of interest is that this early onset of the menstrual cycle is associated with future risk of breast and other types of cancers (Nightingale & Giovannucci, 2006). So then cancer risk increases with body weight in adults and young people. The mechanism is likely tied to metabolic and hormonal changes such as increased circulating sex hormones, insulin, and insulin-like growth factor (IGF). These are now recognized as powerful vectors for cell differentiation, proliferation and apoptosis. Human studies have shown that high serum IGF-1 and insulin are strongly linked to colon cancers in the more prosperous populations (Giovannucci, 2001). These findings suggest then that weight loss should be associated with a decline in cancer risks. This however, has not been investigated very thoroughly in the human population. Nevertheless, one prospective study (Parker & Folsom, 2003) had found that women, who had purposely lost at least 20lbs, experienced a significant reduction in breast cancer risk.

7.4. COLON CANCER & THE U.S. DIET

Colon cancer is third most prevalent form of cancer, in both men and women, in the U.S., and is responsible for as many as 51,000 deaths/year (ACS, 2010); but most interesting, 90% of colorectal cancers are diagnosed after 50 years of age, and the risk of a genetic predisposition is only weighted at 5% (NCI, 2014E). This means that most colorectal cancers are the result of either endogenous or exogenous factors that damage genes, and therefore are considered preventable (ACS, 2010). A colonoscopy is the preferred method of screening for colonic polyps which could be benign or malignant. From a preventative perspective, it is best to consider polyps as potentially cancerous. Polyps found in the colon are generally raised (**Figure 7.5**) or flat, and should be surgically removed in order to decrease the risk of the polyp becoming cancerous. Research conducted at the Memorial Sloan-Kettering Cancer Center, reported a 53% decline in death rates when all polyps were systematically removed from subjects during standard colonoscopies (ACS, 2012B).

It was this study that helped establish the extent to which early detection of polyps with colonoscopies could help reduce the risk of colon cancer. Findings from long term epidemiological prospective studies, over the last 10 years, reveal that individuals at risk of developing polyps regularly consume fatty foods; they tend to have a diet high in red and processed meat; they consume few fruits and vegetables, exercise very little, smoke and drink alcohol excessively, and tend to be either overweight or obese (DHHS, 2008; ACS, 2010). Moreover, high fruit and vegetable intake tends to decrease risks of oral, esophageal, stomach and colorectal cancers. Indeed, those who tend to eat more abundant fruits and vegetables will also be more likely not to consume as much fatty foods. The research findings are not always consistent since not all vegetables are equal. Those studies that have found vegetables to be anticarcinogenic, almost unfailingly point towards carotene-rich vegetables

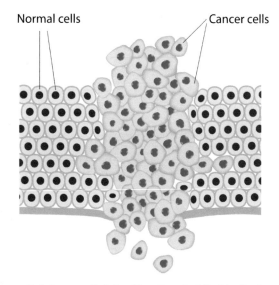

Figure 7.4 Cancer Cell Proliferation © Alila Medical Media/shutterstock.com

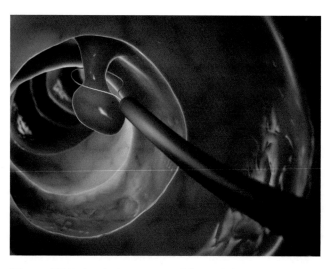

Figure 7.5 Polyp being removed from Colon. © Sebastian Kolitzski/shutterstock.com

that contain a vast array of carotenoids such as lutein, zeaxanthin, criptoxanthin, lycopene, ß-carotene and α-carotene. Visually this means the lunch and dinner plate must be loaded up with yellow/red and yellow/orange vegetable combinations—a dramatic shift from the dreary monotonous brown and beige plates often seen throughout popular restaurant chains. In fact, the ß-carotene rich fruits and vegetables appear to inhibit cancer-induction events. But be warned that ß-carotene supplements have been shown, in the beta-Carotene and Retinol Efficacy Trial, published in the high impact New England Journal of Medicine (Omenn, et al. 1996), to increase lung cancer risks among smokers. It becomes clear that the full protective effect of phytochemicals can be better felt using minimally processed vegetables and fruits, not supplements. The prevalence of colon cancer has declined considerably since screening for patients >50 years of age became a more common practice by physicians since 1998. Consequently, the prevalence declined from 63.3 to 45.5 /100,000 people over age 50, but did increase since 1994 in those men and women younger than 50 (ACS, 2010).

Experts believe that it is the routine colonoscopies, conducted in men and women over 50 years of age, that have led to lowering the incidence rates in the > 50 years age group through early detection and treatments. The main reason is that the early phases of colon cancer are virtually asymptomatic or without noticeable symptoms (DHHS, 2008). By the time the polyp has evolved to a cancerous stage-4 (**Figure 7.6**) and caused more frequent and noticeable lower abdominal cramping in addition to bloody stools, the cancer has more likely begun to spread systemically throughout the body. In that sense the cancer is said to have metastasize or spread to other tissues.

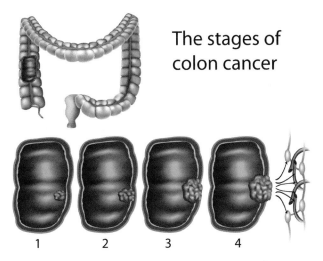

The stages of colon cancer

1   2   3   4

Figure 7.6 Colon Cancer © Alila Medical Media/ shutterstock.com

7.5. BREAST CANCER & THE U.S. DIET

The National Cancer Institute predicts that there will be an estimated 232,670 new cases of invasive breast cancer in the U.S. in 2014 that will lead to approximately 40,000 deaths. Ductal breast carcinoma represents about 70% of invasive breast cancers (**Figure 7.7**) and is the leading cause of cancer deaths in women (NCI, 2014D; CTCA, 2014). There are a few non-modifiable factors that heighten the risk of breast cancers in women, starting with an early age at menarche or late onset of menopause, and a family history of breast cancer. The breast cancer susceptibility genes (BRCA1 and BRCA2) are very rare, representing between 5-10% of all breast cancer cases (ACS, 2010). It is however encouraging to note that between 1999 and 2006 the incidence of breast cancer has been declining at a rate of 2% per year, and experts believe this decrease is likely the result of two events: first, a 2002 publication that came out of the Women's Health Initiative (WHI) which was a 15 year NIH study program that followed 161,808 post-menopausal women. Researchers, in that study, had successfully linked hormonal menopausal therapy (HMT), consisting of a combined use of estrogen and Progestin, to higher risks of breast cancer (ACS, 2010); second, there has also been a decline in the use of mammography as an early screening tool for cancer which may have simply delayed early breast cancer detection and falsely brought down incidence rates. The findings from the WHI study persuaded professional medical bodies to change therapeutic approaches for managing menopausal women.

It is hopeful that breast cancer incidences can be reduced in the population by modifying medical therapies. But even more encouraging is the fact that there are lifestyle and diet changes that can be embraced by women in order to greatly decrease their risk of developing breast cancer in future years. The main risk factors for breast cancer that can be modified include, first, significant weight gain after the age of 18; second, becoming overweight or obese; third, adopting a physically inactive lifestyle; fourth, the intake one or more alcoholic drinks per day; sixth, recent consumption of oral contraceptives; seventh, never having children; or eighth, delaying having the first child until after the age of 30 (ACS, 2010). In order to further decrease risks women are encouraged to breastfeed, engage in moderate to vigorous exercise, and maintain a healthy body weight (ACS, 2010). The good news is that 5 years survival rates have significantly improved since the 1960s, going from a mere 63% to an impressive 90% today. If the cancer is localized in the breast and has not spread, the survival jumps to 98%. By contrast, patients with breast cancer that metastasize to

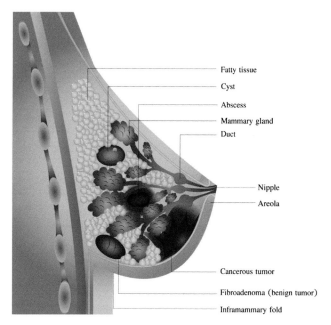

Fatty tissue
Cyst
Abscess
Mammary gland
Duct

Nipple
Areola

Cancerous tumor
Fibroadenoma (benign tumor)
Inframammary fold

Figure 7.7 Breast cancer and other breast anomalies
© GRei/shutterstock.com

the lymph nodes, have a 5 year 84% survival rate, however, metastatic cancer that invades other organs brings survival rates down to 23% (ACS, 2010).

7.6. ASSESSMENT OF CANCER PATIENTS

A little over 50% of all newly diagnosed cancers in women are lung, breast and colorectal, whereas in men, 55% are lung, prostate and colorectal. These four types of cancers are responsible for more than 50% of the half million cancer deaths reported every year in the U.S. Moreover, the direct cost to manage cancer is estimated at $40 billion a year, and the forecast is for health care costs to continue to rise as the absolute number of cancer patients is expected to increase (Shattener and Shike, 2006). There is a clear incentive to improve cancer management strategies, because rates have not declined in a manner consistent with the 1970's National Cancer Institute goals of halving cancer mortality rates by the year 2000 (Sporn, 2006).

One of those possible strategies is to improve the nutritional status of cancer patients undergoing treatments. There are several factors that need to be considered in assessing the nutritional status of cancer patients. First, the primary goal is to accurately provide a prognosis or in other words, a reasonable forecast of the patient's ability to fare well physically during the treatment process. A poor nutritional status translates into a poor prognosis for patients undergoing chemotherapy, and therefore a

poor outcome. Malnutrition is so prominent in cancer, that among the 1.3 million patients newly diagnosed with invasive cancer in 2003, 80% were malnourished and experienced significant weight loss (Shattener & Shike, 2006). In fact between 54 to over 80% of patients suffering from prostate, lung, pancreatic, colon, and gastric cancers, experienced moderate to severe weight loss about 6 months prior to the official cancer diagnosis. It is generally accepted that an involuntary weight loss greater than 10% of usual body weight, over a 6 month period, is concerning, and needs to be addressed (Shattener & Shike, 2006).

The reasons for the weight loss are multifactorial, but the most significant contributor is a decline in caloric intake, generally attributed to an early sense of satiety in 71% of patients, anorexia in 56% of cases, and a change in taste perception 60% of the time (Komurcu et al. 2002).

The second most influential cause of weight loss are metabolic alterations that affect the way the body metabolizes carbohydrates, proteins and lipids (Shattener & Shike, 2006). There is indeed a distinct metabolic pattern in cancer patients that contrasts with the metabolism seen in patients suffering from simple starvation. Carbohydrate metabolism, during weight loss that is tied to carcinogenesis, for instance, favors a heightened glucose turnover as depicted by an increased endogenous production of glucose, thus leading to hyperglycemia; this is likely the consequence of glucose intolerance, insulin resistance and possibly a decline in pancreatic release of insulin. In simple starvation, by contrast, weight loss is intimately associated with a decline in glucose turnover. What does this mean? In starvation, the lack of food intake leads to a decline in food and sugar ingestion, and therefore sugar absorption. Likewise, insulin secretion from the beta cells of the pancreas also decreases, which normally leads to an increased secretion of hormone-sensitive lipase, and to an ensuing increase in lipolysis or breakdown of fat via oxidative metabolism. In cancer patients, this process is altered, thereby leading to a rate of glucose oxidation that increases proportionally with the tumor size, and that never really completely relents, even when exogenous glucose is infused through the veins of these patients. Still, endogenous glucose production persists maximally first, through the continued breakdown of hepatic glycogen reserves—maximal output lasts 12-14hrs after the start of fasting—followed by a persistent gluconeogenesis that catabolizes protein in order to form glucose. Researchers have also noted a persistent Cori cycle (**Figure 7.8**), that is metabolically inefficient as it costs the body a net 4 ATPs to revert anaerobically-produced muscle lactate via glycolysis back to glucose using a gluconeogenic pathway in the liver. In cancer, the body can relentlessly breakdown muscle

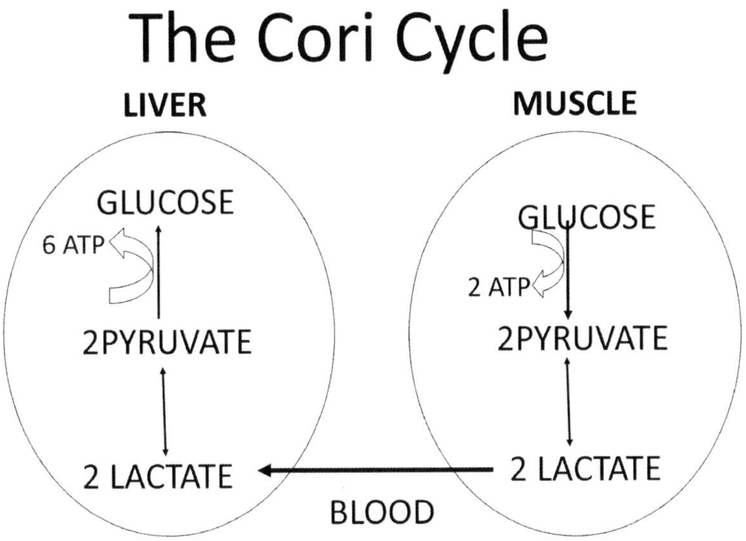

The Cori Cycle

LIVER   **MUSCLE**

GLUCOSE   GLUCOSE

6 ATP   2 ATP

2 PYRUVATE   2 PYRUVATE

2 LACTATE ← ← 2 LACTATE

BLOOD

Figure 7.8 The Cori cycle.

lactate, via the Cori cycle, which eventually comes to an end with the depletion of muscle glycogen stores. The body then more completely reverts to the degradation of skeletal muscle protein for glucose production, and to the inhibition of muscle protein synthesis, both causing, over time, a visible wasting of the skeletal muscle mass that so characteristically reflects the state of cachexia (advanced wasting), seen in advanced cancer.

Also, concomitantly, liver protein synthesis increases during this time, perhaps to produce C-reactive proteins and other stress-related proteins. Interestingly, the relentless muscle protein breakdown, observed during carcinogenesis, is not naturally diminished over time, as in simple starvation, nor is it completely prevented with nutritional support, whether it be given parenterally (veins) or enterally (gut). In other words, hyper-alimentation is not capable of completely preventing continued muscle breakdown in cancer-generated anorexia. Concomitantly, fat reserves are also depleted in cancer patients, in part because of a lipid-mobilizing factor (LMF) generated from the tumor, which causes a persistent lipolysis, and in part by insulin resistance, and a heightened catecholamine secretion due to metabolic stress (Shattener & Shike, 2006). In ordinary starvation, by contrast, the body's reliance on glycogen quickly changes to gluconeogenesis within about 12 to 14hrs, then by about 2 days, 90% of the body's glucose needs is derived from protein, and about 10% from glycerol in order to maintain neurological function (**Figure 7.9**). Afterwards, dependency on protein rapidly shifts again, so that by the 10th day of starvation the nervous system's reliance on ketone bodies, rather than glucose, is at its peak (Rolfe et al 2009). In this manner, long term dieting leads to a high reliance on fat and thus spares protein. However, because fat is effectively oxidized in the flame of carbohydrate metabolism,

the production of ketone bodies becomes more prominent during fasting because precisely of the absence of dietary carbohydrates. This is nicely depicted in **Figure 7.9** with the TCA cycle's downward arrow which occurs with a less active glycolysis. The abundant fat being broken down for energy (lipolysis), rather than get oxidized through the TCA cycle, is diverted towards the synthesis of ketone bodies. The upside is that the brain can use ketones instead of glucose. Fortunately, gluconeogenesis, by this time, has dropped by 67% in light of this adaptation. Carcinogenesis, contrariwise, persistently taxes both muscle protein and adipocytes, causing a significant depletion of both body reserves; in this way, the body appears cachectic, or severely emaciated.

7.6.1 Nutritional Assessment of Cancer Patients:

A proper determination of the patient's nutritional status should be established by the dietitian. This information is vital to the medical team who must assess the patient's prognosis or likelihood of recovery or enduring a difficult chemotherapy. The understanding here is that the dietitian has two possible roles: first, determine the patient's ability to tolerate the chemotherapy and/or radiation therapy and recover if the physician wants to pursue and aggressive treatment protocol; or second, determine the kind of nutritional support that will be needed to help meet the patient's needs for hospice.

Patients aggressively treated for their cancer need to receive strong nutritional support. The baseline nutritional status, before medical treatments, is important to establish, as it will help the medical team determine pre-treatment nutritional support in order to increase

CATABOLIC METABOLISM

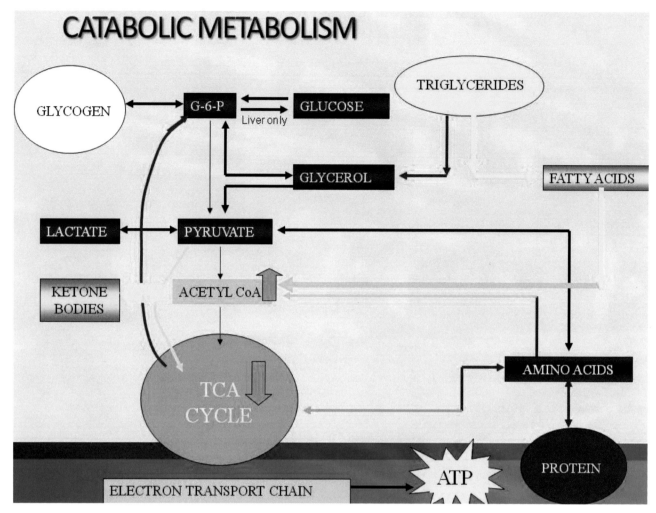

Figure 7.9 Catabolic Pathways during Fasting.

the likelihood of the patient tolerating and successfully getting through the chemo and radiation relatively unscathed. The nutrition support prevents complications that may arise from surgery, chemotherapy or radiation therapy and increase survival rate (NCI2014G). The Prognostic Nutritional Index (PNI) and the Patient-Generated subjective Global Assessment (PG-SGA) are prognostic nutritional indicators, currently in use, that assist medical teams in establishing reliable and accurate patient prognosis (NCI,2014G).

The Prognostic Nutritional Index (PNI) equation is depicted here and represented as a percent:

PNI = 158 - 16.6(Alb) - 0.78(Ts) - 0.20(Trn) - 5.8(DH)

Used as a method of predicting the occurrence of complications in patients that are undergoing non-emergency surgery, this method relies on: serum albumin (Alb) expressed in g/dl; delayed hypersensitivity (DH), with assessment ranges represented here: (no reaction = 0, < 5mm induration =1, and > 5mm induration = 2) (Dempsey et al. 1983); triceps skinfold (Ts) measured in

mm; and serum transferrin (Tns). The major limitation is that the index has difficulty differentiating between the effects of malnutrition and those of disease. Therefore this technique can only be effectively applied to patients that are not suffering from trauma, sepsis and disease states that increase metabolism significantly. The criteria, utilized to interpret the PNI percentages, are represented below (Gibson, 1990).

PNI > 50% = High risk
PNI= 40-49% = Intermediary risk
PNI=<40% = Low risk

Patient-generated Subjective Global Assessment (PG-SGA), on the other hand, was specifically developed for assessing the nutritional status of specifically cancer patients (Laky, et al., 2008; Bauer et al. 2002). This method does not utilize a numeric system for quantifying risk, such as PNI, but purely a subjective approach as indicated in Figures 7.10A and 7.10B. The most sensitive indicator of

PATIENT-GENERATED SUBJECTIVE GLOBAL ASSESSMENT

NAME:_____; AGE:_____; DATE:___/___/_____

Complete this form by questioning the patient or selecting the most likely option

WEIGHT HISTORY

Current Weight_____ Kg Percent usual weight: _____

Usual Weight _____ Kg

Weight 3 Months Ago: _____ Kg % weight loss:____

Weight 6 months Ago:: _____ Kg % weight loss:____

Goal Weight to Achieve:____ Kg

DIET ASSESSMENT

My FOOD INTAKE compared to 1 month ago:

□ I am eating more

□ I am eating the same

□ I am eating less

The type of FOOD I am eating:

□ Normal diet

□ Very little solid food

□ Only liquids

□ Only nutritional supplements

□ Very little food of any kind

ACTIVITY ASSESSMENT

Daily activity level over the last month:

□ Normal

□ Less than usual

□ Don't feel like doing anything

□ I spend half of the day in bed or sitting down

ABILITY TO EAT/TOLERATE FOOD

I have problems eating:

□ YES

□ NO

If the answer is "YES" indicate below the problem (s) you are having

□ I have no appetite

□ I have nausea

□ I am Vomiting

□ I have constipation

□ I have gas /bloating

□ I have diarrhea

□ Smells bother me

□ Foods are tasteless

□ Foods have funny taste

□ I feel full quickly

□ I have problems swallowing

□ I have problems with my teeth

□ I have pain. Where is the pain located? _____

_____

□ I have depression

□ I have money problems

□ I am worried

□ I am anxious

□ I am nervous

Figure 7.10A. A patient-generated Subjective Global Assessment (PG-SGA) form-1 for the nutritional assessment of cancer patients. (Source: adapted from Gomez-Candela et al 2012.)

PATIENT-GENERATED SUBJECTIVE GLOBAL ASSESSMENT

THIS PART OF THE FORM WILL BE FILLED OUT BY YOUR DOCTOR

DISEASE ASSESSMENT

CURRENT DISEASES: _____

_____

ONCOLOGICAL TREATMENTS:_____

_____

OTHER TREATMENTS:_____

_____

SERUM ALBUMIN before oncological treatments:

_____g/dl

PRE-ALBUMIN after oncological treatments:

_____mg/dl

PHYSICAL EXAM

Body fat deficit: □ YES □ NO

If YES rate: ___mild to moderate ___severe

Body muscle deficit: □ YES □ NO

If YES rate: ___mild to moderate ___severe

Body edema/ascites: □ YES □ NO

If YES rate: ___mild to moderate ___severe

Pressure sores: □ YES □ NO

Fever: □ YES □ NO

% weight loss over 3 months:_____%

% weight loss over 6 months:_____%

Current weight as a % usual weight:_____%

ASSESSMENT CRITERIA & GUIDELINES

A. **WELL NOURISHED**: A well nourished patient will have <5% body weight loss. In addition, the patient will not experience any loss of muscle or fat tissue. There will be no observable gastrointestinal problems or symptoms, nor will there be any documented decline in physical activity levels

B. **MODERATELY MALNOURISHED**: A mild to moderately malnourished patient will experience a 5%-10% weight loss over the previous 3-6 months. The patient will have had a mild loss of fat and muscle tissue, and will report having digestive problems and /or difficulties consuming adequate amounts of food.

C. **SEVERELY MALNOURISHED**: A severely malnourished patient will experience > 10% weight loss over the previous 6 months. There will also be a severe loss of fat and muscle tissue, a significant loss of physical function (activity level will be low), many gastrointestinal problems, and edema in extremities and possible ascites.

A serum albumin <3.0g/dl is a poor prognostic indicator and is tied to poor tolerance of treatment and poor survival independent of nutritional status (Lien et al, 2004)

(Source: Rolfes et al 2008; Gibson, 1990; Gomez-Candela, et al. 2012)

Figure 7.10B. A patient-generated Subjective Global Assessment (PG-SGA) form-2 for the nutritional assessment of cancer patients. (Source: adapted from Gomez-Candela et al 2012; Rolfe et al. 2008; Gibson, 1990)

poor nutritional status and increased risk of not tolerating cancer treatments is significant weight loss 5%—10% or >10% of ideal body weight within a 6 month period.

NUTRITION THERAPY

The overall goal of any nutritional intervention is to optimize the patient's quality of life whether active treatment or palliation is being pursued. Specific goals have to do with preventing or reversing nutrient deficiencies, impeding the loss of lean body mass, preserving strength and energy levels so as to better tolerate the cancer treatments, minimizing infections and preventing complications arising from malnutrition (ACI, 2014H). Nutritional support in the form of oral supplemental nutrition or oral nourishment is recommended as the method of choice as it preserves gut function by maintaining GI integrity of the villi. A high protein and calorie meal plan is provided to patients who are at 80% of their healthy weight, or who have unintentionally lost >10% body weight within a narrow span of time; perhaps 3-6 months. This kind of therapeutic meal plan in combination with appetite stimulants is prescribed to patients who have been unable to eat or drink adequately for more than 5 days, probably because of alteration in taste, xerostomia, mucositis, nausea, and/or diarrhea following cancer therapy (ACI, 2014H). The dietitian is usually in charge of determining the degree of malnutrition using various assessment techniques, and, based on the findings, a type of nutritional support is usually recommended.

Total parenteral nutrition (TPN) is considered as a viable strategy of providing much needed nutrition through the veins, in instances when the gastrointestinal tract is compromised either from injury, resection or inflammation often resulting in malabsorption or short bowel syndrome (ACI, 2014H). There is, however, insufficient data to support the consistent use of TPN for patients receiving anti-cancer therapy at this time; more studies are required to further investigate if there are notable benefits. Otherwise, enterally administered nutritional support through the gut, in the form of a nasogastric tube, gastrostomy or jejunostomy are popularly given precedence in order to minimize atrophy of the GI villi, and infections that would otherwise occur through TPN (Shattener & Shike, 2006).

Enteral Nutrition Tube Feedings: A polyurethane or silicone tube is place up the nose and down the back of the throat (nasopharynx) until it reaches the gastric pouch—this is a nasogastric feeding or NG feed—in order to facilitate the delivery of a liquid nutritional supplement, often over the short term (<2 weeks). The tube, which is 30-43 inches long, can also be positioned

in the duodenum (nasoduodenal feeding), or the jejunum (nasojejunal feeding) depending on the risk of aspiration. Patients, prone to aspiration, will be particularly vulnerable to aspirating stomach contents into the trachea, causing the patient to choke. The preferred alternative would be the duodenum or jejunum which are locations, along the GI tract, less likely to cause aspiration. In instances, when the vulnerability to aspiration is very high, TPN will be prescribed. If the long term plan (>2 weeks) involves enteral nutrition, then it is customary to implement **percutaneous endoscopic gastrostomy tubes (PEGs)** and **percutaneous endoscopic jejunostomy tubes** (PEJs). A patient with a PEG (**Figure 7.11**) can conceal the tube better than with an NG tube feeding.

These methods are particularly suitable for patients who are unable to tolerate tubes in their mouths, noses and throats because of mucositis, esophagitis, or some kind of fungal lesions in the mouth or throat (ACI, 2014H). The PEG tubes tend to be wider and placed through the abdominal wall in order to allow liquid nutrition to flow directly into the stomach (gastrostomy) or jejunum (jejunostomy).

The school is still out as to whether aggressive nutritional support is warranted for patients with malignant tumors as the increased calories may promote tumor growth. Quality of life most certainly improves with nutrition but not necessarily longevity. There is also the problem of **refeeding syndrome** which takes place when infusion rates of enteral nutrition, and even TPN, are too elevated, causing rapid and fatal cellular shifts in

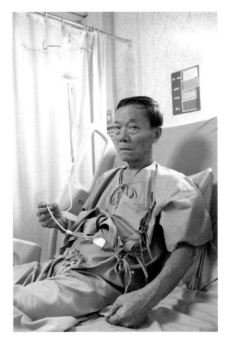

Figure 7.11 Percutaneous endoscopic gastrostomy (PEGs) tubes © Stockphoto Mania/ shutterstock.com

fluid and electrolytes such as potassium, magnesium and phosphorous (Mehanna, et al. 2008).

7.7 PATIENT WITH CANCER EXPERIENCES WEIGHT LOSS

Background: 46 year old female presents with 6 month history of gradually worsening fatigue, appetite loss and weight loss. In the last 2 weeks has developed some shortness of breath (SOB) with exertion and family members think she looks pale. Over the course of the last 6 months she has lost some weight and has noticed her clothes fitting loosely but she has not weighed herself.
Pertinent negatives: no diarrhea, melena, or chest pain.
Exam: Adult female, in no distress, appears mild to moderately ill and tired, and somewhat older than her stated age. Skin is pale but turgor is normal, and there is no rash. Heart and chest exam is normal. Abdominal (ABD) exam is also normal. Rectal exam is normal except for hemo-occult positive stool indicative of a possible malignant tumor, confirmed by colonoscopy.

Lab Results Interpreted: low hemoglobin is observed most likely because of bleeding from the colon; this will be confirmed with a colonoscopy. The elevated liver enzymes (ALT, AST, alkaline phosphatase), reveals the possibility of metastases in the liver. This should prompt the physician to further explore this likelihood.

Serum albumin is low, indicating an overall advanced disease state, and a poor prognosis. Elevated glucose is typically seen in an advanced catabolic state. It is specifically a failure of the balance between glucose production and clearance that is really taking place (Schlichtig & Ayres, 1988). Catabolism means a metabolic breaking down of tissue which occurs concomitantly with

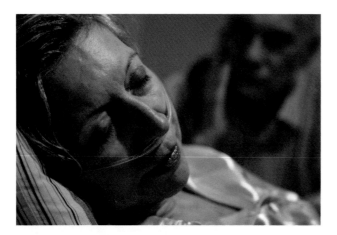

Figure 7.12 Jennifer F is a 46 year old wife and mother of 4 who presents with 12% weight loss, anorexia, occasional nausea credit line © CandyBox Images/shutterstock.com

TABLE 7.1 Patient Chart Information

Jennifer F. CHART INFORMATION		
Female Age: 46; Current Weight: 189lbs has poor appetite. Usual Weight: 230lbs; Height: 5 feet 9 in. Patient lost 25lbs in last 3 months from anorexia. She has a long Hx of chronic constipation; she has frequently dieted for weight loss. Regular BP: 100/69		
TESTS	ACTUAL	GOAL
*Glucose (mg/dl)	175	≤100
Albumin (g/dl)	2.3	3.9-5.0
Creatinine (mg/dl)	1.3	0.8-1.4
BUN (Blood Urea Nitrogen) (mg/dl)	38	6-20
Sodium (Na) (mEq/L)	138	136-144
Hemoglobin (g/dl)	7.8	12-18
Alkaline Phosphatase (IU/L)	152	44-147
ALT (Alanine Aminotransferase) IU/L	54	8-37
AST (Aspartate aminotransferase) IU/L	47	10-34

Source: MedlinePlus: comprehensive metabolic panel: http://www.nlm.nih.gov/medlineplus/ency/article/003468.htm

MedlinePlus: Hemoglobin: http://www.nlm.nih.gov/medlineplus/ency/article/003645.htm * Fasting plasma glucose

significant wasting as evidenced by the 25lbs weight loss in 3 months; it is also tied to a higher mortality rate (Pakhetra et al 2011). This represents an 11.7% weight loss, which is clinically significant. Again the general assessment guidelines recognize that involuntary weight loss is clinically significant when more than an 8% weight loss occurs over 3 months, and when there is a greater than 10% weight loss over 6 months. Increased circulating catecholamine, cortisol and glucagon, in concert with cytokines such as tumor necrosis factor-α (TNF-α) cause blood sugars to soar and insulin resistance to become more prevalent in this kind of acute catabolic state (Pakhetra et al. 2011). The increased secretion of glucagon from the α-cells of the pancreas favors a heightened glycogenolysis. This is the biochemical step that breaks down the glycogen reserves of the liver into glucose, which is then abundantly released as glucose into the blood. The low insulin also promotes lipolysis which can lead, in catabolic states, to lipotoxicity and an aggravation of the inflammatory state.

The high levels of BUN reveals an unusually elevated urea synthesis occurring in the liver from the breakdown of large amounts of amino acids which lead to ammonia and then to urea. The urea moves into the blood as BUN and enters the kidney where it is expelled in the urine. This overabundance of amino acids can come from large dietary protein—likely via intravenous feedings like TPN—or from extensive muscle erosion or break down, the consequence of metabolic stress—the largest proteolysis is seen in burn patients. The implications of catabolizing protein and creating a negative nitrogen balance environment are that wound healing can be impaired and susceptibility to infections heightened (Pakhetra et al. 2011). Not even nutritional support can completely reverse the negative balance.

The creatinine is only slightly elevated, indicating no real kidney dysfunction. So then the BUN is not elevated because of decreased renal function, but rather from increased proteolysis (breakdown of protein in the body).

Nutritional Assessment of Patient:
The first part of a nutritional assessment involves determining the actual dietary intake of the patient. Here there are three goals the dietitian will attempt to achieve: first, assess the amount of calories, protein, carbohydrates and fat consumed; second, determine how long the patient has been eating this way; and third, establish if dietary patterns have changed significantly for her usual intake (Table 7-2).

The next step is to establish the patient's resting energy requirements using the Harris Benedict equation for hospitalized patients and then, using the appropriate activity and metabolic stress factors, determine total energy needs. The equation, found in **Table 7.3** below will assist the students in determining the patient's resting energy expenditure (REE)

$\female$REE = [665 + 9.56 W (kg) + 1.85 H (cm)] – 4.6 A
REE = [665 + 9.56 (85.81Kg) + 1.85 (175.26)]-(4.6 x 46)
REE = [665+820.34+324.23] – (211.6)
REE = 1812.23-216.2
REE= 1597.97 kcal ~1598 kcal

The patient is bedridden while in hospital, and is therefore assigned a 1.0 activity factor.

REE x AF = 1596 kcal x 1.0 = 1596 kcal

Work done by Vernon Young out of Cambridge, MA, showed that cancer patients, taken as a whole, require upwards of 10% all the way to 120% of normal energy requirements with various types of cancers (Young, 1977). Assigning a stress factor (SF) is not a hard and exact science. The stress factor is indeed difficult to predict, as energy needs will depend on the stage of the cancer, the size of the tumor and the location of the cancer (NCI, 2014I). Applying an approximate stress factor of 1.25 based the published work of Kohr and Mohd (2011) would appear reasonable and conservative for this patient's possible GI malignant tumor. The patients total energy expenditure (TEE) would then be the resting energy expenditure (REE) multiplied by an activity factor (AF) of 1.0 since she is bedridden and then multiplied again by a stress factor (SF) of 1.25:

TEE = REE x AF x SF
TEE = 1596 kcal x 1.0 x 1.25
TEE = 1596 x 1.25 = 1995 kcal/day

This is the patient's total daily energy requirements. Based on her recent usual intake reported on the **usual food intake form** (Figure 7.2), in which she reports a daily intake of 1186 kcalories, it is not surprising to find that she has been experiencing weight loss.

Her protein intake is 54g which is deficient when expressed per kilogram body weight:

54g / 85.8Kg = 0.63g/kg body weight. This does not meet the minimal physiological requirement of 0.8 g/kg body weight. Moreover, there is evidence that additional protein may be needed because of the persistent catabolic state that is often seen in cancer patients—Long (1984) recommends 1.5-2.0g/kg for moderately stressed patients. Also fat intake represents only 16.7% of her actual caloric intake and only 10% of her DRI calories, which is far below the 20%-35% recommended by Healthy Eating Guidelines for Americans. Carbohydrate intake equals 193g or 38.6% of DRI calories, a value that is much below the 45-65% of DRI calories recommended by Healthy Macronutrient Range Guidelines.

Treatment of Recommendations of Patient:
The persistent nausea and red blood found in her stool, in concert with the colonic tumor found by colonoscopy suggests a cancer. Slightly elevated liver enzymes raise suspicions of possible metastases which must be confirmed by oncologist. Even if the patient's BMI of 27.9 (85.81 Kg / (1.753 meters)^2) is classified as overweight, the recent weight loss of 11.7% over a 3 month period reveals a high likelihood of malnutrition. Patient will be given 1995 kcalories per day through TPN because of a likely obstruction in the colon from the tumor. In this instance, intravenous nutrition makes good sense, as her GI tract will be compromised until after the surgical removal of the tumor. This amount of calories will prevent further weight loss, and is not intended to allow weight gain. Moreover, the nutritionally complete supplement will regenerate nutrient stores and decrease risks of complications from surgery.

TABLE 7.2 Usual Food Intake Record of Recent Past

PATIENT NAME: **Jennifer F.**	USUAL FOOD INTAKE	
FOODS CONSUMED	**QUANTITY CONSUMED**	**PLACE**
BREAKFAST: TIME: 7:00 am		
Porridge (homemade)	1 cup	Kitchen
AM SNACKS TIME: **10:00 am**		
Applesauce (Mott's Natural)	1 cup	Dining room
LUNCH TIME: 12:30pm		
Egg sandwich on white bread (Homemade) Milk skim	1s/w 1 cup	Hospital Cafeteria
PM SNACK TIME: **2:15 pm**		
Pudding (vanilla) Jell-O pudding cup	1 cup	home
DINNER TIME: 7:00 pm		
Strawberry Milkshake (McDonald's)	medium	restaurant
ENEVING SNACK TIME:		
None		

NUTRIENT BREAKDOWN OF USUAL FOOD INTAKE	
Kcals recommended: 1996 kcal/day (1796--2196 Kcals/day) Carbohydrates recommended: 299g/day (60% DRI Kcals) (224-324g) Protein recommended: 75g/day (15% DRI Kcals) (50g-175g) Fat recommended: 55g (25% DRI Kcals) (44-78g) Total Maximal Sugar: <125g (25% DRI Kcals) Total Maximal Sodium: <2400 mg/day	Kcals eaten: **1186 kcals** Carbohydrates eaten: **193g** Protein eaten: **54g** Fat eaten: **22g** Total Sugar eaten: **60g** Sodium eaten: **1189 mg**

Calories measured using the www.myfitnesspal.com website

TABLE 7.3 Total Energy Expenditure in health and disease.

Equations	Descriptions
♂REE= [66.47 + 13.75 W(kg) + 5 H (cm)]– 6.76 A ♀REE = [665 + 9.56W(kg) + 1.85 H (cm)] – 4.6 A	Harris-Benedict equation for hospitalized patients with disease
♂REE= [10W(kg) + 6.25 H (cm)] – (5A -5) ♀REE =[10W(kg) + 6.25 H (cm)] – (5A +161)	Mifflin equation for non-hospitalized patients without disease. Mifflin, M.D. *Am.J.Clin.Nutr.1990;51:241-7*
♂REE = 879 + 10.2 WT (kg) ♀REE (non-athletes) = 795 + 7.18 WT (kg) ♀REE (athletes) = 50.4 + 21.1 WT (kg)	Owen equation for the estimation of caloric requirements in healthy lean and obese men, healthy women. Owen, OE et al. *Am.J.Clin.Nutr.1986; 44:1-19;* Owen, OE. *Mayo Clin Proc 1988; 63: 503-510*
♂REE = 1 kcal/kg/Bwt/hr · 24 hrs (subtract 0.1 kcal/hr sleep) + activity increment + spec dynamic action (10%) ♀REE = 0.95 kcal/kg/Bwt/hr · 24 hrs (subtract 0.1 kcal/hrs sleep) + activity factor + specific dynamic action of food (10%)	Rule of thumb method for estimating energy needs

Activity Factors	Injury Factors

Confined to bed: **1.0-1.2**
Ambulatory, low activity: **1.11-1.12**
Average Activity: **1.25-1.27**
High activity: **1.45-1.48**
TEEs equal to 1.55, 1.78 and 2.10 × BMR were proposed for men with light, moderate and heavy occupational activities, respectively (FAO/WHO/UNU, 1985). The corresponding factors suggested for women were 1.56, 1.64 and 1.82.\
Source: Khor, SM & Mohd, BB (2011) Assessing the Resting Energy Expenditure of Cancer Patients in the Penang General Hospital. Mal J. Nutr 17(1): 43-53
	1. Surgery. – Minor: **1.0-1.1**
	  -- Major: **1.1-1.2**
	2. Infections –Mild: **1.0-1.2**
	  --Moderate: **1.2-1.4**
	  --Severe: **1.4-1.8**
	3. Skeletal Trauma: **1.2-1.35**
	  + Head injury + steroids: **1.6**
	4. Burns. 20% BSA: **1.0-1.5**
	  20-40% BSA: **1.5-1.85**
	  >40% BSA: **1.85-1.95**
	5 Cancer: severely aggressive: **1.5-1.7**
	......Tumor & leukemia: **1.20-1.36**

Adapted from: Long, CL The energy and protein requirements of the critically ill patient. 1984. In: Nutritional Assessment. Wright, RA and Heymsfield, S. (eds), Blackwell Scientific p: 157-181; Vernon Young, Cancer Research 1977; 37:2336-2347; Khor, SM & Mohd, BB (2011) Assessing the Resting Energy Expenditure of Cancer Patients in the Penang General Hospital. Mal J. Nutr 17(1): 43-53.

REFERENCES

1. American Cancer Society (2014). What is Cancer? Retrieved May 7, 2014 from: http://www.cancer.org/cancer/cancerbasics/what-is-cancer

2. American Cancer Society (2014B). Lifetime Risk of Developing or Dying from Cancer. Retrieved May 8, 2014 from: http://www.cancer.org/cancer/cancerbasics/lifetime-probability-of-developing-or-dying-from-cancer

3. American Cancer Society (2012) Guidelines on Nutrition & Physical Activity for the Cancer Prevention. Retrieved May 12, 2014 from: http://www.cancer.org/healthy/eathealthygetactive/acsguidelinesonnutritionphysicalactivityforcancerprevention/acs-guidelines-on-nutrition-and-physical-activity-for-cancer-prevention-summary

4. American Cancer Society (ACS, 2012B). Colon/Rectum Cancer, Prevention/Early detection. Removing Polyps Prevents Colon and Rectal Cancer Deaths. Retrieved May 12, 2014 from: http://www.cancer.org/cancer/news/news/removing-polyps-prevents-colon-and-rectal-cancer-deaths

5. American Cancer Society (ACS, 2010). Cancer Facts & Figures 2010. Retrieved May 12 from: http://www.cancer.org/acs/groups/content/@epidemiologysurveilance/documents/document/acspc-026238.pdf

6. Anand, P et. al. (2008). Cancer is a Preventable Disease that Requires Major Lifestyle Changes Pharmaceutical Research 25(9)

7. Bauer J, Capra S, Ferguson M (2002): Use of the scored Patient-Generated Subjective Global Assessment (PG-SGA) as a nutrition assessment tool in patients with cancer. Eur J Clin Nutr 56 (8): 779-85

8. Bissonnette, D (2014) It's All About Nutrition: Saving the Health of Americans. Lanham, MD: University Press of America, 232pp

9. Cancer Treatment Centers of America (CTCA, 2014). Breast Cancer Types. Retrieved May 13 from: http://www.cancercenter.com/breast-cancer/types/tab/invasive-breast-cancer/?source=GGLPS01&channel=paid%20search&c=paid%20search:Google:Non%20Brand:{campaignName}:invasive+breast+cancer:Exact&OVMTC=Exact&site=&creative=36290882721&OVKEY=invasive%20breast%20cancer&url_id=190113679&adpos=1s2&device=c&gclid=COnhpseZqb4CFaY-MgodbXUAXQ

10. CDC. National program of Cancer Registries (2014). About United States Cancer Statistics reported from 1999-2010. Retrieved May 6, 2014 from: http://www.cdc.gov/cancer/npcr/about_uscs.htm

11. CDC. Chronic Disease Prevention and Health Promotion (2013). Cancer: Addressing the Cancer Burden at a Glance. Retrieved May 6, 2014 from: http://apps.nccd.cdc.gov/uscs/toptencancers.aspx

12. CDC. Cancer Prevention and Control (2013B). Cancer Among Women. Retrieved May 6, 2014 from: http://www.cdc.gov/cancer/dcpc/data/women.htm

13. Dempsey DT, Buzby GP, Mullen JL (1983). Nutritional assessment in the seriously ill patient. J Am Coll Nutr. 2: 15-22

14. Gibson, R.S. (1990). Principles of Nutritional Assessment. New York: Oxford University Press, 691pp.

15. Giovannucci, E. et al. (2003). A Prospective Study of Cruciferous Vegetables on Prostate Cancer. Cancer Epidemiol. Biomarkers Prev. (12): 1403-9

16. Giovannucci, E (2001). Insulin, insulin-like growth factors and colon cancer: a review of the evidence. J. Nutr. 131:3109S-20S

17. Gomez-Candela, C et al. (2012) Nutrition intervention in onco-hematological patient. Nutr. Hosp. 27(3): 669-680

18. Khor, SM & Mohd, BB (2011) Assessing the Resting Energy Expenditure of Cancer Patients in the Penang General Hospital. Mal J. Nutr 17(1): 43-53

19. Komurcu, S, Nelson KA, Walsh D, et al (2002) Gastrointestinal symptoms among inpatients with advanced cancer. *Am J Hosp Palliat Care.*19:351-355.

20. Laky, B. et al. (2008) Comparison of different nutritional assessments and body composition measurements in detecting malnutrition among gynecologic cancer patients. Am J Clin Nutr 87:1678–85.

21. Lien, Y.C et al. (2004). Preoperative serum albumin level is a prognostic indicator for adenocarcinoma of the gastric cardia. J. Gastrointest Surg 8(8): 1041-8

22. Long, C.L. (1984). The Energy and Protein Requirements of the Critically Ill Patient. In: Nutritional Assessment, (R.A. Wright and S. Heymsfield, eds). Boston: Blackwell Scientific Publication, p: 157-181

23. Mehanna, H.M et al (2008). Refeeding syndrome: What is it? And how to prevent and treat it. BMJ; 336(7659): 1495–1498.

24. Merck Manual for Health Professionals (2013). Modalities of Cancer Therapy. Retrieved May 6, 2014 from:

25. http://www.merckmanuals.com/professional/hematology_and_oncology/principles_of_cancer_therapy/modalities_of_cancer_therapy.html?qt=CANCER&alt=sh

26. National Cancer Institute (NCI) (2014). What is Cancer? Retrieved May 7 2014 from: http://www.cancer.gov/cancertopics/cancerlibrary/what-is-cancer

27. National Cancer Institute (NCI) (2014B). Antioxidants and Cancer Prevention. Retrieved May 8, 2014 from: http://www.cancer.gov/cancertopics/factsheet/prevention/antioxidants#r8

28. National Cancer Institute (NCI, 2014C). Leukemia. Retrieved May 12, 2014 from: http://www.cancernet.nci.nih.gov/cancertopics/types/leukemia

29. National Cancer Institute (NCI, 2014D). Breast Cancer. Retrieved May 12, 2014 from: http://www.cancernet.nci.nih.gov/cancertopics/types/breast

30. National Cancer Institute (NCI, 2014E). Colorectal Cancer Prevention. Retrieved May 12, 2014 from: http://www.cancernet.nci.nih.gov/cancertopics/pdq/prevention/colorectal/HealthProfessional

31. National Cancer Institute (NCI2014F). Nutrition in Cancer Care. Nutrition Implications of Cancer Therapies. Retrieved May 20, 2014 from: http://www.cancer.gov/cancertopics/pdq/supportivecare/nutrition/HealthProfessional/page3

32. National Cancer Institute (NCI2014G). Nutrition in Cancer Care. Nutrition Screening and Assessment. Retrieved May 20, 2014 from: http://www.cancer.gov/cancertopics/pdq/supportivecare/nutrition/HealthProfessional/Page4#Section_50

33. National Cancer Institute (NCI2014H). Nutrition in Cancer Care—Nutrition Therapy. Retrieved May 21, 2014 from: http://www.cancer.gov/cancertopics/pdq/supportivecare/nutrition/HealthProfessional/page4#Section_50

34. National Cancer Institute (NCI, 2014 I). Nutrition in Cancer—Tumor Induced Effects on Nutritional Status. Retrieved May 23, 2014 from: http://www.cancer.gov/cancertopics/pdq/supportivecare/nutrition/Health Professional/page2

35. National Cancer Institute (NCI) (2010). Chemicals in Meat Cooked at High Temperature and Cancer Risk. Retrieved May 9 2014 from: http://www.cancer.gov/cancertopics/factsheet/Risk/cooked-meats

36. National Center on Health, Physical Activity, and Disability (NCHPAD) (2014). Retrieved May 7, 2014 from: http://www.nchpad.org/163/1257/Cancer~and~Exercise

37. National Cancer Institute (NCI) (2012). Cruciferous Vegetables and Cancer Prevention. Retrieved May 9, 2014 from: http://www.cancer.gov/cancertopics/factsheet/diet/cruciferous-vegetables

38. Omenn, GS. et al. (1996) Effects of a combination of beta-carotene and vitamin A on lung cancer and cardiovascular disease. N. Engl. J. Med. 334(18): 1150-155

39. Pakhetra, R. et al. (2011) Management of Hyperglycemia in Critical Illness: Review of Target and Strategies. MJAFI. 67: 53-57

40. Parker, ED & Folsom, AR (2003). Intentional weight loss and incidence of obesity-related cancers: the Iowa Women's Health Study.Int J. Obes. Related Metab. Disorder. 27: 1447-52

41. Rolfes, S.R., Pinna, K., and Whitney, Ellie (2009). Understanding Normal and Clinical Nutrition. 8th Edition, Belmont, CA: Wadsworth, Cengage Learning, 925pp

42. Schattner, M and Shike, M. (2006) Nutritional Support of the Patient with Cancer. In: Modern Nutrition in Health and Disease. 10th edition (Shils, ME., Shike, M. et al. Eds). New York: Lippincott, Williams & Wilkins. p: 1290-1313.

43. Schlichtig, R. and Ayres, S.M. (1988) Nutritional Support of the Critically Ill. Chicago: Yearbook Medical Publishers Inc. 223pp

44. Sporn, M.B. Chemoprevention of Cancer (2006). In: Modern Nutrition in Health and Disease. 10th edition (Shils, ME., Shike, M. et al. Eds). New York: Lippincott, Williams & Wilkins. p: 1280-89

45. Suzuki M et al. (2001) Oxidative Stress and Longevity in Okinawa and investigation of blood lipid peroxidation and tocopherol in Okinawa Centenarians. Asia Pac J Clin. Nutr. 10(2):165-71. Retrieved May 8, 2014 from: http://www.ncbi.nlm.nih.gov/pmc/articles/PMC3068305/

46. U.S. Cancer Statistics Working Group (USCS). *United States Cancer Statistics: 1999–2010 Incidence and Mortality Web-based Report*. Atlanta: U.S. Department of Health and Human Services, Centers for Disease Control and Prevention and National Cancer Institute; 2013. Available at: www.cdc.gov/uscs.

47. U.S. Department of Health & Human Services (DHHS) (2008). National Digestive Diseases Information Clearinghouse (NDDIC). What I need to know about colonic polyps. NIH Publication No. 09–4977, retrieved May 12, 2014 from: http://digestive.niddk.nih.gov/ddiseases/pubs/colonpolyps_ez/

48. Willcox BJ et al. (2006) Siblings of Okinawan centenarians exhibit lifelong mortality advantages. J Gerontol A Biol Sci Med Sci. 61:345-54

49. Willcox, C., Willcox, BJ, Hsueh, W-C, and Suzuki, M. (2006B) Genetic determinants of exceptional human longevity: insights from the Okinawa Centenarian Study. AGE 28(4): 313-332

50. Willett, W. and Giovannucci, E. (2006) Epidemiology of Diet and Cancer Risk. In: Modern Nutrition in Health and Disease. 10th edition (Shils, ME., Shike, M. et al. Eds). New York: Lippincott, Williams & Wilkins. p: 1267-79

51. Young, VR (1977). Energy Metabolism Requirements in the Cancer Patient. Cancer Research 37:2336-2347

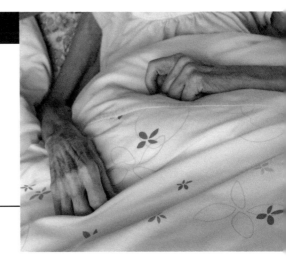

CHAPTER 8

THE PROBLEM OF MALNUTRITION

8.1. UNDERNUTRITION IN DEVELOPING COUNTRIES

The ability to access, pay for and consume adequate amounts of nutritious foods, on a daily basis, in order to support a healthy and active life, is referred to as **food security**. It is however, specifically food insecurity—the inability to access nutritious foods daily—that was responsible for limiting regular access, of an estimated 840 million people worldwide, to nutritious foods between 1990 and 1992 according to the 6th World Survey administered by the WHO. Moreover, despite the millennium development goals, of reducing by half the prevalence of hunger and poverty in the world, formulated by the WHO in 2000, the number of hungry jumped to 1.023 billion by 2009. But it was mostly the preschool children in addition to the women and girls that were the most vulnerable to malnutrition. In fact, it has been estimated that up to 60% of people suffering from hunger are female (Pinstrup-Andersen & Cheng, 2007). Malnourished women of reproductive age pose a particular risk to their offspring by increasing the chances that they will be born underweight. There is an estimated 20 million babies born every year from undernourished mothers. These underweight infants are at risk of chronic disease later in life (Caballero, 2006).

Internationally, the WHO has identified **vitamin A**, **iodine** and **iron** as the three most prominent nutrient deficiencies, in underdeveloped and developing countries. Together, they affect up to 33% of the world's population (WHO, 2006). Ever since 1992 the Health and Nutrition Monitoring System, established from the World Health Resolution WHA45.33, has been set up to assess the degree to which these three nutrient deficiencies are affecting populations, and to what extent control programs have been effective in containing the magnitude of the threat (WHO, 2006). What has become evident since that time is that it is dictatorships, wars, sectarian violence, famines, earthquakes, droughts, poverty, and social conflicts of various types that compromise population access to nutritious foods and water. It is especially the mass migration and individual poverty that is behind the selloff of properties and livestock in order to access the money necessary to purchase food. Contrary to popular belief, it is not the lack of food, but rather the poverty itself that becomes the greatest threat for undernutrition. More recently, greater emphasis on the economic development of countries, aimed at boosting the gross national product (GNP) of underdeveloped nations, has been recognized as having the potential of greatly decreasing world hunger (Quandt, 2006). Indeed, the **economic development approach** suggests that greater family income can translate into improved pur-chasing power, thus better food and improved nutrition. The paradox and contention here is that an enhanced GNP does not necessarily translate into better food pur-chases and nutrition. Adherents of the **world systems theory**, advance that greater GNPs invariably translate into a lowering of living standards and heightened nu-trition problems such as obesity (World Bank, 1993). The main problem is that while countries may be able to increase their GNP by transitioning from subsistence-based farming to cash cropping, they also appear to cause an important drop in the nutritional status of the population (Quandt, 2006). Traditional farming prac-tices, consisting in multi-plot and multi-crop farming, provide a diverse assortment of agricultural products to the food supply. This accomplishes two goals: first, it manages to smooth out anomalies in nutrient content in the food supply, and second, it protects the farmer from the devastation that could come from crop failure (Feuret and Fleuret, 1980). Transitioning to a cash crop-based agriculture necessitates greater imports of diverse foods in order to feed the population. These imports invariably create a dependency on the surplus grains that influx into these countries from the industrialized west. The cash earned from this kind of singular crop agriculture does not necessarily translate into better nutrition because of two main phenomena: first, the money earned is usu-ally paid in two annual bulk sums that do not always go towards nutritious foods, but often towards competing non-food needs; second, the influx of cash usually drives up food prices, thus making nutritious foods more dif-ficult to obtain, and thus subjecting the population to the dangers of significant market price fluctuations (Fleuret and Fleuret, 1980).

Historically, between 1950 and 1960 international relief had been primarily preoccupied with protein de-ficiency in children identified as kwashiorkor. However, in the 1960s and 70s interest shifted towards protein and energy malnutrition (PEM). At the 1974 World Food Conference in Rome, economists took over from nutritionists and pediatricians as the main policy makers, with a focus placed on food security. The World Bank strategically began promoting increased income genera-tion as a solution to poverty and malnutrition. This was the main thrust of the WHO international relief efforts right up until 1985, at which point the International Monetary Fund (IMF) began to make structural adjust-ments at around the same time that the WHO and UNI-CEF renamed the Applied Nutrition Program (ANP), the Joint Nutrition Support Programs (JNSPs). No long after, in 1990s nutritionists successfully set the stage for the interest to shift towards micronutrient deficiencies in response to goals that were set by 1989 World Summit

on Children and the 1992 International Conference on Nutrition (FAO, 1997). Suddenly, PEM got pushed to the background, while an urgent need to eradicate three of the most prevalent micronutrient deficiency diseases—vitamin A, iron and iodine—rose to the top of the international agenda (FAO, 1997). These were deficiencies that demanded quick fixes as it was clearly recognized that retinol, iodine and iron deficiencies in combination with vitamin D, folate and zinc were linked to 7.3% of human diseases worldwide, and thus repre-sented a significant threat to human health in developing countries (WHO, 2006).

The result of a broad analysis of malnutrition inter-nationally, concluded that there were 6 key factors that were in play. Notably, **agricultural production** became a critical component in the discussion, for indeed, the shift from subsistence agriculture to cash cropping will tend to impoverish population diets. Also, the question of **food preservation,** as it pertains to processing after harvest, plays a significant role in population nutrition because of excessive wastage. In fact, roughly 25% of grains and 50% of fruits, vegetables and roots are lost in post-harvest storage in developing countries. There is also the question of over processing which leads to poor nutri-tional food quality and a greater susceptibility to nutrient deficiencies of thiamin (vitamin B1) and niacin (vitamin B3). **Overpopulation** has been argued as central to the discussion in so far as child spacing and the financial bur-den felt by families that have too many children. **Poverty** of the family has now been recognized as a determinant of nutritional status. When the purchasing power of the family becomes constricted because of economic strife, then access to food is limited with direct consequences on the health of family members. The **geopolitical landscape** will also influence population nutrition as it becomes central to political stability. Dictatorships are infamous for creating strife, poverty and social upheaval. In the midst of social unrest, lawlessness, and poor government policies, food production can be hampered. Finally the prominence of certain **pathologies**, especially infections can seriously devastate the nutritional status of a population (FAO, 1997).

More recently, since the turn of the new Millennium, there has been an important reduction in the prevalence of undernutrition and mortality among children younger than 5 years of age. Yet, despite this improvement, there are still 170 million undernourished children worldwide of which about 3 million indirectly die from diseases that are worsened by undernutrition. However, the paradox is that overnutrition also afflicts populations of under-developed transitioning countries at the same time. Of particular concern are the 1 billion overweight adults in addition to the 300 million clinically obese adults around the world who are emerging because of a nutrition transition (Caballero, 2006).

8.1.1 The Nutrition Transition

The concept of a nutrition transition was first proposed in the 1990s by Dr. Barry Popkin, a leading epidemiologist and obesity researcher out of the University of North Carolina, Chapel Hill (Popkin, 1994). The premise was that food consumption, over the last 50 years, in developing countries, such as Egypt, Mexico and South Africa, was changing and fueling a rise in chronic diseases. The transition refers to **technological**, **economic** and **demographic** changes taking place in developing countries that increase population access to cheap vegetable oils, animal foods such as meats and dairy products, in addition to soft drinks, all of which have contributed to a spike in obesity rates that begin to rival those of the U.S. (Caballero, 2006). It is specifically demographically significant **population shifts** that describe rural agricultural workers moving to cities to find work. This occurs with the disappearance of small subsistence farming and the emergence of cash crop mega farms. It also describes populations, immigrating to westernized countries, looking for opportunities. The improved technology transforms what used to be, heavy labor, into more mechanized work with few calories expended on a daily basis. The other factor coming into play here is greater **urbanization**. The city dweller produces very little food products, but actually becomes a great purchaser of commodities. He also drives everywhere and walks very little. Moreover, access to cheap and affordable high calorie foods is facilitated by a **globalization** of the food production and marketing (Caballero, 2006). The end result is a 600 kcal/day increase in energy availability per capita in many developing countries, with China exhibiting as much as 1000 kcal/day jump in available energy per person. The biggest culprit appears to be a dramatic increase in caloric sweeteners which takes place with urbanization (Caballero, 2006). Hence, the face of malnutrition is changing in a dramatic way, as it now includes a preponderance of overnutrition alongside much undernutrition in intermediate-income countries. The repercussions are mostly observed in the form of spikes in many secondary diseases such as type-2 diabetes, cardiovascular disease and hypertension (Caballero, 2006)

8.1.2 Protein Energy Malnutrition

Protein intake has been historically central to the discussion on malnutrition since the 1950s, because of the role of protein in the maintenance of lean tissue, the synthesis of new lean body mass, and in ensuring the competence of the immune system which is also referred to as immuno-competence. Protein foods of high biological value (BV) tend to be of limited availability in underdeveloped countries, especially during famines, droughts and during periods of war and civil unrest. The role of protein cannot be overestimated at the international level. A Jamaican pediatrician by the name of Dr. Cicely Williams, introduced, in 1935, the medical term, "**kwashiorkor**," to describe cases of prolonged protein malnutrition observed in Ghana. Derived from the African Ga language of coastal Ghana, the term refers to the sickness that the baby contracts after the birth of the newborn (Williams, 1935). The infant develops red wiry hair, enlarged fatty liver, dermatitis, no visible erosion of fat or skeletal muscle mass, but a noticeable drop in visceral protein (blood proteins), with a concomitant development of edema (water accumulation in the extremities) and ascites (water accumulation in the peritoneal cavity), causing a protruding belly (Bissonnette, 2013). The predominantly starch-based diet, derived mainly from the cassava root, abundant in Ghana, is very poor in protein, and thus compromised the protein status and the immune system which leads to increased infections, diarrhea and higher death rates. A second form of malnutrition, called **marasmus**, occurs when both calories and protein are deficient in the diet (Lee and Nieman, 1996). This condition results in advanced emaciation, the consequence of suboptimal calories and protein leading to both fat and muscle erosion, but with no edema or noticeable change in blood proteins. In this situation, the person experiences emaciation and a significant decline in body weight (Lee and Nieman, 1996).

Both kwashiorkor and marasmus emphasize the importance of protein and calories in survival. To ensure that amino acids from protein are appropriately used for tissue maintenance and growth, it has been determined that calories be independently provided from carbohydrates and fats, that an adequate amount of essential amino acids be present in addition to a quantity of protein that can meet the body's need which is estimated at 0.83g/Kg body weight for adults (WHO, 2007).

The aim of nutrition relief was to originally provide protein in adequate amounts to quell the negative nitrogen balance that is so prominent in malnutrition. The notion of nitrogen balance stemmed from original work by Rose (1957) in the 1950s that identified nitrogen excreted from the urine and feces as byproducts of protein. The main assumption was that protein was certainly the most significant nitrogen-based compound in the body— about 95% of all nitrogen is derived from protein—and thus, any losses or gains had to be attributable to protein losses and gains in the body. Nitrogen balance is a method still used today to assess protein requirements.

8.1.3 Key Vitamin and Mineral Deficiencies in Developing Countries.

There is an estimated 2 billion people around the world who are affected by micronutrient deficiencies, and subject to greater risk of diseases, disabilities and death (Pisciano, 1999). Vitamins A, folate and D, have been identified as most prominent and treatable vitamin deficiencies in the population of underdeveloped and developing countries.

8.1.3.1 Vitamin A Deficiency

Vitamin A's active form "retinol"—known as **pre-formed vitamin A**—is strictly found in the animal components of the diet such milk, cheese, eggs, and chicken and beef livers. Consequently, it is not surprising that developing countries, with difficulties accessing meat protein of high biological value, such as in South East Asia and the Middle East, might experience retinol deficiency. The WHO estimates that there are 250,000 to 500,000 cases per year of blindness—**xerophthalmia** and **keratomalacia**—resulting from vitamin A deficiency with most of the incidences occurring in young children. Interestingly, the WHO considers vitamin A deficiency as the most preventable cause of blindness in the world (UNICEF, 2003). There are non-animal sources of precursors to vitamin A called **pro-vitamin A**, that are found in vegetables such as carrots, sweet potatoes, cantaloupes, apricots, spinach, broccoli and kale. Found in the form of carotenoids, pro-vitamin A is transformed, in the body, to retinol, only to the extent that it is needed. There is never a concern that toxic amounts of retinol would be formed from beta-carotene. Of the hundreds of carotenoids present in our food supply, beta-carotene is the most easily transformed into the active form of vitamin A, called retinol. For retinol deficiency to become a serious threat to a population, there has to be a very impoverished diet with limited access to both animal protein and to a broad assortment of fruits and vegetables.

At the international level children, suffering from measles and diarrheal disease have been identified by the WHO as being at high risk of vitamin A deficiency. Consequently, supplementation has been recognized as an acceptable treatment protocol (COID, 1993). It is noteworthy to point out that when diets are also suboptimal in calories, protein, and zinc, vitamin A deficiency tends to also be prominent. This is because the synthesis of the transport protein, retinol binding protein (R BP), requires proteins, calories and zinc (COID, 1993).

8.1.3.2 Folate Deficiency

At the international level, folate and B12 deficiencies have been identified as a potential public health problem that could possibly affect several millions of individuals (de Benoist, 2008). Folate, which tends to be high in green leafy vegetables—the name folate is derived from foliage—legumes and a variety of fruits, will tend to be deficient in populations that consume suboptimal diets containing unfortified wheat, maize, or rice, and poor in legumes and folate-rich vegetables and fruits (de Benoist, 2008). Countries such as India and Chile have a high prevalence of folate deficiency because of the heavy reliance on processed white flour. This tends not to be a problem in Mexico, Guatemala or Thailand where erythrocyte folate levels were found to be elevated (WHO, 2006). This poor form of nutrition can be found in both developing and developed nations alike. Low blood erythrocyte folate concentrations—the most reliable indicator of long term folate status—have been tied to high risk of low birth weights. Moreover, there is strong evidence in support of a direct link between suboptimal maternal folate intake or status, measured by blood values, and the risk of megaloblastic anemia and neural tube defects (NTD) such as spina bifida in the offspring (de Benoist, 2008). Large scale supplement studies in China in addition to post-fortification trials in Canada, Chile and the United States have successfully confirmed this association. By contrast, the evidence in support of orofacial clefts and heart defects and poor folate intake is modest at this time (de Benoist, 2008).

8.1.3.3 Vitamin D Deficiency

Historically, vitamin D deficiency was prominent in the U.S, Canada, western Europe and Asia in the early years of the 20th century. However, despite quelling the prominence of rickets in the Northern hemisphere (**Figure 8.1**) with improved food fortification and understanding of the role of ultra violet light on vitamin D synthesis, rickets has still become a public health problem in some developing countries (Pettifor, 2004) and developed nations such as France and China (WHO, 2006). The problem however, does not appear to be tied solely to poor vitamin D status necessarily, but rather to a suboptimal intake of dietary calcium, a position for which there has been growing support (Pettifor, 2004). About 80% of vitamin D (calciferol) is synthesized subcutaneously from UV sunlight directly interacting with 7-dehydrocholesterol—the precursor

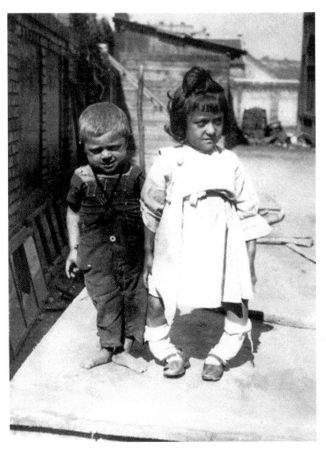

Figure-8.1 Children with rickets in the 1940s presented here with bowed legs. Credit line © Getty Images

to naturally occurring vitamin D_3. The diet provides a vitamin equivalent called vitamin D_2. Both D_3 and D_2 are metabolized in the liver to 25-hydroxyvitamin D (25-OH-D3), and then in the kidney to the biologically active form of 1,25-dihydroxyvitamin D (1,25-(OH)2-D3), also called calciferol (WHO, 2006). Because vitamin D plays a central role in regulating calcium and phosphorus homeostasis in the body, it should not be a surprise that a deficiency of this vitamin could cause devastating bone malformation in infants called rickets (Figure 8.1), and osteomalacia in adults, which leads to osteoporosis and frequent bone fractures (WHO, 2006). Rickets characteristically presents with a poor calcification of femoral, tibia and rib matrix, thus resulting in soft bone that bends to the growing weight of the child (Figure 8.1). The typical risk factors for rickets, have been well accepted, and include: living in a temperate environment above latitudes 40°N and below 40°S, poor sun exposure, dark skin pigmentation, exclusive breast feeding, and mothers with a deficient vitamin D status (WHO, 2006). Infants particularly vulnerable to rickets and adults susceptible to osteomalacia are those with complete skin covering, typically seen in the Middle East. The surge in the

international prevalence of rickets appears to be mostly tied to both exclusive breast feeding and to shielding the skin from the sun. The problem is particularly exacerbated by the immigration of individuals with heightened skin pigmentation coming from non-European countries and settling in the northern hemisphere with shorter daylight hours during winters (Pettifor, 2004; WHO, 2006)). In this context, full body garments that shield the sun completely in combination with prolonged exclusive breastfeeding practices have made infants and young children susceptible to rickets and the elderly to osteomalacia (WHO, 2006). Also, surprisingly, there are some countries, in which calcium intake is suboptimal, that exhibit a surge in rickets, despite having adequate vitamin D status with blood 25(OH)D concentrations that are >10–12 ng/mL (Pettifor, 2004). These would be cultures with limited dairy intake in combination with elevated cereal-based phytate consumption which tends to bind available calcium (Williams, 1998). The lower calcium intake also defines the important shift from traditional food habits to a more impoverished urban nutrition high in sweetened beverages that displace dairy out of the diet (Popkin, 1994). The most reliable method of determining poor vitamin D status is measuring low plasma 25-OH-D and elevated parathyroid hormone (PTH).

8.1.3.4 Key Micromineral Deficiencies.

Internationally, **iodine**, **iron**, and **zinc** have contributed most significantly to the onset of disease worldwide (WHO, 2006). The devastating impact of iron and iodine deficiencies on the prevalence of anemia and mental retardation worldwide respectively, has forced the international community to prioritize the elimination of iodine deficiency and the reduction of the prevalence of anemia by one third. Iron status, specifically, is of great interest as it is the prominent nutrient deficiency in the world, and because it is linked to national productivity and health.

Since the WHO identified iodine deficiency as the most preventable cause of mental retardation in the world, there has been a strong impetus to eliminate this deficiency. The fortification of salt with iodine—a process called iodization—has been helpful in eradicating the problem in western industrialized countries. However, there are still developing countries that have not yet fortified their food supply with iodine, and that rely too heavily on cassava as a main carbohydrate staple, even though it is a goitrogen that binds iodine, thus making it unavailable for absorption. Iodization is a priority as many countries have iodine-impoverished soil, the result of the leaching effect of heavy rain, snow fall and past glaciation (WHO, 2006).

Roughly 20% of the world's population is at risk of zinc deficiency with countries like Bangladesh and India, Africa and the western Pacific being particularly prone to deficiency (WHO, 2006). Zinc's roles in cell division and protein synthesis mean that it can directly impact the growth and maturation of children, and so when deficient in the diet, stunted growth becomes prominent in the children. About 33% of children in developing countries are reported to be stunted. The causes can vary, but suspicions run high that poor dietary zinc intake, compromised absorption because of parasitic infestations, or high prevalence of phytates, which bind both iron and zinc and diminish its bioavailability are somehow involved. However, recent work on zinc bioavailability in diverse diets has not shown conclusively that phytates bind zinc to the extent of limiting availability (WHO, 2006). While the symptoms of severe zinc deficiency are overt and easy to document such retarded growth, dermatitis, and diarrhea, mild to moderate deficiencies are more difficult to track. Nevertheless, zinc supplementation directly reduced the frequency of pneumonia and diarrhea, in addition to the duration of diarrheal episodes (WHO, 2006). Iron and zinc deficiencies tend to occur concurrently as they are found in similar foods.

8.1.4 Other Varied Nutrient Deficiencies in Developing Nations

Although not as prominent as iron, retinol, iodine and zinc deficiencies on the global stage, there are still numerous types of vitamin B deficiencies prominently reported internationally among nations that consume little meat, eggs, and dairy products, where cereals and wheat are over processed through extensive millings, and where fruits and vegetables are not abundant and varied (WHO, 2006).

8.1.4.1 Cyanocobalamin (B12) Deficiency

The prevalence of B12 deficiency is widespread internationally with 15% of German women of reproductive age, 31% of the elderly in the United Kingdom, and 11-12% of Venezuelan pre-school and school aged children with reported suboptimal serum values. The highest prevalence was found in among 46% of Indian adults and 40% of Kenyan school-aged children, whereas the lowest incidences were reported in the U.S. (0-3% of the population), Botswana, Japan and Thailand. A vitamin B12 deficiency is determined by serum levels that drop to <150 pmol/L. In developing countries it appears that the infestation of *Helicobacter pylori* infection and growing old are at the source of the gastric atrophy

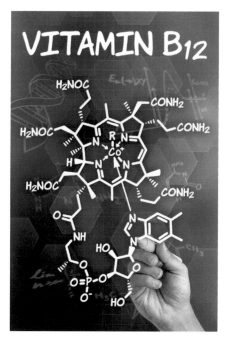

Figure 8.2 Cyanocobalamin (vitamin B12) molecule/ Credit line © Zerbor/shutterstock.com

that compromises the secretion of intrinsic factor (IF) from parietal cells of the stomach. The IF is a transport protein that is necessary for the absorption of B12 in the ileum. The main symptom is pernicious megaloblastic anemia (See chapter 9 for more details about the deficiency). Blood levels are also low among strict vegetarians but surprisingly even among lacto-ovo-vegetarians. Only those who consume meat have adequate plasma concentrations of B12 (WHO, 2006).

8.1.4.2 Thiamin (Vitamin B1) Deficiency

Although thiamin deficiency—beriberi is the deficiency disease—has been mostly eliminated in industrialized nations with the enrichment of the wheat and cereal supplies, thiamin deficiency disease, beriberi, is still documented in Asian and African countries such as Ethiopia, Guinea, Nepal and Thailand where refined and unenriched white rice is a staple of the diet, and in countries afflicted with civil unrest, or torn apart by war and compromised by famines (WHO, 2006). Thiamin is richly abundant in wheat germ, yeast extracts, legumes, dairy, meat and green vegetables. In diets that rely on the refinement or processing of wheat, rice and other cereals, in addition to including alcohol and frequent raw fish that contain the thiamin agonist, thiaminase, the risk of thiamin deficiency greatly increases (WHO, 2006). Beriberi can present as a wet cardiomyopathy which can lead to heart failure, or as a dry peripheral neuropathy. The overconsumption of alcohol can lead to a neurological-based

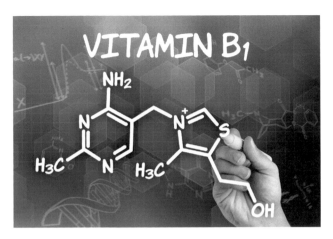

Figure 8.3 Thiamin (Vitamin B1) molecule/credit line © Zerbor/shutterstock.com

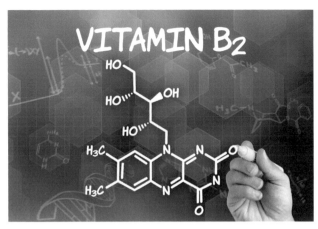

Figure 8.4 Riboflavin (Vitamin B2) molecule/credit line © Zebor/shutterstock.com

cognitive dysfunction involving memory loss and confabulation called Wernicke–Korsakov syndrome; this is a disease typically observed in alcoholics (WHO, 2006). Erythrocyte thiamin transketolase activity (ETKA) and thiamin pyrophosphate effect (TPPE) are two enzymes involved in carbohydrate metabolism that are sensitive indicators of tissue concentrations of thiamin, and thus should be used together in confirming thiamin deficiency (Gibson, 1990; WHO, 2006).

8.1.4.3 Riboflavin (Vitamin B2) Deficiency

Riboflavin is a key precursor to two important nucleotides, flavin mononucleotide (FMN) and flavin adenine dinucleotide (FAD) that function as coenzymes in beta oxidation, the tri-carboxilic acid (TCA) cycle and in the electron transport chain located in the walls of the mitochondria (Newsholme & Leech, 1983). Erythrocyte FMN + FAD are regarded at the most accurate measure of riboflavin status (WHO, 2006; Gibson, 1990).

The WHO has conducted several international assessments of riboflavin status, and has reported a surprisingly elevated prevalence in over 90% of pregnant Gambian women, 50% of elderly Guatemalans and 70% of lactating women. Urinary flavin concentrations, which reflects recent intake more than status, were low in 90% of China's adults (WHO, 2006).

The implications of a deficiency are serious as it interferes with iron absorption and utilization thus leading to iron deficiency anemia. The milder symptoms of fatigue, weakness, mouth pain, burning eyes and itching are truly non-specific but nevertheless influences the quality of life of individuals. The more advanced deficiency symptoms characterized by dermatitis with cheilosis and angular stomatitis, brain dysfunction and microcytic anemia are more visually recognizable (WHO, 2006).

8.1.4.4 Niacin (Vitamin B3) Deficiency

Structurally niacin is known as nicotinic acid and nicotinamide. It is specifically nicotinamide that is an important component of the nucleotides nicotinamide adenine dinucleotide (NAD) and nicotinamide adenine dinucleotide phosphate (NADP). They are heavily involved in oxidation reduction reactions within the TCA cycle involving the oxidation of carbohydrates, proteins and fats (Bourgeois et al. 2006). Niacin deficiency, if not contained, leads to pellagra, which is recognizable by the four D symptoms of **dermatitis**, **dementia**, **diarrhea** and **death**.

It is usually seen in populations that rely a lot on cereal-based diets that are low in both niacin and tryptophan. This is the only known vitamin that can be synthesized from protein. Indeed, tryptophan, an essential amino acid, can convert to niacin through the involvement of vitamins B2 and B6, in addition to iron and copper. In a protein poor diet that is based on overly processed wheat or cereal, there is a propensity to

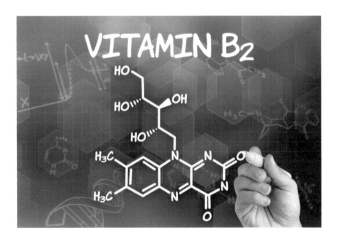

Figure 8.5 Niacin molecule (Vitamin B3). Credit line © Zebor/shutterstock.com

develop pellagra. This deficiency can seemingly occur when either copper, iron, riboflavin or pyridoxine are suboptimal or missing, within the context of poor quality protein and unprocessed maize or overly processed non-enriched cereal products (Bourgeois, 2006). Internationally, pellagra can still be found in countries such as India, in some regions of Africa, and China, where the diets of maize, sorghum and polished rice predominate. Pellagra also rears its ugly head in refugee camps such as the one for Mozambicans in Malawi (WHO, 2006). Interestingly, abundant coffee consumption in Latin America may be playing a significant role in why pellagra is absent those countries. The roasting of the coffee bean appears to greatly increase the bioavailability of nicotinic acid. Moreover, the soaking of maize, in a mild alkali solution of lime water, helps release the niacin from the maize for absorption. Pellagra is a deficiency disease which should not be thought of in a linear fashion, in that, unlike other nutrient deficiency diseases, this one does strictly take place when there is poor intake of niacin (WHO, 2006). The inclusion of both milk and rice in the diet, for instance, ensures a proper ingestion of tryptophan which will invariably convert to niacin in amounts considered sufficient to ensure a recovery or a prevention of pellagra, and this despite the fact that both foods are poor in niacin (Bourgeois, et al., 2006).

8.1.4.5 Pyridoxine (Vitamin B6) Deficiency

Vitamin B6 is naturally found in three distinct forms: pyridoxine (PN), pyridoxal (PL) and pyridoxamine (PM). This vitamin in a phosphorylated form of pyridoxal phosphate (PLP) will serve as a coenzyme in protein and amino acid metabolism (WHO, 2006).

A singular deficiency of this vitamin is relatively rare since it is widely spread throughout the food supply.

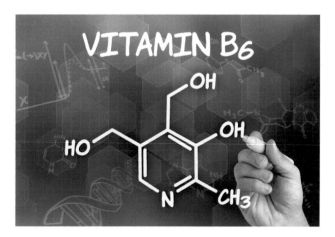

Figure 8.6 Pyridoxine molecule (Vitamin B6). Credit line © Zebor/shutterstock.com

Hence, a deficiency usually takes place concomitantly with other suboptimal nutrients. For instance, the activation through phosphorylation of B6 is done with the help of zinc. Conversely, niacin, folate and carnitine require pyridoxine for their biosynthesis. Despite these complex and intricate links with other nutrients, there are indications of suboptimal blood levels in about 40% of Indonesian children in rural and 10% in urban centers. In Egypt, vitamin B6 concentrations in about 40% of the milk of breastfeeding mothers were low (WHO, 2006). Epidemiologically, diets that rely extensively on refined grains with very little meats, vegetables and nuts will be prone to be deficient in B6. Chronic forms of alcoholism will also increase the risk of deficiency (WHO, 2006). Severe cases of B6 deficiency typically show symptoms of dermatitis, glossitis and cheilosis because of its ties to other nutrients such as niacin. But the link to anemia is related to the critical role played by pyridoxal phosphate (PLP) on hemoglobin synthesis. In the absence of PLP a microcytic hypochromic anemia ensues (Mackey et al. 2006). Elevated blood homocystein is generally thought to occur in folate deficiency, but should not be unexpected also in vitamin B6's deficiency as its role in folate metabolism is well documented (See chapter 9). What is unclear is whether B6 plays any significant role in carnitine metabolism in humans (Mackey et al, 2006)? The fact that B6 is a critical step in neurotransmitter synthesis explains the impact of deficiency on convulsions (Mackey, et al 2006).

8.1.4.6 Ascorbic Acid (Vitamin C) Deficiency

Severe ascorbic acid deficiency has been almost completely eradicated in industrialized nations, but remains a brutal reality for populations that are displaced into refugee camps, because of civil unrest, for periods of 3-6 months as recently seen in places like Ethiopia, Kenya, Somalia, Sudan and Nepal. Somalian refugees in the mid-1980s had scurvy outbreaks that affected between 7 and 44% of refugees (WHO, 2006). All it takes is consuming 3–4 consecutive months of a vitamin C-impoverished diet (<2mg per day) to cause the scorbutic symptoms to appears.

The W.H.O, using 1988-1994 data from the National Health and Nutrition Examination Survey (NHANES) in the U.S., which showed that about 9% of women and 13% of men had a mild form of ascorbic acid deficiency, concluded that there was a likely mild vitamin C deficiency prevalent worldwide (WHO, 2006). Although the symptoms of scurvy, which include follicular hyperkeratosis, hemorrhagic manifestations, swollen joints, swollen bleeding gums and peripheral edema, with a risk of death, have been well documented, the milder form of deficiency, which could be referred to as subclinical

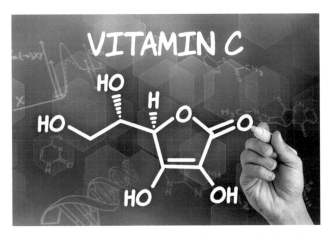

Figure 8.7 Ascorbic acid molecule (Vitamin C). Credit line © Zebor/shutterstock.com

vitamin C deficiency, does not have such clearly defined symptoms. There are some suspicions that poor bone mineralization—because of poor or slower collagen synthesis—lassitude, fatigue, anorexia, muscular weakness and increased susceptibility to infections could very well be the most common subclinical symptoms. Understanding ascorbic acid's involvement in enhancing non-heme iron absorption could very well help explain the fatigue and lassitude typically observed in people that ingest inadequate vitamin C (WHO, 2006).

8.2. UNDERNUTRITION IN HOSPITALS

8.2.1 Basic Concepts of Starvation

There is no doubt that starvation represents a state of crisis for the body as it forces it into a sort of metabolic emergency that involves the rapid breakdown of endogenous tissues in order to provide vital fuel for oxidative phosphorylation and energy production. There is, in fact, a shift from a reliance on exogenous sources of food for energy to an internal breakdown of fat and protein stores to keep the body alive. Total starvation and semi-starvation both restrict sufficient calories to cause weight loss. The rate of weight loss is, however not linear, in that the body does not experience weight loss at rates that are proportional to the degree of restriction or the length of the caloric restriction. Early experimental work by Benedict and colleagues in 1912 investigated this paradox. They held a man in an enclosed area for 31 days, feeding him only distilled water. He lost 16.7% of his original body weight within the first three weeks, yet experienced a 30% drop in bodily heat production, clearly demonstrating that the body metabolism had dropped more sharply than the body weight. Hence, it was not only the lower body weight that

accounted for the decline in basal metabolic rate, but some other unknown factor (Kinney, 2006). The question was picked up again, during WW-II, by Ancel Keys and his colleagues at the University of Minnesota. Wanting to emulate the semi-starvation diets imposed by the Nazis in concentration camps, they fed young healthy men 1600 kcal/day over a 6 month period. They found that while the men lost 24% of their body weights, they lost on average 39% of basal metabolic rate (BMR). Interestingly, at the end of the 6 months the BRM ceased decreasing and stabilized (Kinney, 2006).

Metabolically, the body has an ability to adapt to fasting or reduced food intake. This is likely related to how our primitive genes saved our ancestors from death during the many prolonged famines throughout history. After several famines the body becomes more efficient at preserving valuable fuel reserves in the body, and does this by making significant metabolic readjustments. About 12-24 hrs after beginning a fast, the drop in insulin concentrations signals the secretion of glucagon from the alpha cell of the pancreas and catecholamines like epinephrine. These endocrine compounds in combination with the increased glucagon: insulin ration enhance the breakdown of liver glycogen stores for the release glucose into the blood in a biochemical process called **glycogenolysis**. It takes between 48-72 hrs of fasting for the complete depletion of liver glycogen to take place (Hoffer, 2006). This release of glucose is necessary to keep to blood sugars homeostatic, as the nervous system, renal medulla, erythrocytes and leukocytes rely on glucose for normal activity. Slowly, as liver glycogen concentrations become depleted, gluconeogenesis will account for a greater percent of the glucose released. Gluconeogenesis will contribute 64% of the glucose released into circulation by the 22 hour of fasting; that percentage jumps to 80% by the 40th hour; indeed, all of the hepatic glucose produced will originate from gluconeogenesis once hepatic glycogen reserves are fully depleted. Interestingly, serum glucose concentrations only modestly decline because there is a concomitant reduction in glucose absorption as well (Hoffer, 2006). Following 3.5 days the brain's reliance on glucose drops 25% as it shifts to an adaptive uptake of ketone bodies for fuel. It is common to expect to smell acetone—a prominent ketone—in the breath of patients who have fasted for 3-4 days (Hoffer, 2006). Leading up to that time, the overall hepatic glucose output declines 40-50% by the 24-48th hour (Rothman et al 1991) as the synthesis of ketone bodies begins to gradually increase as a fuel utilized by the brain and muscles. In fact between days 4 and 7 of a fast, the body relies on 30-40% of its energy needs from the oxidation of ketone bodies in the mitochondria (Hoffer, 2006). Gradually, however, over the following week, the muscles entirely shift from ketones to fatty acids a source of calories. This means that by week-2 of a fast, the breakdown of fat—a process called known as lipolysis—begins to gain in importance, resulting in the increased release of free fatty acids (FFA) into the blood which remain relatively stable over the remainder of the fast. The release of FFA is further aided by the fall in insulin early on. The glycerol fractions of the triglycerides that are being broken down along with glucogenic amino acids, catabolized from protein, are used for glucose production through **gluconeogenesis**.

Translated into a practical concept, the state of starvation will cause a 75 kg man to breakdown 160 g of fat and 180 g of glucose per 24 hour period in the early stages of the fast. The glucose is primarily coming from hepatic glycogenolysis early on, whereas after about 1 day gluconeogenesis begins to supply glucose to the blood from lactate, glycerol, pyruvate, and from about 75 g of catabolized protein coming mostly from skeletal muscle. This loss of protein translates into increased content of urinary nitrogen (Schlichtig & Ayres 1988). Based on the fact that 1 g of nitrogen is found in 6.25 g of protein, it can be assumed that these 75 g of protein would result in 12 g of urinary nitrogen. Overall, the quantity of skeletal muscle protein catabolized during pure starvation is approximately the same during metabolic stress (Schlichtig & Ayres 1988); the difference is that nutritional support is effective in suppressing protein catabolism in pure starvation, whereas it is not in situations of metabolic stress (Gibson, 1990). In the late phase of starvation—about 5-6 weeks of fasting—the need for glucose is downsized from 180 g to a mere 80 g/d, thus conserving muscle mass. This shift takes place because of a greater reliance on fat from adipose tissue. Consistent with this shift, there is a decrease in urinary nitrogen loss from 8g/d to 3g/d within about 2 weeks (Schlichtig & Ayres 1988). The drop in the amount of lost nitrogen resulting from a decline in protein erosion is also attributed to a downward shift in metabolic rate. This is a kind of adaptation process that allows people on semi-starvation and starvation diets to survive a long time before dying. This downward adjustment in metabolic rate with fasting, translates into a 15% decline in resting energy expenditure (REE) by 2 weeks, and another 25-35% by the third and fourth week of fasting (Hoffer, 2006). Death can be precipitated by a 40% loss of body weight in non-stressed starvation. In a situation of stressed starvation, a 25 % loss of body weight or a 70-94% loss of adipose tissue is considered to be associated with a high risk of mortality (Schlichtig & Ayres, 1988; Bistrian, 1984).

8.2.2 Prevalence of Hospital Malnutrition

Malnutrition is defined, as a nutritional imbalance that becomes observable as either over-nutrition or under-nutrition. In many developed and developing nations over-nutrition is on the rise and has led to an increased prevalence of obesity in many countries worldwide in which excessive calories and nutrients such as cholesterol, saturated fat, sodium, salt, and sugar are over consumed, but key nutrients are under-consumed (Via, 2012). Under-nutrition, in contrast, is typically seen in underdeveloped and developing nations, and in western hospitals and long term care facilities and residences (Barker et al 2011). Here in the U.S., suboptimal protein intake is almost never seen except as protein-energy malnutrition (PEM) in hospitalized patients suffering from cancer, AIDS, gastrointestinal diseases, alcoholics, and drug abuse (Lee and Nieman, 1996).

The prevalence of hospital malnutrition was documented as far back as the 1970s by Bruce Bistrian and colleagues, who reported a 44% prevalence of malnutrition among general medicine patients (Bistrian et al. 1976). It is shocking that this level of malnourished patients has not declined over the decades with improved nutritional support protocols and nutritional supplements widely available in the market. Currently, the prevalence of hospital malnutrition is estimated at between 20-50% with the majority of clinical studies showing a tighter cluster varying between 30-36% (Barker et al, 2011). The medical implications of such an elevated prevalence of malnutrition are worrisome, as they translate invariably into more frequent infections, slower wound healing, greater loss of muscle mass and mortality, and hospital stays that are on average 3-6 days longer. Others have reported 43% longer hospital stays when patients were malnourished (Barker, et al 2011).

8.2.3 Assessment of Hospital Undernutrition

The degree to which hospitalized patients are undernourished before entering or while under hospital care, especially in acute and chronic care settings, necessitates nutritional risk screening as the best strategy to decreasing the problem (Charney and Marian, 2008). Those patients found to be at risk are then referred to a clinical dietitian for a more complete nutritional assessment (Barker et al. 2011).

First, in a nutritional risk assessment the health professional is interested in monitoring the patient's weight, height, non-desired weight changes, food allergies, dietary practices, recent changes in appetite, whether they have recently experienced vomiting or nausea, bowel habits that may intimate constipation or diarrhea, the presence of chronic disease, a compromised ability to chew or swallow. In instances when laboratory turnaround time is fairly rapid, then serum albumin or hematocrit can used in screening patients at risk (Charney & Marian, 2008).

A patient would be classified nutritionally at risk if he meets at least one of the following criteria:

a. Weight loss or gain that is >10% of the usual body weight within 6 months
b. A Weight loss or gain >5% of the usual body weight within 1 month
c. A body weight that is either at 80% or less or 120% or more of the patient's health weight.
d. Recently affected by disease, surgery or trauma
e. Affected by some kind of chronic disease or an change in metabolic requirements
f. Has not ingested adequate amounts of food or nutrition supplements for > 7 days
g. Has experienced difficulty swallowing or absorbing food for > 7 days

(Source: Charney & Marian, 2008)

There is also a rapid nutritional screening tool, popularly used by nurses in hospitals in order to quickly and efficiently identify patients who are at risk of malnutrition, that is popularly used in American hospitals. The **Rapid Nutrition Screen for Hospitalized Patients** is made up of a three question scoring questionnaire that can be completed promptly; a numeric value can be generated that will position the patient on a nutritional risk scale (Charney & Marian, 2008).

a. Have you lost weigh recently without trying: NO (0) / Unsure (2)
b. If yes, how much weight (Kg) have you lost?
    1. 1-5 kg (1 point)
    2. 6-10 kg (2 points)
    3. 11-15 kg (3 points)
    4. >15 kg (4 points)
    5. Unsure (2 points)
c. Have you eaten poorly because of poor appetite
    1. YES (1 point)
    2. NO (0 point)

A score that is ≥ 2 implies the patient is at risk of malnutrition, and a nutritional assessment is advised (Charney and Marian, 2008).

The **Malnutrition Universal Screening Tool** is also popularly used by medical professionals because it uses familiar weight parameters. Using this screening technique, the nurse or physician can signal a moderate problem if the patient's BMI is between 18.5-20 or a more serious risk if the BMI<18.5. In a second step, the nurse can assess any unexpected weight loss by assigning a numerical value to weight loss of between 5-10% or > 10%. The patient would be categorized, depending on the score as low, medium or high nutritional risk. In the third step the nurse needs to estimate if the patient has been or is at risk patient of going without food for more than 5 days because of illness (Charney & Marian, 2008). These examples illustrate the fundamental reliance on both body weight and appetite in screening patients for nutritional risk.

Once the screening is complete, then a dietitian can engage in a more thorough nutritional assessment of the patient. This step will rely on medical, nutritional, and medication histories; physical examination, anthropometric measurements and laboratory data to complete a more comprehensive understanding of the patients nutritional status (Charney and Marian, 2008); The assessment will also likely be able to assign a prognostic risk based on the nutritional status (Busby and Mullen, 1984). A prognosis is an estimation of a patient's risk of morbidity or mortality. A poor nutritional status is likely to increase the risk of post-surgical complications. This is because the prognosis determination is based on four important measures: first, serum albumin levels which when low (< 2.5 g/dL) indicate a high risk of mortality; second, triceps skinfold which measure the degree of subcutaneous fat; it is a measure of emaciation which when low correlates poorly with good health; third, serum transferrin is a measure of both iron status and protein status. When low, it can be an indirect measure of poor protein status, however, elevated transferrin is expected in anemia; fourth, delayed cutaneous hypersensitivity. It is a skin reactivity skin test to three antigens. The idea here, is when nutritional status is compromised so will the immune system (Busby and Mullen, 1984). Students can review more details of the Prognostic Nutritional Index in chapter 7 section 6.

8.2.4 TREATMENTS OF HOSPITAL UNDERNUTRITION

8.2.4.1 Energy Determination

Following a complete assessment of the patient's nutritional status, it is possible for the clinician to prescribe an appropriate strategy to enhance or rebuild the nutritional status if it is suboptimal. The first thing to consider is the type of nutritional support needed by the patient. In hospital settings, patients are in a disease state and may have undergone some kind of trauma such as a bone fracture, or multiple bone fractures as seen in an automotive accident. The patient may have experienced burns to a broad surface area of the body. All these are traumas and are responsible for increasing both the energy and protein needs of the patient. De-Souza and Green (1998) report that, on average, burn patients require 40-45 kcal/kg body weight /day. The burn patient's energy needs works out to be about 1.47 times the resting energy expenditure (REE) calculated using the Harris-Benedict formula. According to Long (1984) this upward caloric adjustment is typically seen in patients with about 20% burned surface area (BSA). And so with a greater BSA that is 40 to 100%, then the energy needs jump 1.85-2.05 times the value of the REE or the basal metabolic rate (BMR) (Long, 1984).

There are traumas of lesser intensities that carry decreased injury factors. Energy estimations using the Harris-Benedict formula and a set of injury factors were previously described by Long (1984) and represented in **table 8.1**.

TABLE 8.1 Energy requirements of hospitalized patients.

Women's BMR Formula	
$(665.10 + 9.56 \times W_{kg}) + (1.85 \times H_{cm} - 4.6 \times A_{years})$	
Men's BMR Formula	
$(66.47 + 13.75 \times W_{kg}) + (5.0 \times H_{cm} - 6.76 \times A_{years})$	
Total Energy Expenditure	
BMR x AF(Activity Factor) x IF (Injury Factor)	
Activity Factor	Injury Factor
1.2 (confined to bed)	Surgery: 1.0-1.2
1.3 (out of bed)	Infection: 1.0-1.8
	Skeletal Trauma: 1.2-1.35
	Multiple Traumas + Steroids: 1.6
	Blunt Trauma: 1.15-1.35

Source: Adapted from Long, CL. (1984)

8.2.4.2 Protein Requirements

Traumatic injuries and sepsis (systemic infection) produce a hypermetabolic state in which energy and protein requirements are heightened in the body (Frankenfield, 2006). Protein requirements will vary depending on whether the injury is classified as mild, moderate or severe, because of the impact of trauma/injury on body proteolysis and lipolysis. Indeed, the greater the trauma

or the infection the greater the protein catabolism and fat breakdown (De-Souza & Greene, 1998).

Historically, research from the 1980s espoused the notion that significant protein ingestion was necessary during trauma in order to offset the greater negative nitrogen balance observed in the post-traumatic period. The therapeutic recommendations for protein are outlined below:

a. Elective surgeries: 1.1 g/kg/day
b. Fractures & infections: 1.5-2.0g/kd/day
c. Multiple fractures, injuries, infections, and burns greater than 40% BSA: 2.0-4.0g/kg/day (Long, 1984)

Despite the higher protein prescription, no amount of protein appears able to completely halt the rate of protein catabolism that occurs during injury; large ingestion of protein can mitigate somewhat the protein erosion, but not stop it entirely. Overfeeding protein does however leave the body with a high nitrogen burden that needs to be excreted. This paradox has created some controversy and a lack of agreement with respect to protein needs during critical illness. Graham Hill's group out of Auckland New Zealand studied this problem more closely by implementing nutritional support protocols with varied protein levels on 18 trauma and 8 sepsis patients. Researchers found that, by increasing protein intake from 1.1 to 1.5g/kg fat free mass (FFM), protein losses declined by 50%. However they reported that further increases up to 1.9g/kg FFM did not continue to abate nitrogen losses from the body. The group concluded that the current practice of prescribing protein to between 1.2-2.0g/kg bodyweight, is likely excessive, especially if post-traumatic body weights—which tend to be overhydrated—are used in the calculation (Ishibashi et al. 1998). Assuming exaggeratedly high weight estimations because of edema and ascites, then the most efficient prescription of 1.5g/kg FFM is adjusted to 1.0g/kg body weight/day after correcting for a water and fat mass (FM) totaling 33%. The team recommended a prescription of 1.2g/kg body weight/day to critically ill patients using pre-illness body weights (Ishibashi et al. 1998). In the instance when body weights prior to illness are unknown then the conservative 1.0g/kg body weight/day prescription is advised. This lower protein recommendation has, however, been disputed by others who argue that protein intakes > 2.0g/kg body weight/day can indeed heighten the rate of protein synthesis. Frankenfield (2006) contends that very elevated protein prescriptions are necessary in order to achieve nitrogen balance in critically ill patients; some of the data is convincingly linked with greater survival (Frankenfield, 2006). A review by Hoffer and Bistrian (2012) could not find, however, strong enough studies that favored clinical recommendations for elevated protein intakes above 2.0 g/kg body weight in critically ill patients. Consistent with these findings, the Canadian Clinical Practice Guidelines (CCPG), considered the most thorough data base on best practices in critical care management, also concluded that the data available in 2013 prevented the committee from making formal recommendations for high or escalating protein doses in critical illness (CCPG, 2013). Nevertheless, although the most common practice in the U.S. is to prescribe on average 1.5g/kg body weight/day of protein in critical care medicine (Wolfe, 1996; Hoffer & Bistrian, 2012), the few good studies that have been published do nevertheless suggest some benefits like better survival rates with protein intakes between 2.0-2.5 g/kg/day (Hoffer & Bistrian, 2012).

8.3 PREVALENCE OF MALNUTRITION IN THE U.S.

Worldwide there is an estimate 200 million pre-school aged children that are afflicted with chronic undernutrition, causing stunted growth, and representing 35.8% of pre-school children in developing countries. Geographically, about 80% are located in Asian countries, 15% in Africa and 5% in Latin America (de Onis et al, 1993). By contrast nobody is really undernourished in the U.S or Canada, but paradoxically, the malnutrition of obesity affects increasing numbers of the U.S. population (Via, 2012).

8.3.1. Obesity as a Form of Malnutrition

It is controversial that an obese person could suffer from malnutrition. The classic image of an emaciated child or adult comes to mind when trying to conceptualize what a malnourished person looks like. As previously discussed, there are many in our hospitals. The commercialization of our food supply has led to an abundant processing of food in order to sell and distribute large volumes of stable and safe food to the population. The problem is that much of what we eat has undergone an extrusion process that uses thermal heat and therefore destabilizes vitamins A, E, D and C especially (Riaz et al. 2009).

8.3.2. Prevalent Micronutrient Deficiencies in the U.S.

8.3.2.1 Vitamin D Deficiency and its History

The fortification of the U.S. milk supply with vitamin D, by the 1930s, caused the prevalence of rickets to begin to decrease (Holick, 2006); it was considered eradicated by the late 1960s. This was a public health success because in the early 1900s about 90% of children living in the North Eastern United States and in large Northern European cities suffered from rickets (Holick, 2006). This was a devastating bone disease (Figure 8.1) that left the children disabled because the pronounced bowing of the legs and curvature of the spine disturbed their gait. Weakened muscles and beaded ribcages were also common symptoms (Holick, 2006).

Rickets, although documented by Glisson among the city dwelling children of 17th century Europe, its cause did not begin to be understood until 1822, when Sniadecki observed that the disease was prominent inside of Warsaw and absent outside the Polish capital. This raised suspicions about the need for sunlight in order to cure the disease, a recommendation that Sniadecki began to promote (Holick, 2006). However the medical establishment continued to pay little attention to the environment as the cause of rickets. Meanwhile, French physician, Bretonneau was able to quickly heal a 15 month child with rickets in 1827 by administering cod liver oil, a practice thought to be more folkloric than true medical science (Holnick, 2006). Nevertheless cod liver oil, the use of fish oils in general in combination with exposure to sunlight became medical recommendations which Bretonneau's student, Trousseau, began to advocate.

Still, this belief that the environmental conditions played no real role in the onset of the disease was further promoted in light of an 1889 epidemiological study, conducted by the British Medical Society, in which a lack of sunlight did not appear as a risk factor. A cure for rickets continued to evade the larger sphere of scientists and medical researchers despite another epidemiological survey in 1890 by Palm that pointed again at the importance of sunlight for prevention. His team found that children of middle class families living in industrialized cities of Britain had the greater prevalence of rickets, whereas those in Chinese, Japanese and Indian cities showed no signs of the disease. Still, it would seem the evidence was not convincing enough to alter medical practice (Holick, 2006). The world would have to wait until 1920, some thirty years later, for Huldschinsky to demonstrate the curative effect of mercury vapor arc lamps on rachitic bones of children.

Meanwhile, the curative features of fish oil, nevertheless, continued to interest a researcher by the name of Edward Mellanby who, in 1918, created a dog model of rickets which he produced using a strict oatmeal diet, and cured with butter fat, but he observed that cod liver oil cured the disease more effectively (Wolf, 2004). He concluded that either vitamin A, which had been discovered a few years earlier or some other factor was the curing agent. McCollum, the discoverer of vitamin A, which his team isolated from butter fat in 1914, wondered whether the curative factor in the butter and cod liver oil was vitamin A. After treating the cod liver oil in order to oxidize the vitamin A and feeding it to rachitic rats in 1922, his team found that although the rats developed xerophthalmia—blindness due to vitamin A deficiency—it still held its rachitic curative properties thus concluding that another factor, other than vitamin A, was healing the animals of rickets (Wolf, 2004). The next major finding occurs in post-WW-I Vienna where Hariette Chick and her team successfully cured rickets in children by feeding them either whole milk or cod liver oil (Wolf, 2004).

At this historical junction, the race to uncover the cure for rickets was taking place in two fronts: The first was the role of sunlight and the second was the food factor apparently present in cod liver oil, butter, and whole milk. It was the work of Huldschinsky on sunlight that was gaining some attention. It was perhaps the bold clinical trial of the doctors Hess and Unger who brought irrefutable evidence, in 1922, that sunlight was able to cure rickets. They placed seven kids with rickets on the rooftop of a New York City hospital where they remained daily for various lengths of time, exposed to sunlight; the epiphyses of the bones began to calcify (Holick, 2006). These two avenues of investigation made it particularly difficult to fully understand the cause of rickets, for indeed, both diet and sunlight were curing rickets, but no researcher was able to find the common factor that linked both treatments. It was in 1924 that this dichotomy began to be unraveled with key observations made by three distinct laboratories (Wolf, 2004). First, Hess's lab showed that the irradiation of linseed oil with U.V light activated some kind of antirachitic factor. A second lab demonstrated, by irradiating, not only, rachitic rats with U.V. light, but also the air inside the empty jar, after removing the rats, that rats were cured of rickets. A third lab further explored the impact of U.V light on the rats. What was going on that had a curative effect? The team killed standard non-irradiated rats, extracted their livers and irradiated them with UV light. Researchers minced up the irradiated livers to create an additive to the standard rat meal. They found that non-irradiated rats with rickets fed the irradiated livers also were cured of rickets symptoms.

What was going on that irradiating liver gave it an increased antirachitic potency? It was this question that eventually led to uncovering, in 1937, the cholesterol derived precursor to vitamin D, 7-dehydrocholesterol, which is formed under the skin of humans and some animals when exposed to U.V light or sunlight (Wolf, 2004; Carpenter, 2003).

In recent times, vitamin D insufficiency has been reported to be alarmingly high in the obese and type-2 diabetics in U.S population, with prevalence rates of 80-90%, prompting some epidemiologist to recommend vitamin D supplementation to improve glucose metabolism and insulin sensitivity in type-2 diabetics (Via, 2012). The problem however is more widespread than originally thought. Up until 2003, the FDA had given the okay for only milk, a few cereals and bread to be fortified with vitamin D (Holick, 2006); without exposure to sunlight the U.S. population had access to very few foods rich in vitamin D. This was especially true within geographic areas where dietary shifts of young people toward greater soft drink consumption meant that there was less milk consumed by children and young adults. Women of color have been identified as particularly at risk. Indeed, NHANES-III reported that 43% of African women between the ages of 15 and 49 had suboptimal vitamin D levels in their blood. In Boston at the end of the winter of 2001, nutrition researchers documented that 32% of Caucasians between the ages of 18 and 29 were vitamin D deficient (Holick, 2006). Those individuals over the age of 50 are also prone to insufficient vitamin D. It is currently estimated that 50% of Americans and Europeans over 50 years of age are likely at risk of a poor vitamin D status. Stratifying by ethnicity really brings out the disparity. Among free living elderly, living in the Boston area in 2001, 84% of African American elderly, 42% of Hispanics, and 30% of whites were found to be vitamin D deficient (Holick, 2006). These findings raised concerns, among public health officials, that something was not right. In 2003, the FDA approved vitamin D fortification of orange juice and other juice products in order to counter the dietary shift away from milk (Holick, 2006). Is this enough of a measure, or is soft drink consumption more widespread and insidious than originally believed?

8.3.2.2 Vitamin E Deficiency and its History

Isolated from wheat germ in 1936, its main role, documented in monkeys, pigs and dogs, appeared to be the prevention of necrotizing myopathy in these and many other animals. However, after 80 years of research, vitamin E remains, in humans, the vitamin without a disease (Traber, M.G., 2006). In the 1950s and 60s, researchers could only find that erythrocytes, taken from men that were induced with vitamin E deficiency, were more susceptible to hemolysis. No other symptoms were evident, until 1960s when cholestatic liver disease and abnormal lipid profiles became evident in children with malabsorption syndrome. It was clearer, by the 1980s, that peripheral neuropathy defined the main symptom of vitamin E deficiency. There were much longer and potentially more devastating implications around chronically suboptimal vitamin E status. By the turn of the new millennium, vitamin E's involvement in antioxidant activity became a game changer. The vitamin interrupted the free radical chain reactions that threatened biologic membranes. Seen as a peroxyl radical scavenger, vitamin E, also known as α-tocopherol, protected the polyunsaturated fatty acids (PUFAs) that made up the phospholipid layer of the cellular membranes. In this manner, the vitamin prevents the oxidation of the fatty acids that made up the cellular membrane (Traber, 2006). Absorbed within the chylomicron during digestion, it circulates to the liver via the chylomicron remnant where it is taken up by hepatic cells and then recirculated to the tissue again as VLDLs, LDLs and HDLs (Traber, 2006). Only but rarely is vitamin E deficiency, resulting from suboptimal dietary intakes, ever reported in humans. The individuals most susceptible to outright vitamin E deficiency are those with fat malabsorption syndromes. Whenever there is an inability to properly secrete adequate amount of bile into the intestine to form micelles, which is part of the normal emulsification process of fat, then malabsorption occurs. This is referred to as a hepatobiliary disorder. Cystic fibrosis, in children, usually involves poor pancreatic secretions of lipase enzyme, therefore leading to steatorrhea, which is when a significant amounts of fat remains in the stool. There is a tendency here for the child to develop vitamin E deficiency even when supplements of pancreatic enzymes are administered orally (Traber, 2006). Intramuscular injections of vitamin E are a preferred treatment option as these patients with malabsorption are unable to absorb the actual vitamin. The other instance of vitamin E deficiency has been documented in patients receiving total parenteral nutrition. Here the lipid component of the intravenous feeding is generally made up of soybean emulsions that contain γ-tocopherol and not the preferred α-tocopherol. In these patients there is evidence of higher than normal levels of lipid peroxidation. This means the fat oxidation is occurring too easily because it does not have enough of vitamin E's antioxidant protection (Traber, 2006).

8.3.2.3 Vitamin C Deficiency in the U.S and its History

Although scurvy—having long plagued sea explorations to the new world, as far back as the 15th century—has been considered eradicated certainly since the late 19th to early 20th century, there have been concerns that people in the U.S. may be at risk of vitamin C deficiency or depletion because of a growing trend in poor dietary practices (Hampl et al., 2004). Because vitamin C (ascorbic acid) is a water soluble vitamin, and is thus not stored in the body for long periods of time, it is important to regularly consume adequate amounts—the RDA is 75mg/day—through the regular consumption of a broad assortment of fruits and vegetables. Smokers in particular have higher needs—about 110-125 mg/day—because smoking causes increased oxidative stress in the body (Hampl et al. 2004). Jeffrey Hampl a nutrition researcher from Arizona State University, Mesa, and his colleagues, in reviewing the literature, described previous studies done in the late 1970s that found that 25% of nonsmoking men and up to 50% of adult male smokers had depleted vitamin C reserves (Hampl et al 2004). Internationally this groups notes that when fruit and vegetable intakes are low in a population, the prevalence of vitamin C deficiency tends to be elevated. Here in the U.S. they write that even though many Americans do meet the 5-A-DAY recommendation from the American Cancer Institute for fruit and vegetable intake, it turns out that the quality and variety of the produce consumed is not actually elevated in ascorbic acid. The truth of the matter is that Americans have a rather narrow intake, with about 30% of all produce consumed in the U.S. being primarily iceberg lettuce, raw tomatoes, French fries, bananas, and orange juice, in descending order of importance (Hampl, et al 2004).

The problem is that vitamin C is the least stable of the vitamins and thus prone to be destroyed by heat, air, alkali and metals. Consequently, cooking and long storage time can cause a significant drop in vitamin C content. For instance, once orange juice is exposed to air, the rate of vitamin C degradation approaches 2% per day (Hampl et al. 2004).

The growing prevalence of obesity has raised some concern about the caloric and nutrient densities of the food consumed by the obese. It has been established that between 35-45% of obese individuals tagged for gastric bypass surgery in the U.S. are likely deficient to some degree in vitamin C. Diabetics are also more predisposed towards suboptimal vitamin C compared to healthy controls (Via, 2012). Although fruits and vegetable consumption continues to be encouraged by health professionals, Vitamin C supplementation has been proposed, in recent years, for vulnerable groups like poor eaters and smokers (Hampl et al, 2004).

Ascorbic acid deficiency causes scurvy, which is characterized by weakness and lassitude, swollen, receding bleeding gums, perifollicular hyperkeratosis, petechial hemorrhage, bleeding into the skin, subcutaneous tissues, muscles and joints. In its severe form, scurvy can cause the loss of teeth, bone damage, internal hemorrhage and infection (Levine et al., 2006). Historically, there is evidence from Egyptian hieroglyphs that scurvy existed at least as far back as 3000BC. The great Greek physician, Hippocrates described the condition in 500BC. But it is really in reading the history books recounting sea explorations to the new world in the 16th and 17th centuries, that most became aware of the condition for the first time. Long term travel at sea, lasting more than 1 month, was responsible for causing many sailors to succumb to the scourge of the sea because of the poor vitamin C content of their diet and of the inability of the ship cargo bays to hold fruits and vegetables, rich in vitamin C, for extended periods (Bissonnette, 2013). It was also a prominent condition that developed in northern European cities during the 19th century because of the city dweller's limited access to fresh fruits and vegetables (Bissonnette, 2013). It wasn't until 1753 that James Lind wrote the first treatise on scurvy in which he proposed that acidic fruits could heal scurvy, and yet, despite his findings, scurvy continued to devastate maritime travel. The main reason was that his discovery went against popular beliefs of the time that scurvy was caused by things like cold climate, dampness, foggy weather and lack of fresh air (Levine et al., 2006). Despite Lind's treatise, it took until 1795, before the British Royal Navy, under advisement by Scottish physician Sir Gilbert Blane, ordered that all British sailors at sea for more than 2 weeks take one ounce of citrus juice—eventually adapting lime juice as a stable—on a daily basis. This practice resulted in British sailors being nicknamed "limeys." Interestingly, there were still cases of scurvy that persisted among sailors and the merchant navies until the Merchant Shipping Act of 1854 which made it mandatory for all ships to carry citrus fruits (Levine, et al., 2006).

Surprisingly, soldiers during the American Civil War and WW-I were widely affected by scurvy. It wasn't until Albert Szent-Gyorgyi managed to isolate antiscorbutic principle in 1928, a feat for which he received the Nobel Prize in 1937, that scurvy vanished from the national landscape (Levine, et al., 2006). It was specifically the Harvard School of Medicine's surgeon who placed himself on a diet containing no vitamin C for 26 weeks that clinically proved the medical efficacy of the vitamin C supplement. During that time he ensured that all other nutrients and micronutrients were supplemented. The terrible hemorrhaging from his legs, physical exhaustion and poor wound healing were quickly reversed with vitamin C supplements (Carpenter, 2003).

Frank scurvy, eradicated from industrialized countries since the early 20th century, has not been considered a threat except in cases of hospital malnutrition often seen in cancer cachexia, malabsorption, alcoholism and drug addiction; subclinical forms of vitamin C deficiency have, however, been seen in recent years in individuals with inadequate and idiosyncratic diets (Levine et al., 2006). Unfortunately, non-specific symptoms make detection more difficult; in fact clinicians have mistaken early signs of scurvy in children for rickets as both are known to impair bone growth (Levine, et al. 2006). Strategies to help maintain a good ascorbic acid status consist of helping the population consume greater varieties of fruits and vegetables on a daily basis. Both the U.S. Department of Agriculture (USDA) and the National Cancer Institute encourage the consumption of a minimum of 5 servings of a wide variety of fruits and vegetables daily. Despite such a minimal target, NHANES data from between 1988 and 1991 reveals that 37% of men and 24% of women in the U.S. take in less than 2.5 servings/day, with French fries representing a large proportion of the intake. Moreover, between 10-25% of the Americans met or fell below the DRI for vitamin C (Levine et al., 2006). Typically excellent fruit sources of vitamin C are fortified grape juice (120mg), strawberries (95mg), papaya (85mg), kiwi (75mg), oranges (70mg) and cantaloupe (60mg), whereas the best vegetable sources of vitamin C are fresh broccoli (60mg), kale (55mg), raw green or red peppers (60mg) and Brussels sprouts (50mg). Cabbages of various types and preparations contain between 10-25 mg per serving (Levine, et al., 2006). Vitamin C supplementation is of course a less preferred alternative by dietitians. Nevertheless the popularity of vitamin C supplementation really began with Linus Pauling's 1970 bestselling diet book: *Vitamin C and the Common Cold*. In it, he recommended daily mega-doses of 3,000 milligrams of vitamin C to stop the common cold Three time Nobel prize laureate, his book began to sell amazingly well with two reprints: one in 1971 and the other in 1973 (Bissonnette, 2013). It did not take too long before the scientific community discredited him, after his claims were tested by acclaimed research centers and shown to be unfounded. It soon became evident that Pauling, now in his seventies, had actually not done any scientific research on vitamin C (Bissonnette, 2013).

8.3.2.4 Thiamin Deficiency in the U.S and its History

Thiamin deficiency, although documented in Chinese texts as early as 2700BC, and then again in 1611 by the first Governor General of the Dutch East Indies, and by European physician, Bontius in 1642, has only sporadically occurred. Thiamin deficiency, also known as beriberi did not become a public health problem until wheat and cereals like rice were being highly processed in the 19th century. Numerous cases began to emerge in two separate geographic areas: First, in Japan around

1880, and a second cluster, around that same time, was reported in the Dutch West Indies among native army recruits in the vicinity of Djakarta.

Many sailors in the Japanese navy were developing a disease known as "kakké" which characteristically presented as a polyneuritis with symptoms of weakness in the lower limbs, heart failure, shortness of breath and edema (Carpenter, 2003B). The degeneration of the peripheral nerves (polyneuritis) was a condition which led essentially to a paralysis of the hands and feet. An English-trained naval surgeon by the name of Kanehiro Takaki was commanded to resolve the problem. After investigating European and Japanese naval practices, he concluded that the only really noticeable difference was that the Japanese naval diet was significantly lower in protein. He ordered the menu on a ship headed to New Zealand to be readjusted to include more meat, condensed milk, bread and vegetables. A year earlier, this same voyage resulted in 25 dead sailors and numerous others sick with beriberi. This second voyage resulted in no death an in only a few cases of beriberi that were limited to sailors who refused to eat the newly adapted diet (Carpenter, 2003B). Takaki concluded that a protein deficiency was the primary cause of the disease. Consequently, his dietary recommendations, which were implemented throughout the Japanese fleet, eventually led to the resolution of the problem. Still in Japan another problem was mounting among its newborn babies and their mothers. A disease called "taon" appeared to poison the mothers' breast make and thus endangered the newborn Japanese infants with alarming symptoms of vomiting, edema, low urination rates and unusually high death rates.

At same time, back in Djakarta Indonesia, a different approach was being proposed. The Dutch government sent a medical team, headed by bacteriologist, professor Pekelharing, for an 8 month investigation. He concluded that the disease had to originate from some unknown bacteria, and proposed that his assistant, Dr. Christian Eijkman, a young army physician, continue the investigation. Eijkman was relieved of military duties and assigned to an army hospital that had many beriberi cases, just outside of Djakarta, Indonesia, where he became research director. Eijkman's first approach was to thoroughly investigate the contagion of the disease using an affordable animal model that would allow him to study large numbers. This was particularly important given the inter-animal variability in symptoms that had been typically observed until that time. His choice of chicken was a rather lucky one as he was able to duplicate the polyneuritis symptoms in chickens by injecting them with blood of infected human patients. This was a logical step as he assumed the disease to be infectious.

The problem was that his control chickens, also kept in the same compound were also developing similar symptoms. Suspecting that the infection had jumped from the infected group to the controls, he repeated the experiment, this time keeping the control chickens in another separate facility; this time the symptoms did not develop in either of the controls or infected animals, causing Eijkman to doubt the validity of using chickens as an experimental animal. He later discovered, by chance, that a cook, several months previously, was supplementing the chickens' diet with leftover polished rice from the hospital compound, but that a recent cook, who had begun his work a few weeks earlier, no longer requested leftover rice to supplement the chicken feed. Eijkman then began to test the leftover rice and was able to duplicate the disorder repeatedly. He suspected that cooked rice, stored overnight caused the proliferation of bacteria-producing toxins that generated the polyneuritis. However he later found that feeding raw polished rice also caused beriberi. This left him in a bit of a quandary, as his experiments were not consistently proving microbial infestation as the cause of the degenerative polyneuritis. This became even more evident when he discovered that feeding brown unprocessed rice healed the condition in the birds. Another set of experiments that tested tapioca versus meat, demonstrated that tapioca caused the disease and that meat cured it; this finding raised suspicions that starches in general were likely the problem not just rice. He hypothesized that starch was possibly fermenting in the intestine and producing a bacterial toxins that was behind the polyneuritis. Adding the rice bran back to the starches also healed the birds, confirming that the bran contained an antidote to the starch toxin. Having lost his wife and contracted malaria, while in Indonesia, he had to promptly conclude his research. Eijkman's work however, never really evolved to include human experimentation, which was a great weakness that prevented him from uncovering the truth. Upon submission of his final report, the scientific community was critical of his work, questioning whether the disease he produced in the chickens was even beriberi.

It is at this point that a recent acquaintance, Dr. Adolphe Vorderman with whom he had discussed his work before departing, was going to attempt to build on Eijkman's unfinished research. Working as a medical prison inspector in Java, he realized that there was already a human experiment in progress within the vast 101 prisons on the island of Java. He observed that the disease beriberi was rampant among prisoners that consumed the white rice and relatively rare in the prisons serving brown rice, thus confirming Eijkman's work. However, the Dutch government did eventually send Eijkman's replacement, a bacteriologist named Gerrit

Grijns, who manage to disprove that starch was the culprit. Rather, he demonstrated, in a 1901 published paper, that a nutrient located in the outer bran layer of the rice in addition to some legumes was necessary to cure and prevent the disease (Butterworth, 2006; Carpenter, 2003B). This finding was not well accepted in other parts of Asia where beriberi was prevalent. It took excellent work, by the Malaysian Institute for Medical Research, to decidedly produce convincing evidence that the white rice was deficient in some kind of factor. They showed that an alcoholic extract of the rice bran when added to white rice, prevented beriberi, and that brown rice from which alcohol extract had been taken actually caused the disease (Carpenter, 2003B).

Following the Spanish-American war of 1898, the U.S. had a sizable proportion of native troops, stationed in the Philippines, who had contracted beriberi. The Philippine government called a meeting, which experts from the U.S., Japan, and many other countries attended, in order to find a solution. Agreement had been reached that it was indeed the populations that had white polished rice as a stable that were at greater risk of developing beriberi. The solution for the Americans was to recommend banning the rice all together or taxing it so heavily that the poor, who were most vulnerable, would abandon it from their daily menu. Around that time, American Medical Corp physicians found that the symptoms of "taon," documented several years earlier in Japan, looked suspiciously similar to those adult with beriberi, and thus began to investigate. Using alcohol extracts from the bran of brown rice which they added to the breast milk, the babies quickly recovered. The Asian populations adopted the white rice so readily because brown rice would become rancid too quickly when stored in tropical conditions. By 1911, the Polish chemist, Casimir Funk (**Figure 8.8**), who had been working at the Lister institute in London, was the first to isolate the thiamin crystal (Carpenter, 2003B).

In the U.S., the adulteration of the food supply had become a significant problem by the 19th century so that with the advent of sophisticated food processing technology, a safer and more hygienic food supply began to appear but at a cost. Indeed, with processing many food ingredients were devoid of nutrients. Three things were occurring that hinted that this pure American food was scandalously compromised nutritionally. First, by the 1930s and 40s, as the U.S. continued to manufacture and market cheap processed foods, food chemists were identifying sizable amounts of food products that were nutritionally deficient. At the same time, cases of malnutrition were popping up everywhere in the early 1930s as the U.S. reliance on bleached white bread continued to grow (Bobrow-Strain, 2012). Second, the FDA in the United States and Health and Welfare Canada, proposed a number of bills intended on regulating the food industry, which had, prior to WW-II, been increasingly producing refine foods that had lost much of their nutrients. The goal of one of the bills was intended to force the food industry to "enrich" the foods they were manufacturing. The bill was, however, defeated in the U.S., where the enrichment of flour and cereals became voluntary after World War-II. Eventually, by 1964, Canada passed legislation, requiring the food industry to enrich its foods with thiamin, riboflavin, niacin and iron. Even today, the U.S. government still does not enforce enrichment, although much of the flour in the U.S. is enriched.

Today, the obesity crisis in the U.S. is setting off alarm bells, as the evidence seems to be pointing to a population with extremely poor eating habits that is being fed by a food supply made up of cheaper calories but a food quality that is more nutrient impoverished (Bissonnette, 2013). It is however among the obese population that a prevalence of thiamin deficiency of 15-25% has been reported, with prevalence rates as high as 79% observed among type-2 diabetics (Via, 2012). It is also found among hospitalized patients, who are ill with anorexia nervosa, alcoholism, HIV-AIDS, G.I. and liver diseases, and persistent vomiting (Butterworth, 2006).

The RDA for adults is 1.1 mg/day and there is no known toxicity concern. Normally it is fairly easy to meet the RDA for this vitamin since it is abundantly found in the U.S. flour supply, breads, breakfast cereals, and grains such as polished rice, whole brown rice, peas, legumes of various types (soy beans, lentils, navy beans, kidney beans, etc.), beef and lamb. So long as the diet is varied, and there are no absorption problems, then there should be little concern for the risk of being deficient in this nutrient. However, the heavy use alcohol has raised some concerns, as there is a tendency to eat poorly, experience diminished absorption, and a reduced hepatic storage of the vitamin because of frequent cases of steatosis and fibrosis that are reported (Butterworth, 2006). One of the diseases derived from abusive intakes of alcohol is called, Wernicke-Korsakoff syndrome which consists of two separate disorders. First, Wernicke Encephalopathy (W.E.) and the second is Korsakoff Psychosis (KP). W.E. is a disease that affects the activities of all three of the enzymatic reactions—transketolase in the monophosphate shunt pathway, pyruvate dehydrogenase in glycolysis and alpha-ketoglutarate dehydrogenase in the Tricarboxilic cycle—that have needed the co-factor, **thiamin diphosphate** (TDP) which was previously called thiamin pyrophosphate (Butterworth, 2006). This cofactor has been found to be suboptimal in the brain of deceased alcoholics with W.E. Medical students are

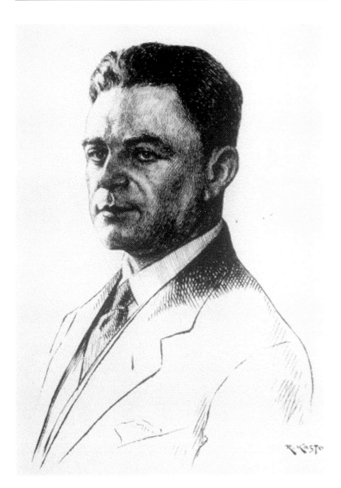

Figure 8.8 Casimir Funk © Getty Images

classically taught to look for a triad of symptoms consisting of ophthalmoplegia, ataxia and confusion, which do not frequently occur in W.E. Rather, the condition is often missed because although it does involve ocular palsies, nystagmus, ataxia of gait, and a decline in mental processing, it will more likely present as apathy and a psychomotor fatigue or slowness (Butterworth, 2006). Korsakoff psychosis is a confabulatory syndrome that involves amnesia, loss of spontaneous initiatives, and abnormal conceptual functions (Butterworth, 2006).

8.3.2.5 Riboflavin and Niacin Deficiencies in the U.S and their History

Beginning in 1905 the niacin deficiency disease, pellagra became more prominent in the American south, and by 1909 pellagra had widened its grip, spreading to several southern states (Carpenter, 2003). The problem became widespread and so persistent that a physician by the name of Goldberger had been put in charge of the U.S. Public Health Service's pellagra program by 1914. The medical community was convinced that the cause was some kind of pathogenic fungi that had gotten into the food supply, or the consequence of excreta from flies that invaded outdoor food storage facilities. These ideas arose from a long standing pellagra problem in Italy, where moldy corn was suspected to be the cause.

When Goldberger became head of the investigation, he quickly ruled out the suspected infectious nature of the disease on the basis that none of the healthcare practitioners were getting ill from treating the sick patients. Suspecting an inadequate diet was at the source of the disease, he persuaded Mississippi authorities to allow him to recruit 12 prisoners from their prison system, who he intended to make sick with the disease. The motivation to participate was that if the prisoners survived 6 months they would be set free. He fed them a diet poor in protein and elevated in maize, which was the staple of the southern poor. By the 6th month the volunteers had developed dermatitis in several regions of the body—a typical symptom seen in pellagra—but escaped from the hospital before Goldberger could confirm with other colleagues that he had produced pellagra in the prisoners. He studied whole families afflicted with the disease and found, after comparing to healthy families, that the difference was that the control families that did not have pellagra, had a dairy cow, from which they extracted daily rations of milk. His group eventually developed a dog model of pellagra that exhibited black tongue after feeding them cornmeal, no milk, milk powder or meat. Most surprising, the animals were healed very rapidly upon feeding them yeast. It took until 1937 before researchers conducted assays on fractions of yeast that allowed them to identify nicotinic acid as a key co-factor in the yeast reaction. Even though researchers were confident at that point that niacin deficiency was at the source of the pellagra, recent reports out of India created some confusion. Polished rice, which was heavily consumed in India, where pellagra was far from being a public health problem, actually contained much less niacin than in the maize consumed in the American south. Why then were they not afflicted with pellagra? The other problem, which deepened the mystery, was that pellagra was not prominent in Mexico where the Indian maize was heavily used (Carpenter, 2003C). In attempting to unravel this paradox, researchers discovered that the amino acid tryptophan, which is an essential amino acid, found in protein of high biological value (meat, poultry, fish and dairy), could become niacin. Though the conversion rate of tryptophan to niacin is low (60g tryptophan creates 1g niacin), it was sufficient to prevent pellagra from occurring. There is however a catch, as this reaction requires vitamin B6 (pyridoxine), B2 (riboflavin), iron and copper to complete the biotransformation. So then, a diet deficient in any one of those additional nutrients could increase the risk of pellagra in the population (Bourgeois, et al. 2006). Also, the native people in Mexico knew to soak their maize in lime or some other kind of alkaline, which helped release the niacin from the maize for absorption. The problem in the southern U.S. was that the maize was not soaked in lime and the overall diet was poor in protein. Those two things created a medical catastrophe; the poor began developing gastrointestinal malabsorption and **diarrhea, dermatitis**, followed later by **dementia** and finally **death**; these are commonly referred to as the 4 D symptoms (Bourgeois et al., 2006). This is not surprising given niacin is involved as a key biochemical co-factor in so many biochemical reactions within the TCA cycle and the electron transport chain, notably as nicotinamide adenine dinucleotide (NAD), and all of the metabolite derivatives such as NADH, NADP and NADPH (Bourgeois, et al., 2006).

The RDA for niacin in adults varies between 14-16 mg/day or niacin equivalents (NE)/day. Now-a-days the good and excellent sources of niacin are well known; nuts, fish and meat, along with enriched breads and cereals (**Figure 8.9**), when regularly consumed as part of a well-balanced diet, prevent deficiency. Additionally, regular consumption of milk and eggs, even though their niacin content is low, still are considered good sources of niacin because of the elevated tryptophan content in the high quality proteins of these foods (Bourgeois et al., 2006). Niacin is also used therapeutically in the management of hyperlipidemias. Medical prescriptions of 2-6g of nicotinic acid have been effective in reducing the ratio of LDL: HDL and so has been considered as an effective alternative to the statins which are popularly used in hypercholesterolemia. It has been advanced that by inhibiting lipolytic reactions in adipose tissue—this decreases the release of triglycerides—and the synthesis of triglycerides in the liver—this process is called lipogenesis—the nicotinic acids prevents the formation of VLDL and LDL. There is, as well in vitro findings that suggest that the vitamin may also promote heightened synthesis of HDL which is the cholesterol scavenger (Bourgeois et al., 2006).

Riboflavin deficiency tended to also occur to varying degrees at the same time as niacin deficiency (Carpenter, 2003). The yeast experiments had also uncovered that riboflavin, like niacin, was part of a rather complex enzymatic system. Indeed, they found that riboflavin was part of flavin adenine dinucleotide (FAD) which acted as a co-factor in numerous enzymatically controlled reactions in glycolysis, the TCA cycle and electron transport chain. The characteristic symptoms of glossitis, angular stomatitis, and cheilosis tended to be documented as well in pellagra patients because the poor quality diet that typically produces pellagra, can and does tend to also generate riboflavin deficiency (Carpenter, 2003).

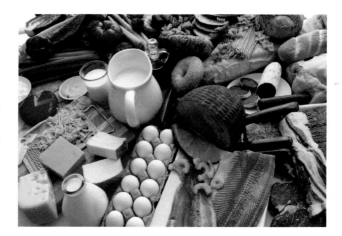

Figure 8.9 Good and excellent sources of riboflavin.
© Hurst Photo/shutterstock.com

Riboflavin is richly found in milk as well as in eggs, lean meat, broccoli and enriched breads and cereals (McCormick, 2006). With an RDA of 1.1 mg/day for women and 1.3 mg/day for men, only very poor dietary selections or disease can compromise somebody's riboflavin status.

Hence those individuals susceptible to a deficiency of this vitamin tend to be patients with anorexia (poor appetite) who eat too little food overall. Vulnerable as well are athletes who restrict energy intake as an unhealthy method of weight loss. Here too, the ingestion of riboflavin tends to be suboptimal (McCormick, 2006).

8.3.2.6 Pyridoxine, Pantothenic and Biotin Deficiencies in the U.S. and their Histories

Pyridoxine—Since its discovery in the 1930s, the understanding of pyridoxine's role in human health and metabolism continues to grow. Low pyridoxal-5'-phosphate (PLP) below the cut-off of 20 nmol/L has been used as the most reliable indicator of poor vitamin B_6 status (Mackey et al. 2006). Abundantly found in meat, poultry, fish, fortified breakfast cereals, starchy vegetables like potatoes and yams, in addition to non-citrus fruits, a deficiency of this vitamin is difficult to find. Nevertheless, lower plasma concentrations have been frequently documented in patients with celiac disease, Crohn's disease and ulcerative colitis (Mackey, et al. 2006). These are classified as malabsorption syndromes which affect not only vitamin B_6 absorption but a multitude of other nutrients and micronutrients. It is believed that the inflammatory responses of these syndromes may also be responsible for the plasma decline of PLP.

Although the symptoms of a pyridoxine deficiency are not well documented and overtly clear as in the cases of scurvy, beriberi and pellagra, there are convincing indicators that suboptimal intakes of this vitamin can lead to some long term diseases. There is epidemiological data that is already between 10 to 30 years old that documents a significant association between low B6 status and increased risk of breast and other cancers. However there is hardly any kind of clinical trial confirming causality (Mackey et al. 2006). It is specifically PLP's role in neurotransmitter synthesis—serotonin and ⊠-aminobutyric acid are sensitive to B6 in rats—that has inspired some to advance a role in cognitive development, but the evidence is not strong in humans, except in the elderly. It seems that getting old may makes us particularly vulnerable to low plasma concentrations of PLP. The reason why levels would drop with aging is not clear, but some have advanced that the lower intake of food typically seen with advanced age, a decline in renal function and perhaps increases in acute phase reactants and inflammation may be behind these changes. What is even more convincing is that large doses of pyridoxine supplementation administered to elderly patients successfully restored biochemical, functional and immunological indices of PLP in the elderly. The fact that plasma levels tend to be suboptimal in cases of rheumatoid arthritis, and Alzheimer's disease gives further credence to the role played by neurological impairment and increased inflammation in B$_6$ deficiency. The involvement of pyridoxine in reducing cardiovascular disease risk is not well documented at this time (Mackey et al. 2006).

Despite not being able to pinpoint a specific deficiency disease, there are non-specific symptoms of peripheral neuropathy and symptoms resembling those of pellagra, along with seborrheic dermatitis, glossitis, and cheilosis in cases of protein-energy malnutrition and in patients receiving anticonvulsant drug therapy (Merck, 2013). Additionally in adults, there is evidence of increased depression, confusion, EEG abnormalities, and seizures when plasma B6 levels are below the cutoff (Merck, 2013). So then, the role of vitamin B$_6$ remains nonetheless well documented and essential for human life with the liver being the principal site of B$_6$ metabolism. The key noteworthy areas of pyridoxine's biochemical involvement are outline below:

a. It acts as a co-enzyme in glucose production via glycogenolysis and gluconeogenesis in the liver.
b. PLP is a recognized co-factor that aids in enzymatic reactions involving amino acid and lipid metabolism (Mackey et al. 2006).

Pantothenic acid—A deficiency is unlikely given that this B vitamin is found in almost every food. Consequently, the only early recorded cases of deficiency were in malnourished prisoners of war found in WW-II Japanese, Philippino and Burmese concentration camps. They experienced strong burning sensations on the bottom of their feet in addition to toe numbness which were reversed with pantothenic acid, and not any other of the B vitamins (Trumbo, 2006). Dr. Lipmann discovered in 1947 that is was a key component of coenzyme A (CoA) in human metabolism. As such it is directly involved in ß-oxidation of fatty acids and in the breakdown of amino acids as they prepare to be oxidized in the TCA cycle. The CoA enzyme plays a critical step in the formation of citrate from oxaloacetate in the TCA cycle. A component of hydroxyl-3-methylglutaryl-CoA, it plays a vital role in cholesterol synthesis (Trumbo, 2006). It is no wonder that a deficiency of this vitamin produced, in subjects tested during the 1950s and 80s, symptoms of irritability, restlessness, sleep disturbances, numbness and gastrointestinal problems. An unintentional acute deficiency caused, in Japanese individuals with mental retardation and suffering from dyskinesia, lactic acidosis, hypoglycemia, and hyperammonemia leading to encephalopathy (Trumbo, 2006). More recently, a 1 g calcium pantothenate supplement, taken daily, was found to be effective in the pain management of patients with rheumatoid arthritis (Trumbo, 2006).

Biotin—the essentiality of this nutrient (**Figure 8.10**) was first suspected back in the 1980s by Velasquez and his co-workers who suspected it in severe cases of pediatric malnutrition based on the activity of the lymphocyte carboxylase enzyme. The certainty, however of its essentiality was documented only by the mid-1990s. Two events clearly outlined the consequences of a deficiency: the first case arose from a prolonged ingestion of raw egg white which contains the biotin binding compound identified as avidin. This was a sequestering agent naturally found in raw egg that bound the biotin thus making it unavailable for absorption. The avidin is deactivated with cooking, thereby no longer posing a threat of deficiency with even abundant egg consumption. The second event that confirmed biotin as an essential nutrient was in cases of exclusive prolonged intravenous nutrition or total parenteral nutrition (TPN) with an infusion mix that contained no biotin. This was administered to patients with short gut syndrome. The patients developed symptoms of periorificial dermatitis, conjunctivitis, alopecia and ataxia (Mock, 2006). There are several other conditions for which biotin deficiency has been proposed as a cause, but only two appear to solidly founded, in good research findings.

The first appears to be in a condition known as "brittle nails." The treatment with 2.5 g/day of biotin reversed the condition, successfully generating increased nail thickness. The second occurrence of biotin

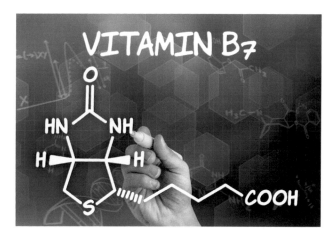

Figure-8.10 This is a chemical structure of vitamin-B₇ or biotin; © Zerbor/Shutterstock.com

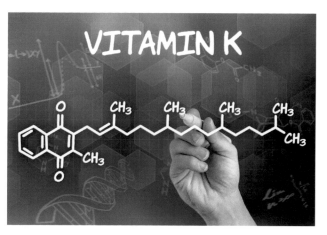

Figure 8.11 Vitamin K chemical structure/© Zerbor/shutterstock.com

deficiency is reliably confirmed in cases of alcoholism and in gastrointestinal diseases (Mock, 2006).

This vitamin plays a key role as a co-factor in the ß-oxidation of fatty acids. It is richly found bound to the protein of meats and cereals (Mock, 2006).

8.3.2.7 Vitamin K Deficiency

Dr. Henrik Dam, working out of Copenhagen in 1929, observed subdural and muscular hemorrhages in chicks that had been fed a diet from which cholesterol had been extracted using a solvent. Subsequent blood extractions from these chicks consistently showed a slowed clotting process. Early in the 1930s, McFarlane and his colleagues, while assessing the nutritive value of various protein sources, also noticed a hemorrhagic disease in chicks that were fed purified diets of fish meal (Suttie, 2006). A new fat soluble dietary factor (**Figure 8.11**) was suspected to be involved in the blood clotting mechanism—at the level of prothrombin synthesis—but it took researchers at the University of California in Berkeley to find, by the mid-1930s, that this factor was present in lipid extracts identified in green plants such as collards, spinach and salad greens. Unexpectedly, bacteria-treated fish meal also had the same factor, a finding which eventually uncovered the existence of vitamin K-producing gut bacteria. This led researcher, Frick and co-workers, in 1967, to demonstrate that prolonged antibiotic treatments, in intravenously-fed starved patients, actually did lead to a decline in gut bacteria production of vitamin K and to significant hypothrombinemia (Suttie, 2006).

Vitamin K's role is also most important in bone metabolism. The most abundant bone-matrix protein, osteocalcin, depends on vitamin K to help catalyze the gamma-carboxylation of calcium in bone, a most critical step in the calcification of bone (Suttie, 2006).

The most prevalent dietary form of this vitamin was identified as "**phylloquinone,**" and it is absorbed into the chylomicrons of the enterocytes of the small intestine and, from there transported to the lymphatic system. Afterwards, it is found in the circulating VLDLs that deposit their triglycerides in adipose tissue and muscle tissue (Suttie, 2006). Pure dietary deficiencies of this vitamin are extremely rare because they are abundantly found in a variety of vegetable oils (soybean, canola, cottonseed and olive oils) and in an assortment of green leafy vegetables (Collards, spinach, salad greens, broccoli, Brussels sprouts and cabbage). The concern with vitamin K deficiency is associated more with newborn babies. In fact, one out of every 100,000 live births (CSPS. 2002), not treated with vitamin K, has hemorrhagic disease of the newborn (HDNB) which is characterized by intracranial bleeding (Suttie, 2006). These babies have a vitamin-K deficient clotting mechanism that shows up, in the classical presentation, about 2-7 days after birth. This is a risk in newborn infants since all newborns are actually deficient in vitamin K because of very poor placental transfer from the mother. This is why intramuscular injections or an oral dose of the vitamin is administered within the first few minutes of birth (CSPS, 2002). In even more rare circumstances, mothers who are taking anticonvulsants place their babies at risk of HDNB within the 24 hrs after birth because these drugs impair the vitamin's action. The third manifestation of this disease is seen about 3-8 weeks after the birth of babies who have been exclusively breastfed by mothers with poor dietary K status. Additionally, this hemorrhagic disease is reported in infants, with neonatal hepatitis, or biliary atresia, who cannot absorb fat or the fat-soluble vitamin K (CSPS, 2002). In adults, vitamin K deficiency has rarely been documented from poor dietary intakes, but is reported more often in patients on long term TPN or with malabsorption syndromes, and gastrointestinal diseases such as celiac disease, ulcerative colitis, and short bowel syndrome to name a few (Suttie, 2006). It would have to take an unfortunate set of circumstances to cause a primary deficiency of vitamin K in a person. For instance, a woman who chronically follows a very low fat weight reducing diet, who does not consume vegetables and who is being treated with wide spectrum antibiotics. In such a case, the dietary intake of vitamin K is not coming from the oils and the green vegetables—touted as the primary sources of K—and nor are there bacteria in the gut producing sufficient amounts of the vitamin either. In theory this could greatly increase the risk of a deficiency.

8.3.2.8 Key Macro-minerals and Micromineral Deficiencies and their Histories

This section will discuss only the relevant and significant minerals and microminerals as they pertain to human health and disease. Calcium, phosphorous, magnesium and potassium will be the main macro-minerals that will be discussed; iron is tackled in a separate section dedicated to anemias. In addition, iodide, copper, zinc and selenium will be discussed as they are most relevant to the formation of Health care professionals.

Calcium, phosphorus and magnesium—calcium is the second most abundant nutrient mineral in the body with 99% of its concentration found in bone and teeth. The rest of the calcium is distributed between blood and also tissue where it functions more specifically in muscle contractions. The body maintains a tight homeostatic control of blood **calcium** levels. Hence a 10% deviance or greater away from the general mean standard blood value, is indicative of either hypocalcemia or hypercalcemia. These are blood conditions that reflect a disease state, and need to be resolved quickly. Understanding the homeostatic mechanism is important in order to have a better grasp of calcium's involvement in the disease process. There are surface receptors located in the parathyroid, thyroid glands, kidney, intestine and bone marrow that monitor the concentrations of calcium in the plasma. Whenever the calcium concentrations begin to rise, less parathyroid hormone (PTH) is released and a greater secretion of calcitonin (CT) takes place. Conversely, when plasma calcium levels begin to decline, there is a greater release of PTH and less calcitonin. In response, the renal tubules begin to reabsorb more calcium, and the same time a greater renal phosphate clearance occurs. In a separate location, the osteoclast cells of the bones become activated thus generating greater bone resorption or breakdown. Concomitantly, the inactive form of vitamin D is activated to 1, 25–dihydroxy vitamin D (1,

$25(OH)_2 D$) also called calcitriol, which is instrumental in increasing intestinal absorption of calcium. Conceptually then, PTH and calcitriol work together to increase calcium renal tubular reabsorption, resorption of calcium from the bone and intestinal calcium absorption. All three processes assist in bringing serum calcium levels back to normal. In contrast, a rising concentration of serum calcium leads to an increase in calcium binding to the receptors on the parathyroid which in turn inhibits the release of PTH. The direct consequence is less calcium tubular reabsorption in addition to a drop in bone resorption rates and a diminished activation of vitamin D in the kidney. At the cellular level, osteoclast activity is diminished and osteoblasts are activated; the latter will translate into less calcium absorption from the intestin. All three of these adjustments will lead to a downward realignment of serum calcium levels (Weaver & Heaney, 2006). It is specifically during the growth period that the bone can become vulnerable to the under mineralized of newly formed bone matrix. Chronically low intakes of dietary calcium can ultimately lead to hypocalcemia even with the hypersecretion of PTH aimed at regaining serum calcium balance. The osteoblasts dysfunction that ensues has been shown to lead to rickets, even without a vitamin D deficiency. Moreover, the hypersecretion of PTH lowers serum phosphate concentration. It is both the low-level of phosphate and calcium in the blood that favor a poor mineralized nation of the bone (Weaver & Heaney, 2006).

A magnesium deficiency will also disturb PTH secretions from the parathyroid glands and the calcium resorption from bone.

Because the dietary requirements for calcium are so elevated—the RDA varies between 1000-1300 mg per day—it is imperative that youth specifically but also adults be judicious in their dietary choices. Dairy products are the richest supplier of calcium in the diet. In fact one cup of milk, 1 cup of yogurt or 1 1/2 ounces of cheddar cheese all contain approximately 300 mg of calcium. This means that 3 cups of milk a day contains about 900 mg of calcium or 69% of the highest RDA value. Regularly consuming milk, yogurt and cheese increases the chances of meeting daily requirement. Indeed 78% of calcium consumption in the U.S. comes from dairy products whereas only a mere 17% of calcium is ingested from fruits, vegetables and grains. There is a good reason why Healthy Eating Guidelines prioritize dairy products. It has to do with both the high calcium content and absorbability. This is especially important for the young who have up to the age of 25 to achieve maximal bone density. Although somewhere between 60 and 80% of the bone mass is genetically determined, it is specifically how the calcium is utilized that is genetically predetermined. So then it is not surprising that calcium intake in adolescent girls is the most significant determinant of bone density. The other reason that dairy products are encouraged in the North American diet is that the overall nutritional quality of the diet tends to increase. In fact, whenever milk is regularly consumed, vitamins A intake jumps 35%, folate increases 38%, riboflavin rises 56%, and there is 22% rise in magnesium intake. Along with an 80% increase in calcium, there is also a 24% jump in potassium compared to non-dairy consumers.

Once the full genetic potential of peak bone density has been achieved there are several things that can be done after the age of 25 to minimize bone loss:

a. regular exercise
b. continued dairy consumption

There is also growing evidence in the literature in support of calcium's role in reducing the risk of colonic cancer in animal models, but still more research is needed before this protective role is confirmed in humans. So far, two prospective studies have shown that neither calcium nor milk influenced the incidence of colorectal adenomas (Weaver & Heaney, 2006).

The role of **phosphorus** in bone is important as 80% of the body's phosphorus is located in the hydroxyapatite structure of bone. It is also a structural component of the phospholipids such a phosphotidyl choline (lecithin). In the form of adenosine triphosphate (ATP) and creatine phosphate it becomes essential in energy production and storage within the cell. Phosphate is abundant in animal protein foods, such as meats, fish, poultry, dairy, and processed foods (Knochel, 2006). In recent years the "acid-ash" hypothesis has been proposed as a mechanism for the advanced prevalence of osteoporosis in North American society. The theory posits that because of the high meat and dairy intake, and the unusually elevated amounts of processed foods consumed here in the U.S., including soft drinks, there is at the same time excessive phosphates ingested that contribute to the diet acid load of the body, which in turn accelerates bone decalcification causing increased urinary calcium losses (Fenton et al. 2009). Although this hypothesis has been embraced as truth, including the Institutes of Medicine, there still remains some debate about the accuracy of the science.

About 60% of **magnesium** in the body is mainly located in bone and the rest in muscle (Rude and Shils, 2006). In the clinical setting, magnesium deficiency usually presents with biochemical, neuromuscular and cardiac abnormalities. The biochemical change that is most common with low magnesium is hypokalemia. Low potassium may be a logical consequence because of the importance of Mg-dependent Na+/K+-ATPase in electrolyte regulation. This is an active energy-dependent cross membrane regulatory system; in the absence of sufficient Mg, there would be insufficient intracellular K released into the extracellular space. Neuromuscular hyperexcitability is one of the repercussions that has been found in patients with low serum magnesium but normal calcium levels. It would appear that magnesium plays a role in modifying the release of the neurotransmitters into the neuromuscular junction, by competitively preventing calcium from reaching the presynaptic terminal. However, when magnesium levels are low more calcium reaches the presynaptic terminal thereby resulting in greater release of neurotransmitters into the synaptic cleft which leads to hyper-responsiveness; this could also translate into a greater propensity to develop leg cramps. Magnesium has also been found in both clinical epidemiological studies to regulate blood pressure. Indeed, hypomagnesemia correlates with hypertension; the DASH study also supported that finding. On the long term a low levels of serum magnesium can also translate into bone demineralization. The mechanism is actually very similar to calcium in that acutely elevated serum magnesium concentrations can prevent PTH secretions from the parathyroid glands, and that acutely suboptimal plasma levels will elicit abundant PTH release leading to bone resorption (Rude and Shils, 2006).

There has been some concern that the U.S. population may not be receiving sufficient amounts of magnesium in the diet, because the food supply is highly processed. The USDA's Continuing Survey of Food Intakes by Individuals, in addition to NHANES-III cross-sectional survey, have both found that 75% of the U.S. population regularly consumes below the RDA for Mg. Although this does not confirm an outright deficiency, it raises some concerns that the population may be at risk. Some have even advanced that it has reached a public health concern. Nobody knows for sure whether there is a nutritional problem here or not. Further studies have been encouraged in this area in light of growing concerns that highly processed foods tend to be low in magnesium (Bissonnette, 2013).

The essentiality of **zinc** in human health was first demonstrated in 1961, when a 21 year old Iranian farmer was diagnosed with anemia, hypogonadism, and dwarfism. His diet had been limited to unrefined flat breads, potatoes and milk (King and Cousins, 2006). As part the glutathione oxidase system, zinc is critical in proving the body with protection against oxidative stress. Richly found in liver and the flesh of beef, fowl, fish and crustaceans, with lesser amounts in eggs and dairy products, deficiencies due to poor dietary intakes would be most rare in affluent societies such as the U.S. that are big meat consumers. Although modest amounts are found in legumes and cereals, their phytate levels are high enough to significantly diminish zinc absorption. It is for this reason that non-meat consuming Middle Eastern countries and those affected by poverty are prone to zinc deficiency. The problem is so widespread that the FAO estimates that close to 50% of the world's population is at risk of being deficient in zinc (King and Cousins, 2006). Here in the U.S. zinc deficiency is encountered in pre-term and low birth weight babies, in instances of chronic diarrhea, and cases of malabsorption disorders such as Crohn's disease, celiac sprue, and short-bowel syndrome. Zinc deficiency especially in children can cause growth retardation, delayed sexual maturation, and hypogonadism; in adults, symptoms of skin lesions adjacent to bodily orifices, poor appetite, impaired taste (hypogeusia), delayed wound healing, and immune deficiencies of various types are observed. In sever enough cases, alopecia and the hypopigmentation of the hair which may take on a reddish hue has been observed (King and Cousins, 2006). The latter resembles the reddish coiling hair seen in kwashiorkor.

Iodine, Copper, and Selenium— Iodine has been briefly covered in a previous section on mineral deficiencies in developing countries. The focus of this section is **iodine** deficiency in the U.S. Historically, in the U.S. iodine deficiency was endemic to certain areas that formed the "goiter belt" in the surrounding regions of the Great Lakes. The soil was impoverished in iodine, therefore causing low iodine levels in the vegetables produced in that region. Consequently the prevalence of goiter was on the rise in that area of the U.S. Characterized by an enlarged thyroid gland—medically termed, goiter—that protruded from the neck like a pouch, goiter was a visible deformity of the neck. In the absence of iodine in the diet, thyroid stimulating hormone (TSH), secreted from the pituitary gland, remains elevated, causing the thyroid to become abnormally large. TSH would normally cause an increased uptake of iodine by the thyroid, the first step before it can synthesize thyroxin (T4) and triiodothyroxine (T3), which are the key hormones secreted by the thyroid. They regulate biochemical processes, metabolism, skeletal and neurological development in the fetus. A severe iodine deficiency can be significantly more compromising when a pregnant mother's intake is suboptimal, as it will invariably lead to hypothyroidism. The low functioning maternal thyroid would be a high risk for cretinism in the newborn. This is a condition involving dwarfism, deaf mutism, and severe mental retardation. While in utero, the fetus experiences irreversible neurodevelopmental deficits because of the hypothyroidism that can be responsible for growth retardation after birth (Bissonnette, 2013; Patrick, 2008). This is because the thyroid hormone plays a critical role in brain development, in as much as it modulates crucial myelination of the central nervous system (Dunn, 2006). In the U.S the most important natural food source of iodine are dairy products, whereas seafood represents a moderate and meats modest sources of the nutrient. There was considerable hope placed on the efficacy of iodized salt in containing the prevalence of goiter and cretinism in the U.S. back in the 1920, when the salt iodization program was implemented. The problem is that in recent years, the has been a population shift towards preferentially consuming much large amounts of processed foods manufactured for the most part using salt that has not been iodized (Dunn, 2006).

Utilized as a therapeutic compound back in 400BC by Hippocrates, **Copper** belonged in the medical pharmacopeia until the 19th century, at which point its therapeutic efficacy could no longer be upheld in light of scientific scrutiny. However, as early as 1912 copper's involvement in human disease was identified in Wilson's disease, which is an autosomal recessive disorder that typically presents with copper accumulation in the liver, brain and cornea of the eyes. Several decades later, in 1962, Menkes disease was also linked back to copper. Trapped with the intestinal mucosa, kidney, spleen and muscle, copper is unable to be transported to organs and tissue thus leading to mental retardation, and poorly pigmented skin and hair (Turnlund, 2006).

Copper's role in iron deficiency anemia began to be suspected in rats that did not improve despite being administered iron supplements. It took until 1930 before scientist began suspecting a link between copper deficiency and anemia in humans, but the mechanism remained obscure (Turnlund, 2006). By the 1980s, it had been found that the copper-containing glycoprotein, ceruloplasmin, was necessary to catalyze the oxidation of ferrous iron to its reduced ferric state. In this way the iron could be stored in the body and ultimately be used in erythropoiesis or the synthesis of red blood cells. So then, if copper is deficient, then iron cannot be oxidized to its active form and be used for the formation of red blood cells; the consequence is a poor production of red blood cells, leading to anemia. It has also been suspected that copper is needed for the normal synthesis of bone marrow, the site of red blood cell production (Turnlund, 2006). Copper is also involved in the **copper/zinc superoxide dismutase**. Located in the cytosol of the cell, this enzyme's role is to shield the cell from oxidative damage by scavenging superoxide radicals (Turnlund, 2006). This process protects cellular integrity and, some suspect it can, over the long term, lessen the disease and aging processes. In the North American diet, copper can be richly found in shellfish, nuts, seeds, legumes, and within the bran and germ factions of the grains. There are only moderate amounts of copper in dried fruits, mushrooms, tomatoes, bananas, potatoes, and meats. Frank outright deficiency of this micromineral is relatively rare. However, in the 1980s, a set of Japanese cases of copper deficiency, involving children and young adults that were mentally retarded, had been documented. Patients consumed a long term enteral diet, deficient in copper. It is important, therefore to make broad food selections that focus on fruits, vegetables and grains, with less attention on meat consumption (Turnlund, 2006).

Selenium's role in human nutrition was documented only 35 years ago, in 1979. Keshan's disease was known to afflict Chinese children and young women with irreversible cardiomyopathy characterized by a diminished heart function. Researchers found that selenium supplements protected the young, living within the northeastern to southwestern regions in China where there was selenium-depleted soil (Burk and Levander, 2006). This specific mineral should be remembered for its biochemical function in glutathione peroxidases (GSHPx), which protects cells against oxidant molecules that threaten the integrity of cells. Abundantly found in all bodily cells GSHPx is the most abundant and widespread antioxidant system of the body.

REFERENCES

1. Barker, L.A., Gout, B.S., and Crowe, T.C. (2011). Hospital Malnutrition: Prevalence, Identification and Impact on Patients and the Healthcare System. Int J Environ Res Public Health. 8(2): 514–527. Retrieved June 28, 2014 from: http://www.ncbi.nlm.nih.gov/pmc/articles/PMC3084475/

2. Bissonnette, D.J. (2013). It's All about Nutrition: Saving the Health of Americans. Lanham, MD: University Press of America, 220pp

3. Bistrian, B. (1984) Nutritional assessment of the hospitalised patient: a practical approach. In: Nutritional Assessment, R. and Heymsfield, S. eds) Blackwell Scientific Publications, Boston, p:183-205

4. Bistrian BR, Blackburn GL, Vitale J, Cochrane D, Naylor J. (1976) Prevalence of malnutrition in general medical patients. JAMA.235: 1567–1570

5. Bobrow-Strain, A (2012). White Bread: A Social History of the store-Bought Loaf. Boston: Beacon Press, 257pp.

6. Bourgeois, C., Cervantes-Laurean, D and Moss. (2006) J. Niacin. In: Modern Nutrition in Health and Disease 10th edition, (Shils, ME et al Eds) Baltimore MD: Lippincott, Williams & Wilkins p: 442-451

7. Burk, R.F. and Levander, O.A. (2006) Selenium. In: Modern Nutrition in Health and Disease 10th edition, (Shils, ME et al Eds) Baltimore MD: Lippincott, Williams & Wilkins p: 312-325

8. Busby, P and Mullen, J.L (1984). Analysis of Nutritional Assessment Indices—Prognostic Equations and Cluster Analysis. In: Nutritional Assessment, R. and Heymsfield, S. eds) Blackwell Scientific Publications, Boston, p:141-155

9. Butterworth, R.F. (2006) Thiamin. In: Modern Nutrition in Health and Disease 10th edition, (Shils, ME et al Eds) Baltimore MD: Lippincott, Williams & Wilkins p: 426-433

10. Caballero, B. (2006). The Nutrition Transition: Global Trends in Diet and Disease. In: Modern Nutrition in Health and Disease 10th edition, (Shils, ME et al Eds) Baltimore MD: Lippincott, Williams & Wilkins p: 1717-1722

11. Canadian Clinical Practice Guidelines (CCPG) (2013). Composition of enteral Nutrition: High Protein vs Low Protein. Retrieved July 2, 2014 from: http://www.critical-carenutrition.com/docs/cpgs2012/4.2c.pdf

12. Canadian Pediatric Surveillance Program (CPSP). 2002. Vitamin K Injection: Best Prevention for Newborns. Paediatr. Child Health 7(8): 588-589

13. Carpenter, K.J. (2003) A Short History of Nutritional Science: Part-3 (1912-1944). J. Nutrition. 133: 3023–3032

14. Carpenter, K.J. (2003B). A Short History of Nutritional Science: Part-2 (1885-1912). J. Nutr. 133: 975–984,

15. Carpenter, K.J. (2003C). A Short History of Nutritional Science: Part-4 (1945-1985). J. Nutr. 133: 3331–3342

16. Charney, P. and Marian, M. (2008) Nutritional Screening and Nutritional Assessment. In: ADA Pocket Guide to Nutrition Assessment. Pamela Charney, and Ainsley M. Malone, (Eds) 2nd edition. Chicago: American Dietetic Association p:1-6

17. Committee on Infectious Diseases (COID). (1993) Vitamin A Treatment Of Measles. Pediatrics. 91:1014-5.

18. De Benoist. B. (2008) Conclusions of a WHO Technical Consultation on Folate and B12 Deficiencies. Food and Nutrition Bulletin, vol. 29, no. 2 (supplement)

19. de Onis, M. et al. (1993) The Worldwide Magnitude of Protein-Energy Malnutrition: An Overview from the WHO Global Database on Child Growth. Bulletin of the World Health Organization—WHO.71(5): 703-712

20. De-Souza, D.A. and Greene, L.J. (1998) Pharmacological Nutrition after Burn Injury. J. Nutr. 128: 797–803.

21. Dunn, J.T. (2006). Iodine. In: Modern Nutrition in Health and Disease 10th edition, (Shils, ME et al Eds) Baltimore MD: Lippincott, Williams & Wilkins p: 300-311

22. FAO (1997). Human Nutrition in the Developing World. FAO Food and Nutrition Series #29. Retrieved June 24, 2014 from: http://www.fao.org/docrep/w0073e/w0073e00.htm

23. Fenton, T.R. et al. (2009). Phosphate decreases urine calcium and increases calcium balance: A meta-analysis of the osteoporosis acid-ash diet hypothesis. J. Nutr. 8(41): 1-14

24. Fleuret, P. and Fleuret, A. (1980). Nutrition, Consumption, and Agricultural Change. Human Organization. 39 (3): 250-260

25. Frankenfield, D. (2006). Energy Expenditure and Protein Requirements after Traumatic Injury. Nutr. Clin. Pract. 21(5): 430-437

26. Hampl, J.S., Taylor, C.A., Johnston, C.S. (2004). Vitamin C Deficiency and Depletion in the United States: The Third National Health and Nutrition Examination Survey 1988-1994. Am J Public Health. 94(5): 870–875

27. Heimburger, D.C. et al (2006). Clinical Manifestations of Nutrient Deficiencies and Toxicities: A Resumé: In: Modern Nutrition in Health and Disease 10th edition, (Shils, ME et al Eds) Baltimore MD: Lippincott, Williams & Wilkins p: 595-612

28. Hoffer LJ, Bistrian BR (2012). Appropriate protein provision in critical illness: a systematic and narrative review. Am J Clin Nutr. 96(3):591-600.

29. Hoffer, J.L. (2006). Metabolic Consequences of Starvation. In: Modern Nutrition in Health and Disease 10th edition, (Shils, ME et al Eds) Baltimore MD: Lippincott, Williams & Wilkins p: 730-748

30. Holick, M.F (2006). Vitamin D. In: Modern Nutrition in Health and Disease 10th edition, (Shils, ME et al Eds) Baltimore MD: Lippincott, Williams & Wilkins p: 376-395

31. Ishibashi, N. Plank, L.D. Sando, K. and Hill, G.L. (1998). Optimal Protein Requirements during the First 2 weeks after the Onset of Critical Illness. Crit. Care Med. 26(9): 1529-35

32. King, J.C. and Cousins, R.J. (2006). Zinc. In: Modern Nutrition in Health and Disease 10th edition, (Shils, ME et al Eds) Baltimore MD: Lippincott, Williams & Wilkins p: 271-285

33. Kinney, J.M. (2006). Human Energy Metabolism. .In: Modern Nutrition in Health and Disease 10th edition, (Shils, ME et al Eds) Baltimore MD: Lippincott, Williams & Wilkins p: 10-16

34. Knochel, J.P. (2006) Phosphorus. In: Modern Nutrition in Health and Disease 10th edition, (Shils, ME et al Eds) Baltimore MD: Lippincott, Williams & Wilkins p: 211-222

35. Lee, RD and Nieman, DC. (1996) Nutritional Assessment.2nd edition. New York: Mosby. 689pp.

36 . Levine, M., Katz, A., Padayatty, S.J. (2006). Vitamin C. In: Modern Nutrition in Health and Disease 10th edition, (Shils, ME et al Eds) Baltimore MD: Lippincott, Williams & Wilkins p: 507-524.

37. Long, C.L. (1984). Nutritional Assessment of the Critically Ill Patient In: Nutritional Assessment, R. and Heymsfield, S. eds) Blackwell Scientific Publications, Boston, p:15-26

38. Lowry, S.F. and Perez, J.M. (2006). The Hypercatabolic State. In: Modern Nutrition in Health and Disease 10th edition, (Shils, ME et al Eds) Baltimore MD: Lippincott, Williams & Wilkins p: 1381-1400

39. Mackey, A.D. Davis, S.R. and Gregory, J.F., (2006). Vitamin B6. In: Modern Nutrition in Health and Disease 10th edition, (Shils, ME et al Eds) Baltimore MD: Lippincott, Williams & Wilkins p: 452-461

40. McCormick, D.B. (2006). Riboflavin. In: Modern Nutrition in Health and Disease 10th edition, (Shils, ME et al Eds) Baltimore MD: Lippincott, Williams & Wilkins p: 434-441

41. Merck Manual for Health Professionals (2013). Nutritional Disorders>Vitamin Deficiency, dependency and toxicity: Vitamin B6. Retrieved July 9, 2014 from: http://www.merckmanuals.com/professional/nutritional_disorders/vitamin_deficiency_dependency_and_toxicity/vitamin_b6.html

42. Merck Manual for Health Professionals (2012). Overview of Undernutrition. Retrieved May 6, 2014 from http://www.merckmanuals.com/professional/nutritional_disorders/undernutrition/overview_of_undernutrition.html?qt=malnutrition&alt=sh#v882493

43. Mock, D.M (2006). Biotin. In: Modern Nutrition in Health and Disease 10th edition, (Shils, ME et al Eds) Baltimore MD: Lippincott, Williams & Wilkins p: 498-506

44. Newsholme, E.A. and Leech, A.R. (1983). Biochemistry for the Medical Sciences. New York: John Wiley & Sons, 952pp

45. Patrick L. (2008) Iodine: deficiency and therapeutic considerations. Altern Med Rev. 13(2): 116-127.

46. Pettifor, J.M (2004). Nutritional Rickets: Deficiency of Vitamin D, Calcium or Both? Am J Clin Nutr, 80(suppl):1725S–9S.

47. Picciano, MF (1999). Iron and folate supplementation: an effective intervention in adolescent females (Editorial). Am. J. Clin. Nutr. 69:1069–1070

48. Pinstrup-Andersen, P and Cheng, F. (2007) Still Hungry: One eighth of the world's people do not have enough to eat. Scientific American297(3): 96-103

49. Popkin, BM. (1994). The nutrition transition in low-income countries: an emerging crisis. Nutr Rev 52:285-298

50. Quandt, S.A. (2006) Social and Cultural Influences on Food consumption and Nutritional Status. In: Modern Nutrition in Health and Disease 10th edition, (Shils, ME et al Eds) Baltimore MD: Lippincott, Williams & Wilkins p: 1741-1751

51. Riaz, M.N. et al. (2009). Stability of Vitamins during Extrusion. Crit Rev Food Sci Nutr. 2009 Apr;49(4):361-8

52. Rose WC. (1957) The amino acid requirements of adult man. *Nutrition Abstracts and Reviews*, 27:631–647.

53. Rothman, D.L. et al. (1991). Quantitation of Hepatic Glycogenolysis and Gluconeogenesis in Fasting Humans with 13C NMR. Science 254 (5031): 573-6

54. Rude, R.K. and Shils, M.E. (2006). Magnesium. In: Modern Nutrition in Health and Disease 10th edition, (Shils, ME et al Eds) Baltimore MD: Lippincott, Williams & Wilkins p: 223-247

55. Schlichtig, R and Ayres, SM. (1988). Nutritional Support of the Critically Ill. Year Book Medical, Publishers, Chicago, pp. 223

56. Suttie, J.W. (2006) Vitamin K. In: Modern Nutrition in Health and Disease 10th edition, (Shils, ME et al Eds) Baltimore MD: Lippincott, Williams & Wilkins p: 412-425

57. Traber, M.G. (2006). Vitamin E. In: Modern Nutrition in Health and Disease 10th edition, (Shils, ME et al Eds) Baltimore MD: Lippincott, Williams & Wilkins p: 396-411

58. Turnlund, J.R. (2006). Copper. In: Modern Nutrition in Health and Disease 10th edition, (Shils, ME et al Eds) Baltimore MD: Lippincott, Williams & Wilkins p: 286-299

59. Trumbo, P.R. (2006). Pantothenic Acid. In: Modern Nutrition in Health and Disease 10th edition, (Shils, ME et al Eds) Baltimore MD: Lippincott, Williams & Wilkins p: 462-469

60. U.N.I.C.E.F. (2003) Micronutrients Iodine, Iron and Vitamin A. Retrieved November 18, 2013 from: http://www.unicef.org/nutrition/index_iodine.html.

61. Via, M. (2012). The Malnutrition of Obesity: Micronutrient Deficiencies that Promote Diabetes. ISRN Endocrinol. 2012: 103472. Retrieved June 30, 2014 from: http://www.ncbi.nlm.nih.gov/pmc/articles/PMC3313629/

62. Weaver, C.M. and Heaney, R.P. (2006). Calcium. In: Modern Nutrition in Health and Disease 10th edition, (Shils, ME et al Eds) Baltimore MD: Lippincott, Williams & Wilkins p: 194-210

63. WHO (2007). Protein and Amino Acid Requirements in Human Nutrition. WHO/ FAO/UNU Joint Report. Technical Report Series 935 United Nations University. Produced by the Agriculture and Consumer Protection Department of the FAO.

64. WHO (2006). Guidelines on Food Fortification with Micronutrients. Lindsay Allen, Bruno de Benoist, Omar Dary, Richard Hurrell (Eds). 341pp.

65. Williams, CD. (1935). Kwashiorkor: A Nutritional Disease of Children Associated with a Maize Diet. Lancet. 226 (5855): 1151-2.

66. Williams, P. (1998) Food Toxicity and Safety. In: Essentials of Human Nutrition. Mann, J. and Trustwell, S. (eds). New York: Oxford University Press p: 379-393

67. Wolf, G. (2004). The Discovery of Vitamin D: The Contribution of Adolf Windaus. J. Nutr. 134: 2015

68. Wolfe, R. R. (1996) Relation of metabolic studies to clinical nutrition—the example of burn injury. Am. J. Clin. Nutr. 64: 800–808.

69. World Bank. (1993). World Development Report. Investing in Health New York: Oxford University Press.

CHAPTER 9

THE PROBLEM OF ANEMIAS

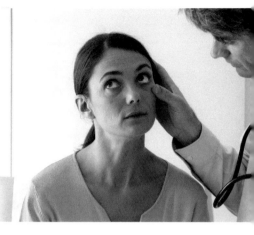

9.1. INTRODUCTION TO ANEMIA

Among hematological defects, anemia is possibly the most common disorder in medical practice. Anemias can be classified as either nutritional or non-nutritional, but, in general, they refer to a defective hemoglobin formation or low concentration in the peripheral blood, which may arise from iron deficiency, B-12 and/or folic acid deficiencies, thalassemic syndromes, sidero-blastic anemia and anemia of chronic disease. The risk of anemia also increases with vitamin A, riboflavin and copper deficiencies, in addition to blood loss and parasite infestation, like hookworm (de Benoist et al, 2008). The most common forms of anemia are the nutritional anemias; specifically, iron deficiency anemia affects an estimated 1.62 billion people globally or 25% of the planet's population, and accounts for about 50% of all anemias, and it is decidedly the pregnant women and children who are the most vulnerable (WHO, 2006; de Benoist, 2008). Moreover, it has been surmised that between 66%-80% of the world's population is at risk of iron deficiency anemia (Bissonnette, 2013). Back in the 1960s the incidence of iron deficiency anemia in England, Canada and the U.S. was three percent in men and 25% in women. That value has not noticeably changed since that time. A 2006 WHO report found that 22.7% of women in industrialized nations suffer from iron deficiency anemia.

Clinically, the iron-deficient patient traditionally presents with low hemoglobin (<13 g/dl for men; <12g/dl for women) (WHO, 2001) accompanied by pallor, lethargy, fatigue, dyspnea, poor physical endurance, faintness, nausea, and anorexia. These symptomatic manifestations and causes of anemia may not always be limited to this classical picture, but could be compounded by other pathologies such as HIV, cancer, malaria and tuberculosis (de Benoist et al, 2008).

The objective is not to become an expert in hematology, rather to increase the recognition of hematological traits of iron, B-12 and folic acid deficiencies as well as to discern between acute and chronic iron deficiency anemias. This is likely the most helpful approach in getting students ready to tackle the assessment of nutrition-related anemias.

9.2 CLASSIFICATION OF ANEMIAS

In addition to being classified as nutritional and non-nutritional, anemias can be subdivided, by automated blood cell counters, into the three categories: i- **hypochromic microcytic anemia**; ii- **normocytic normochromic anemia**; and iii- **normochromic macrocytic anemia**. This classification is based on determining the mean corpuscular volume (MCV), the mean corpuscular hemoglobin (MCH) and mean corpuscular hemoglobin concentration (MCHC) (Gibson, 1990).

Anemias that are hypochromic signify a problem in hemoglobin synthesis. And so it should not be surprising that the association between hypochromia and iron deficiency anemia is very strong. In fact, approximately 25-50% of women and 15% of men, worldwide, are diagnosed with hypochromic anemia, and of these, 90% are iron deficient (Ali, 1976).

Normocytic and normochromic anemia tends to be linked to anemia of chronic disease, whereas macrocytic anemia is tagged to megaloblastic anemia, which originates from folic and/or vitamin B12 deficiency. Macrocytic and megaloblastic anemias are diagnosed using the mean corpuscular volume (MCV). This red blood cell indices, refers to the size of the red blood cell. A small MCV would mean a microcytic cell, which occurs in more advanced forms of iron deficiency, whereas a larger than normal red blood cell would be referred to as macrocytic (Gibson, 1990).

MCV = Hematocrit /red blood count/L

The MCH allows the determination of the hemoglobin cell count in the red cell. When the value is low—something that occurs only in the late phase of anemia (Gibson, 1990)—the red blood cell has a pale or diluted red color, and is therefore referred to as **hypochromic**. The MCHC also will tend to be low in advanced iron deficiency; it refers to the concentration of hemoglobin rather than the cell count. It is the MCH that is most often used to confirm hypochromic anemia (Ali, 1976).

9.3 NON-NUTRITIONAL ANEMIAS

As previously shown, microcytic hypochromic anemia can be caused by iron deficiency, thalassemic syndrome, congenital sideroblastic anemias and anemia of chronic disease. At this stage it may be advantageous to describe some of the non-nutritional anemias in terms of their hematological traits, as it can provide students with a more discerning eye for the accurate identification of the nutrition-based anemias. Students will likely find **Figure 9.6** a helpful algorithm depicting the diagnosis and treatment of a broad assortment of nutritional and non-nutritional anemias.

9.3.1 Thalassemia

Thalassemia is a genetic disorder characterized by a failure in the synthesis of one or more of the globin chains (α,

ß, γ, δ) of the hemoglobin protein, and commonly found in the Mediterranean, African, and Southeast Asian countries (Merck, 1987). The thalassemic syndrome can be expressed following a wide range of clinical variability, depending on whether globin chains are totally or partially affected. The heterozygote form (thalassemia minor) is referred to as the carrier with a mild to moderate microcytic manifestation, whereas the homozygous representation (thalassemia major) has the more severe microcytic and hypochromic anemia symptoms (Hb ≤ 6gm/ dl) primarily resulting from hemolysis (Merck, 2013B). Both the major and minor forms are microcytic as evidenced by the smaller MCVs, however the thalassemia most likely to be confused with iron-deficiency is the heterozygous type (Ali, 1976) because it is the milder form that presents with less pronounced microcytic cells (Merck, 1987). The microcytic and hemolytic red blood cells, observed in thalassemia, are related to an abnormality in hemoglobin production. The clinical features of the homozygous thalassemia, are jaundice, leg ulcers, cholelithiasis, hepato-splenomegaly, hemolysis and absorptive iron overload, and are frequently represented with elevated bilirubin, serum iron and ferritin (Merck, 2013B; 1987). Iron overload will tend to occur because of frequent blood transfusions (Merck, 2013B). Key to differentiating thalassemia from iron-deficiency anemia is that both serum iron and ferritin will increase in thalassemia, a very distinct presentation from the early decline of these markers in iron-deficiency (Merck, 1987).

9.3.2 Sideroblastic Anemias

Congenital sideroblastic anemia is characterized by inherited abnormalities in the production of the hemoglobin protein or in other words a dyserythropoiesis, the consequence of inadequately utilizing iron (Fe) from the bone marrow. This is the reason sideroblastic anemia is often referred to as an iron-utilization anemia (Merck, 2013). The repercussion is a polychromatophilic red blood cells showing up as hypochromic and normocytic which makes it easily confused with iron-deficiency anemia. However, this kind of anemia does not tend to be purely microcytic but rather dismorphic that is to say both large (macrocytic) and small (microcytic) (Merck, 1987; Ali, 1976). So then, despite iron deposits in the mitochondria of the marrow (Wiseman et al, 2013), and an iron overload, this kind of anemia can nevertheless occur through genetic mutations and autosomal disorders. Pyridoxine (vitamin B6) deficiency can increase the risk of developing sideroblastic anemia (Merck, 2013) and B6 has been shown to be somewhat therapeutic in partially reversing the anemia in some congenital cases

(Merck, 1987; Bergmann et al, 2010). If the sideroblastic anemia is secondary to a hematological malignancy, one could expect abnormal leukocytes or thrombocytopenia. In addition, expect to find an elevated plasma ferritin and serum iron, in addition to high transferrin saturation (Merck, 1987). High ferritin occurs when there is excess iron; the unused iron is converted to ferritin and stored in the liver, spleen and bone marrow. High levels of serum iron results from a disproportionally low concentration of hemoglobin for the available iron. This anemia can be distinguished from iron-deficiency anemia because the serum iron can be elevated, the transferrin concentration normal, and the percent iron saturation of transferrin elevated (Merck, 1987; 2013; Ali, 1976).

9.3.3 Anemia of Chronic Disease

On a worldwide basis this is the second most common anemia, and within the hospital medical and surgical settings, this form of anemia is certainly the most common. Anemia of chronic disease is mild and secondary to the acute/chronic response phase to infection, inflammation and malignancy, and should therefore be considered normal for a clinical setting (Merck, 1987). There are several mechanisms occurring that may explain this mild anemia: reduced erythropoiesis and erythropoietin probably from disease-induced reactive oxygen species (ROS) derived from the synthesis of cytokines (Weiss and Goodnough, 2005). Additionally, there is a macrophage iron withholding, shortened red cell life span, a decline in iron absorption from the duodenum, and a small increase in plasma volume. The anemia in this setting acts as a compensatory mechanism to the trauma or infection by increasing the fluidity of the blood. In fact, the sequestration of iron into the reticuloendothelial system—earlier referred to as a macrophage iron withholding—may actually be beneficial as it keeps the iron from microorganisms thus preventing the growth of pathogens (Weiss and Goodnough, 2005). It is therefore important to avoid an inappropriate diagnosis of iron deficiency anemia, but to closely study the multi-factorial dimensions of the problem. This mild anemia is often seen as a normocytic normochromic anemia (Weiss & Goonough, 2005; Ali, 1967) however, in the case of a chronic disease, persisting over many weeks and months, it is more likely to observe a microcytic hypochromic profile. At this advanced stage it becomes quite difficult to distinguish it from iron deficiency; doing a white cell differential and platelet count could help more clearly identify patients in an acute/ chronic phase reaction. The following laboratory markers represent the typical profile found in patients with an acute/chronic phase reaction:

1. MCV: normal or slightly reduced
2. Plasma ferritin: high or normal
3. Plasma iron: low
4. Transferrin: normal to low
5. Serum albumin: mildly reduced
6. Hyponatremia
7. Significant tissue damage: high lactate dehydrogenase
8. Total Iron Binding Capacity (TIBC): low
9. Neutrophilia, lymphopenia and thrombocytosis (Gibson, 1990; Ali, 1967)

In anemia of chronic disease, there is a "***mucosal block***" at the level of the reticulo-endothelial (RE) cells, resulting in a reduced release of iron into the blood even though iron reserves overall may be satisfactory (Gibson, 1990). The reticuloendothelial (RE) system is a phagocytic network of fixed macrophages and monocytes located in the reticular connective tissue that surround the liver, kidney and spleen (Encyclopedia Britannica, 2013; Strum et al. 2007). Because there is less iron released from the RE cells, then the availability of iron to the red blood cells is reduced, therefore causing a buildup in erythrocyte protoporphyrin (EP), a precursor to heme. The reaction describing the role of iron (Fe) in hemoglobin synthesis is shown here:

$$EP + Fe \rightarrow Hemoglobin$$

Hence the rise in EP occurs in the absence of Fe and from the inability to completely form hemoglobin. The elevated EP mimics the response normally seen in iron-deficiency anemia. Contrary to the expected response, serum transferrin levels do not rise since iron reserves are not depleted. It is important to understand that transferrin concentrations generally increase in response to depleted iron reserves; in the anemia of chronic disease the iron reserves have not declined therefore, transferrin synthesis is not stimulated. Also, in anemia of chronic disease, serum ferritin levels are not affected and nor is the MCV (Figure 9.6). Hence, in wanting to differentiate iron-deficiency anemia from anemia of chronic disease, a second level of testing is needed in order to get the desired confirmation before proceeding with treatment. The second step is done in concert with the patient's clinical history, thereby allowing the clinician to assess the impact of secondary underlying pathologies contributing to the patient's anemia. For instance, blood loss from GI inflammation or ulceration would confirm the likelihood of an iron deficiency anemia. The "*four variable model*" has been successfully used to differentiate between anemia cause by inflammatory conditions and iron-deficiency anemia (Gibson, 1990). The four variables are outlined below:

a. Serum ferritin
b. Transferrin saturation & transferrin
c. Erythrocyte protoporphyrin (EP)
d. Mean corpuscular volume (MCV)

Iron-deficiency anemia can be diagnosed fairly accurately when the MCV or serum ferritin decline, concomitantly with one other abnormal parameter such as an elevated EP. A serum ferritin that declines to < 25 ng/ml invariably implies a loss of iron reserves and therefore a high risk of iron deficiency anemia (Killip, 2007). A serum ferritin that varies between 30-100ng/ml could indicate an anemia of chronic disease combined with true iron deficiency, and thus requires a third marker such as an elevated transferrin or low transferrin saturation to confirm iron deficiency anemia, or a normal to slightly reduced transferrin in the instance of an anemia of chronic disease (Weiss and Goodnought, 2005). On the other hand, a patient with a slightly elevated MCV or ferritin and a high EP would NOT be diagnosed with Fe-deficiency anemia since the MCV and ferritin did not decrease. A patient presenting with a profile of low ferritin (<25mg/ml) and elevated erythrocyte protoporphyrin would likely be suffering from Fe-deficiency anemia. The decisive indication in the latter example is the low ferritin, since EP has also been found to increase in anemia of chronic disease (Killip, 2007; Gibson, 1990).

9.3.3.1 Uremia

This condition is seen in chronic renal failure and is associated with a decrease in renal excretory and regulatory function. Typically, anemia tends to develop when plasma creatinine increases to between 12-16 mg/dl or when the glomerular filtration rate (GFR) falls below 10% of normal (Merck, 2013D; Abuelo, et al 1992). There are a number of mechanisms contributing to the moderately severe normochromic and normocytic anemia typically seen in uremia: uremic toxins cause a suppression of bone marrow; the decrease in renal mass causes a deficiency in erythropoietin—a hormone produced by the kidney for the purpose of producing red blood cells in the bone marrow. Moreover, in renal dialysis (**Figure 9.1**), there is consistent blood loss. Hemolytic uremic syndrome and drug therapy can also be responsible for the occurrence of anemia (DHHS, 2014; Merck, 2013D).

9.3.3.2 Liver disease

In 75% of the cases of chronic liver disease, anemia, resulting most often from blood loss, is frequently diagnosed. This is because of the deficiency of coagulation

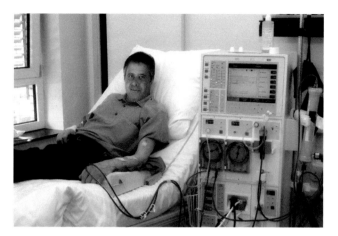

Figure 9.1 Patient undergoing dialysis © gopixa/shutterstock.com.

factors. Portal hypertension is also a common occurrence which generally leads to **splenomegaly** and to secondary hemolysis, increased blood volume, macrocytosis and megaloblastic anemia. Alcohol can suppress bone marrow, and can cause malnutrition which can lead to folic acid deficiency. In addition cirrhosis of the liver can cause a chronic haemorrhage into the GI tract, as well as a slow blood loss from gastric and esophageal varices. Over time the slow loss of blood produces iron deficiency anemia. In liver disease, anemia usually surfaces as a normochromic macrocytic anemia (MCV=100-110fL) (Gonzalez-Casas, et al. 2009).

9.3.3.3 Endocrine disease

In hypothyroidism (myxedema) there is usually a mild anemia of unknown etiology that presents as normochromic and normocytic. A hypochromic anemia can occur that is caused by poor iron intake and absorption in addition to menorrhagia. The latter can go unnoticed or its severity can be masked because of a vasoconstriction, which occurs in order to reduce blood flow, and from a megaloblastic anemia derived from poor folate intake and /or absorption (Merck, 2012).

9.4 NUTRITIONAL ANEMIAS

9.4.1 Iron Deficiency Anemia

On the worldwide stage, iron deficiency anemia is the most common and most treatable of all anemias, affecting 24.8% of the world's population, and representing 50% of all types of anemias (de Benoist, 2008). It is also recognized as the single most import contributor to the burden of disease

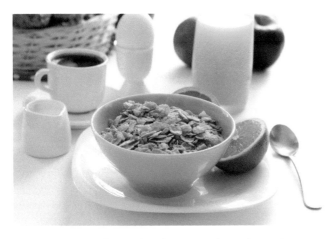

Figure 9.2 Breakfast rich in heme and non-heme iron.
© kiboka /shutterstock.com

worldwide (WHO, 2002). The prevalence in developing countries among children is 46-51% and 42% among women (Pisciano, 1999). Although the preschool children and pregnant women, when expressed as a percent, are most affected by iron-deficiency anemia, it is specially the non-pregnant women who encompass the greatest number of individuals—an estimated 468 million—suffering from iron-deficiency anemia (de Benoist, 2008). The causes appear to be associated with three main problems: 1-blood loss due to chronic bleeding typically seen in menorrhagia, slow GI and urinary tract bleeds, and blood loss from ulcers, colon polyps and cancers; 2- poor dietary intake; and 3-an inability to absorb iron as seen in inflammatory bowel disease (DHHS, 2014). The most common presentation is fatigue, facial pallor, although the absence of pallor in ruling out anemia is not very reliable. Physicians will also check for pale gums and nail beds, irregular heartbeats, uneven breathing, and will conduct rectal and pelvic exams in search of internal bleeding (DHHS, 2014). Other symptoms such as koilonychia (spoon nails), glossitis, or dysphagia are uncommonly observed in the North American population (Killip et al. 2007).

9.4.1.1 Dietary Sources of Fe

Approximately 80% of the iron supplied by the North American diet is in the form of non-heme iron, which is abundantly found in legumes (lentils, soybeans, chick peas, navy beans), some fruits (prunes, apricots, raisins) and vegetables (spinach), grains and cereals (DHHS, 2014), whereas the other 20% comes from animal protein-based heme iron. Breakfast cereals, enriched with iron, are sometime a good source of iron, as they contain at least 10% of the RDA, but more often they are excellent sources of non-heme iron, with one serving containing

25%-50% of the RDA. The cereal brand "Total" enriches many of their cereals with enough iron to meet 100% of the (RDA); this is certainly a strategic way to meet daily iron requirements with very little effort (**Figure 9.1**). Animal sources of protein are elevated in heme-iron, which has a higher absorption rate. Red meats, liver, and eggs are examples of animal proteins rich in heme iron that are commonly found in the North American diet.

9.4.1.2 Those at Risk of Fe-Deficiency

Infants, children and women of child-bearing years are the three groups most vulnerable to iron deficiency. At birth infants have between 4-6 months before the iron reserves of the body are depleted. It is for this reason that an infant cereal fortified with iron is usually introduced at that time. Infant formulas rich in iron is also available, but breast milk, though lower in iron content, has a much greater rate of absorption compared to infant formulas. It is however essential that breastfeeding mothers consume a diet rich in iron. Infants that consume junk food, or too much milk, can become iron deficient. The reason is that soft drinks, candies in addition to cow's milk are particularly poor sources of iron, and so, when consumed in excess, can displace good and excellent sources of iron out of the regular menu (DHHS, 2014). Women, who embrace weight reducing diets, will tend to restrict meats, carbs and fats, in addition to avoiding breakfast in order to accelerate the weight loss process. This puts them particularly at risk of not ingesting sufficient iron. It is estimated that about 12% of women who live in industrialized countries suffer from iron deficiency anemia, and that the prevalence jumps to 43% among non-pregnant women residing in developing countries (Allen, 2000). In the U.S. 11% of women and 9% of adolescent girls and toddlers are believed to suffer from iron deficiency anemia (Looker et al 1997). Surprisingly, as many as 54% of pregnant women living in developing countries, and 18% residing in industrialized nations have iron-deficiency anemia, and thus are at greater risk of delivering low birth weight babies prematurely (DHHS, 2014; Allen, 2000). For this reason, most obstetricians working in the U.S prescribe an iron supplement around the second trimester of pregnancy in compliance with the U.S. Preventive Services Task Force recommendations (USPSTF 1996) which are consistent with current research findings (Killip et al. 2007).

9.4.1.3 Iron Metabolism

Dietary iron is absorbed mostly from the duodenum and combines with a glycoprotein, transferrin, which transports it to the bone marrow for the synthesis of hemoglobin, and for storage in tissue; residual iron is then attached to ferritin and stored in the liver, spleen, bone marrow and reticulo-endothelial system (Gibson, 1990). There is no official excretory route for iron, therefore requiring that absorption be tightly controlled to ensure iron homeostasis and avoid toxicity. The amount of iron absorbed is pretty much dependent on the iron storage capacity and iron status of the body; the greater the deficiency in body stores, the more iron is absorbed from the duodenum. Indeed, up to 15% of non-heme iron and a maximum of 30-35% of heme iron intake can be absorbed when iron stores are low. In a non-deficient state only 5 to 10% of ingested iron (15 mg/d) is actually absorbed overall (Killip et al. 2007). Normally when there is a rich supply of iron stores, the body can slowly draw from this reserve to synthesize iron-rich erythrocytes (red blood cells). There are iron absorption enhancers that can be included in the diet which enhance the non-heme iron absorption, most notably meat and vitamin C; there are also iron inhibitors, such as calcium, fiber, wine, tea and coffee that minimize the absorption of iron from the gut (Killip et al. 2007). It is important to note the slowness at which iron can be mobilized for the synthesis of hemoglobin. In an acute hemorrhage, the rapid loss of iron from the body cannot be easily compensated, by reaching into body iron stores, even though there may be a rich reserve. The end result is the release, from the bone marrow, of a number of iron-deficient hypochromic erythrocytes in an acute blood loss; overall, however, the blood film may show either polychromatic or normochromic cells.

9.4.1.4 The Stages of Iron Depletion

Iron-deficiency anemia can have several causes: i- poor dietary intake, especially in premature infants; ii- menstruation in women and hemo-dilution in pregnancy; iii-occult blood losses in men and postmenopausal women; and iv- decreased iron absorption because of the gut infestation of hookworm, and the presence of phytates and phenolic compounds in the diet (de Benoist, 2008).

There are 3 main stages of iron depletion (**Figure 9.3**) and at each stage specific markers can be used to assess the degree of depletion of body iron reserves. The **first stage** is characterized by the gradual depletion of iron stores with which NO physical symptoms can be associated. Very promptly the serum ferritin decreases. This is considered the most sensitive marker of the depletion of iron reserves, and thus as an early screening for the risk of iron-deficiency anemia, but it is NOT the most specific. The **second stage** is referred to as "*iron deficiency without anemia*". In this stage can be observed,

the beginning of the transferrin saturation-declining phase, the gradual increase in erythrocyte protoporphyrin and a mild decline in hemoglobin; levels may be slightly above or below the cut-off point. The second stage is short-lived, and the changes in blood markers may not be accentuated enough to raise any concern. The **third stage** is the most advanced and is referred to as "*iron deficiency anemia.*" At this stage the hemoglobin has significantly decreased, transferrin saturation is at its lowest, erythrocyte protoporphyrin (EP) is quite elevated, the MCV should be small, indicating a microcytic anemia, and the MCH should also be low, indicating hypochromia. The haematocrit is not all that sensitive and will only tend to decline once hemoglobin levels have plummeted (Gibson, 1990).

9.4.1.5. Markers of Iron-Deficiency Anemia

There are several markers used to assess iron deficiency anemia, however, none of them are specific enough to be used alone to identify iron deficiency with 100% certainty. In the assessment of anemias, the following markers are frequently used (see Figure 9.3 below for marker vs stage of iron depletion).

1. Hemoglobin
2. Hematocrit
3. Serum iron
4. Red cell indices
5. Erythrocyte protoporphyrin (EP)
6. TIBC + Transferrin saturation + Serum ferritin

Hemoglobin and *hematocrit* are considered very good markers of anemia, but abnormal values are not specific to iron-deficiency (Gibson, 1990) and it isn't until the late stages of iron deficiency anemia that abnormal values become visible. In fact, haematocrit concentrations tend only to decrease once hemoglobin synthesis is impaired. The **serum-iron** and total iron binding capacity (**TIBC**) are done by most labs at the same time and from these values **serum-transferrin saturation** can be derived [(s-iron/TIBC) x 100]. The transferrin saturation is by far the most sensitive to iron-deficiency compared to serum iron and TIBC. The serum iron is a measure of the iron bound to transferrin; it is subject to both large day-to-day variability and within-day variability. So much so that serum iron in itself is not regarded as a reliable index as there can be up to 50% variability due to diurnal changes alone. The TIBC, on the other hand, is not subject of diurnal changes; it increases in states of iron depletion and decreases in cases of iron overload and in inflammatory conditions. The TIBC reflects the number of free iron-binding sites located on the transferrin protein. The **erythrocyte protoporphyrin (EP)** is a more stable marker of iron reserves than transferrin saturation. It begins to increase quite noticeably in the third stage of iron depletion. This marker, however, is incapable of differentiating between a depletion of body reserves of iron and the impact of a mucosal block resulting from inflammation (Gibson, 1990).

The American Medical Association (AMA) guidelines recommend monitoring hemoglobin and hematocrit over 4 weeks following the prescription of an iron supplement. This is considered the most cost effective approach. The improvement of these markers (Hg > 1-2 g/dl; Htc> 3%) every 2 to 3 weeks with the iron challenge confirms the iron deficiency anemia. Treatment involves a continuation of iron supplementation for another 2 months and referral to a dietitian for a teaching of nutritional guideline for high iron intake. This is most cost efficient. Should these markers be normal or not influenced by the challenge, consider the possibility of being in the early stage of anemia and monitor s-ferritin; a value < 25 ng/mL confirms a depletion of iron stores. S-ferritin >100 ng/ml is recognized as indicative of normal iron stores. If hemoglobin concentrations remain low and unresponsive to supplements the likelihood of continued blood loss must also be envisioned. Clinicians generally expect a normalization of hemoglobin after 4 months of daily supplement use (Killip et al. 2007). It is however noteworthy that ferrous fumarate is considered a redox-active form of iron that is capable of catalysing free radical production in the form of peroxides. In iron deficient animals, studies have shown the intestine to be particularly susceptible to peroxidative damage with intake of iron supplementation. It appears that the manganese superoxide dismutase activity, the enzyme responsible for free radical detoxification in the mitochondria, tends to drop with iron supplementation (Picciano, 1999).

9.4.1.6. Avoiding the Misdiagnosis of Iron Deficiency Anemia

Some attention must be placed on minimizing the chances of misdiagnosing iron-deficiency anemia. Various pathologies or clinical situations can affect the typical markers that are relied on for the diagnosis of iron-deficiency anemia: *first*, iron-deficiency anemia and anemias resulting from genetic abnormalities (thalassemia, sideroplastic anemia) can influence similar blood markers. *Second*, anemias of chronic disease can often lead to a misdiagnosis of iron-deficiency anemia when, in fact, there can be more serious underlying infections, inflammations or malignancies. Refer back to the earlier section that describes this anemia. The problem is that inflammatory conditions can mimic or mask some of the changes in iron deficiency anemia. *Third*, copper (Cu) deficiency affects a variety of enzyme systems one of which causes a decrease in ceruloplasmin, a key transport protein, which carries iron to erythropoietic sites; the consequence is a hypochromic anemia. This should not be considered a major problem, as Cu deficiency is very rare. Incidences of Cu deficiency have, however, been reported in cases of chronic diarrhea and chronic protein losses (nephritic syndrome, protein losing enteropathy (Gibson 1990). *Fourth*, anemia can result from blood loss. Initially the blood film will be polychromatic (some hypochromic) and the MCV will be slightly elevated because of compensatory reticulocyte activity (reticulocytosis) which is the production of large immature red blood cells. Afterwards hemoglobin concentrations will then begin to fall. As blood loss progresses, the iron stores are gradually depleted, leading to microcytic (small MCV) and afterwards, the MCH begin to fall (low MCH) and finally the MCHC decreases. The anemia profile typically seen in a hemorrhaging patient will also include the following changes:

a. Serum iron: low
b. *TIBC*: high
c. *Plasma ferritin*: low

It is important that an underlying hemorrhage not go unnoticed. Generally this is not a problem as the blood loss is usually associated with pain. However, there are exceptions to the rule, which may cause the blood loss to either be overlooked or delay its recognition: i- in the case of psychiatrically disturbed patients or patients with head injuries, in whom pain and blood loss may not be noticed or reported; ii- an occult G.I hemorrhage may not produce the typical episode of hypotension and the expected melena (black tar-like stool) may be delayed; iii- the initial stages of a retroperitoneal hemorrhage may be silent; iv- in trauma patients undiagnosed occult hemorrhage can go unnoticed as the dark coffee-ground-like blood particulate leak out gradually and imperceptibly. The gastroenterologist will order a fecal occult blood test to confirm the presence of blood; the key concept is that trauma can seize the peristaltic movements of the intestine and greatly lengthen the transit time of the stool creating constipation or fecal impaction; and finally v- it may quite impossible to accurately localize pain in patients with multiple soft tissue injuries.

Fifth, anemia can also be the consequence of hemolysis: the separation of hemoglobin from the red blood cell. This is a tricky domain to move into, yet it is also a very important diagnosis to establish since it may be present in such a wide range of diseases. For this level course, I will briefly review the different settings in

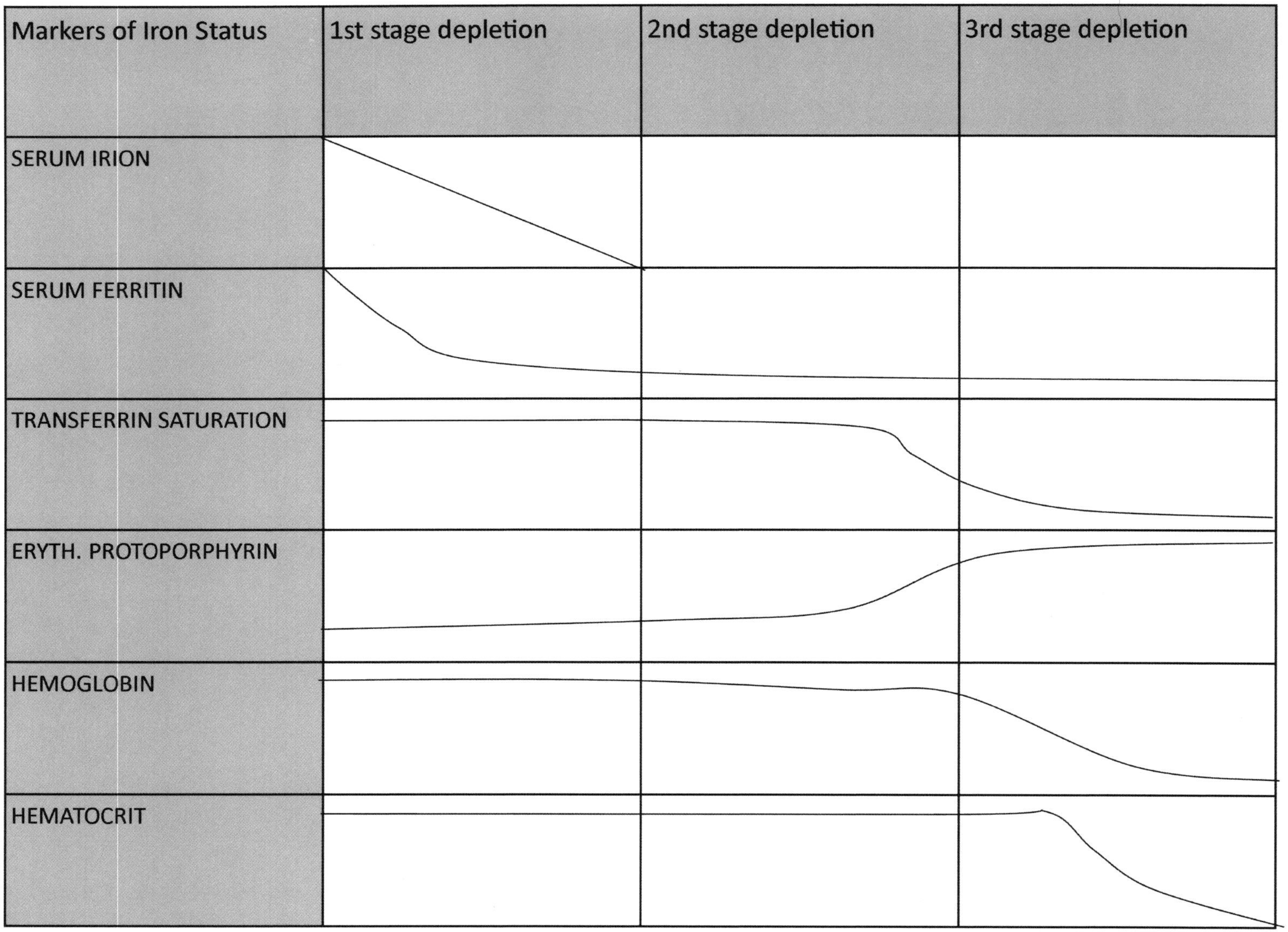

Markers of Iron Status	1st stage depletion	2nd stage depletion	3rd stage depletion
SERUM IRION			
SERUM FERRITIN			
TRANSFERRIN SATURATION			
ERYTH. PROTOPORPHYRIN			
HEMOGLOBIN			
HEMATOCRIT			

Figure 9.3 Effect of Iron Deficiency on Specific Markers of Anemias

Source: Adapted from Gibson, 1990

[1] Serum iron should be taken while fasting in the morning.

which hemolysis can be found. The first indication that hemolysis may be suspected is when the blood film reveals anemia with polychromasia. The presence of red or brown plasma in concert with dark urine suggests hemolysis; likewise, yellow plasma, the result of unconjugated hyperbilirubinemia (liver and biliary functions are normal) with clear urine can also be interpreted as a sign of hemolysis. Acute hemolysis is commonly found in shock or septic patients who have an impaired bilirubin transport. In this scenario the bilirubin becomes conjugated and the blood profile shows a conjugated hyperbilirubinemia. In cases of acute or chronic intravascular hemolysis one should expect to find hemosiderinuria. A high circulating lactic acid dehydrogenase is typically seen when there is red blood cell destruction as is expected in hemolysis or in an ineffective erythropoiesis.

9.4.1.7. Strategic Steps in Diagnosing Fe-Deficiency Anemia

The final diagnosis of iron-deficiency anemia requires some competence in reading the various plasma markers. There are several steps to follow in attempting to diagnose iron deficiency anemia. The *initial screening* (previously described) involves deriving from the complete blood count (CBC) (Hemoglobin, hematocrit, white blood cell count (WBC), WBC differential, platelet count, and red blood cell morphology) information pertaining to the red cell indices. Based on the red cell indices, the anemia can be classified as either microcytic and hypochromic, normocytic and normochromic or as macrocytic and normochromic. The microcytic and hypochromic profile in the red cell indices occurs usually when there is a severe depletion of the iron reserve, which takes place late in the second and into the third stages (Figure 9.3). These changes in the red cell indices can give you the first hint that iron status is part of the etiology, but does not confirm it since thalassemia and

congenital sideroblastic anemia also produce low MCV and MCH (Gibson, 1990).

9.5 INTRODUCTION TO MEGALOBLASTIC & MACROCYTIC ANEMIAS.

The objective of this section is to further explore the nutritional-based anemias and thus, a logical progression is to move towards megaloblastic anemia. However, for the sake of clarity, it is important to point out that megaloblastosis comes under a much larger umbrella of macrocytosis. This is a more generalized state that refers simply to larger than normal erythrocytes. The causes of these large RBC are many, however it suffices for now, to mention that macrocytic anemia can be non-megaloblastic if it is secondary to the following conditions (Snow, 1999):

1. Alcohol, drugs, smoking
2. Liver disease
3. Reticulocytosis
4. Marrow disease
5. Myelodisplastic syndromes
6. Hypothyroidism
7. Dyserythropoiesis

Megaloblastic anemia is represented by large ovalocytic erythrocytes, and arises from defects in DNA synthesis, which affect nuclear maturity by preventing the mitotic division of the cell located in the marrow (Snow, 1999). In contrast, cytoplasmic mass and maturation continue to increase because of uninhibited RNA synthesis. Hence, there is advanced cytoplasmic hemoglobinization in comparison to the nucleus therefore resulting in a greater mean corpuscular volume (MCV). The megaloblastic state is almost always tied to folate and/or B-12 deficiencies. However, they can also result from the

TABLE 9.1 Standard reference ranges for red cell indices.

Red Cell Indices	Calculation	Hypochromic Microcytic	Normochromic Normocytic	Normochromic Macrocytic
MCV	$\frac{\text{HEMATOCRIT}}{\text{RBC}}$	≤80 fL	84-100 fL	> 100 fL
MCH	$\frac{\text{HEMOGLOBIN}}{\text{RBC}}$	low — 5-25 pg	normal -- 26-32 pg	high -- 33-53 pg
MCHC	$\frac{\text{HEMOGLOBIN}}{\text{HEMATOCRIT}}$	20-30%	30-36%	33-38%

Klusek-Hamilton (Eds), H. (1984). Diagnostics: Nurses' Reference. Springhouse PA: Springhouse Corporation, 1133pp

intake of some drugs and inborn errors of metabolism. If megaloblastosis can be established with elevated MCV (fl>130)—above this cut-off there is a greater certainty of low B12, folate or both (Snow, 1999)—then it may not be necessary to do a bone marrow study in order to confirm the diagnosis. However, a bone marrow examination remains a helpful option in cases of multifactorial anemias. For instance, MCV is known to remain quite normal in a state of microcytic anemia combined with megaloblastosis (Snow, 1999).

9.6 ETIOLOGY AND PATHOPHYSIOLOGY OF B12 DEFICIENCY.

The main cause of B-12 deficiency is decreased absorption which, in 90% of patients with B12 deficiency, is reflected by a serum B12< 74 pmol/L (Snow, 1999). However, contrary to most other B vitamins, the body is able to store up to between 2-5 mg of Cbl, and will reutilize the Cbl via the enterohepatic circulation. Consequently, it takes between 2-5 years before neurological symptoms of deficiency begin to appear (Snow, 1999). There are many reasons why absorption could be compromised. From an epidemiological view point, the most likely causes of B-12 malabsorption are:

i.   Failure of gastric parietal cells/mucosa to secrete IF
      — Gastrectomy
      — Chronic atrophic gastritis
      — Myxedema
ii.   Competition for available B-12 and cleavage of IF
      — Blind loop syndrome
      — Fish tapeworm infestation
iii. Destroyed or absent ileal absorptive sites
      — Inflammatory enteritis
      — Surgical resection
iv.   Chronic pancreatitis
v.   Malabsorption syndromes
vi.   Certain drug therapies (oral calcium chelating agents, aminosalicylic acid, biguanadines)

There are two relatively frequent causes of B12 deficiency in North American society. The most prevalent occurrence is seen in gastric-bypass patients, who are now more numerous because of the obesity epidemic. Costing the U.S. $1.3 billion per year, there are about 113,000 bariatric surgeries performed every year (Livingston, 2010); the second most prevalent in Western society is related to an autoimmune disorder called Addisonian pernicious anemia. It is diagnosed mostly in those >50 years of age, who suffer from gastric mucosa atrophy of the fundus which is associated with parietal

cell antibodies seen in 90% of patients. It is noteworthy that very rarely are tests for gastric mucosa atrophy ever indicated. In addition, anti-thyroid antibodies, reported in 50% of patients and anti-intrinsic factor antibodies in 60% of cases characteristically describe this condition, and could help confirm the diagnosis of Addisonian pernicious anemia (Merck, 1987B).

9.6.1 Diagnostic Approaches to Identifying B12 Deficiency

In patients that present with unexplained macrocytosis, either folate or cobalamin (Cbl) deficiencies are generally suspected, but most often the cause is likely a B12 (Cbl) deficiency. Following a normal time line, MCV size would tend to increase before any significant decline in hemoglobin became evident. MCV dimensions equal to or exceeding 100fl tend to indicate macrocytosis, but clinical studies have shown that an MCV>130fl, more accurately predicts low vitamin B12 and/or folate concentrations (Snow, 1999). Caution is advised here, as it is possible to observe normal MCV values despite Cbl or folate deficiency, especially within the context of Fe deficiency anemia or thalassemia. In instances of neurological manifestations such as paresthesias and ataxia, Cbl deficiency is considered as a very likely contributor to the etiology. It is generally accepted that haematological abnormalities show up before the onset of neurological symptoms, however, more than 25% of patients presenting with Cbl based neurological symptoms, have either a normal hematocrit or a normal MCV. In some cases both the MCV and hematocrit are normal (Snow, 1999).

The advent of folic acid supplements, which are biologically active, has masked B12 deficiency in many instances. Whereas it was possible for a physician, upon observing macrocytic erythrocytes to ponder whether the cause was folate or B12 deficiencies or both, it is now more difficult to do so as megaloblastic cells are less prevalent now that folic acid supplements keep the problem of megaloblastosis in check. Nevertheless, folate supplements do not prevent the neurological anomalies associated with B12 deficiency, and so the pernicious nature of B12 deficiency goes unnoticed (Snow, 1999).

Serum Cobalamin: The specificity of low serum Cbl as a predictor of B12 deficiency is variable. Using a cut-off of < 74 pmol/L, some have found a specificity of 90%. Translated into laymen terms, this means that 9 times out 10 a person without Cbl deficiency will not have a serum B12 that is < 74 pmol/L. **Specificity** refers to the proportion of individuals without the disorder who exhibit normal blood values or in other words negative results. This means that, should a patient's serum

Cbl value fall < 74 pmol/L, he would likely have a Cbl deficiency (Snow, 1999).

Schilling Test. This test is recommended once a B12 deficiency has been confirmed, and the clinicians wants to determine if the cause is B12 malabsorption due to the absence of intrinsic factor (IF) (Gibson, 1990). Briefly the technique has two stages: **Stage 1** consists of administering an oral dose of crystalline Cbl, containing radioactive cobalt, and then, measuring the amount of radiolabeled Cbl in a 24hr urine collection. If the value is abnormally elevated, then **stage 2** is implemented. In this second step, an oral administration of labelled Cbl and IF is given 3- 7 days later. If urine values subsequently collected are normal then IF factor was truly missing (Snow, 1999).

Limitations of the Schilling Test: There could still be a problem even if the stage 2 results were normal. In instances of partial IF deficiency or gastric hypochlorhydria, crystalline Cbl—used in the Schilling's test—would likely be more easily absorbed than the protein bound Cbl normally encountered in food; the Schilling's test would, in this situation, be producing false negative results. Inadequate urine collection is another popular reason for false results. In cases of a dysfunctional ileum, caused by Cbl deficiency, the Cbl-IF complex is malabsorbed. This can however be reversed with prolonged Cbl administration. In renal insufficiency there is a delay in the urinary excretion of labelled Cbl, therefore producing again false negative results (Snow, 1999).

Modified Food Schilling test: Rather than using crystalline Cbl, radioactive B12 is incorporated into food products like chicken, eggs or egg albumin and fed to patients. This method can correctly diagnose poor absorption of protein bound Cbl and would be relevantly applied to elderly with low gastric acidity (Gibson, 1990).

The **deoxiuridine (dU) Suppression Test** is capable of determining a B12 and/or folate deficiency using bone marrow. The test is done by adding either cobalamin or methyl-tetra-hydrofolate to bone marrow culture. The vitamin that decreases the suppression of H-thymidine incorporation into DNA is the deficient vitamin (Gibson, 1990). The test can be used to measure chronic B12 and folate status by using lymphocyte rather than bone marrow (Gibson, 1990).

Antiparietal Cell Antibodies: This is a fairly sensitive test as these antibodies are present in 85% of patients suffering from the autoimmune gastritis of pernicious anemia they are very non-specific with detectable concentrations in patients with a variety of autoimmune endocrinopathies (Snow, 1999).

Anti-Intrinsic Factor Antibodies: This is an insensitive test as only 50% of patients with pernicious anemia have detectable levels of these antibodies. It is however very specific, thus it is possible to rule out pernicious anemia using this test. In other words these antibodies are rarely seen in healthy individuals (Snow, 1999).

9.7 CHARACTERISTICS OF FOLATE.

Folic acid is a term that refers to the chemical compound, pteroylglutamic acid which is the synthetic and active form that is added to food by the food industry. Folic acid also refers to the more generalized class of compounds called folates, which exhibit similar nutritional activity. Folates are actively absorbed mostly from the jejunum, although the folic acid from milk tends to be absorbed in the ileum because of a specific folate-binding protein. Folate becomes active when its methyl group is removed; methyl-tetrahydrofolate (MTHFA) becomes active tretrahydrofolic acid (THFA), and vitamin B12 is critical in the removal of the methyl group from THFA. Without B12, folate remains trapped in an inactive form thus interfering with DNA synthesis, which is needed for mitotic red blood cell division. The absence of active folate is responsible for the generation of large immature red blood cells (megaloblastic), typically observed as large MCVs >100 fl, but is not linked to pernicious anemia; the latter is strictly the consequence of B12 deficiency. Interestingly, a B12 deficiency can however cause a deficiency in active folate, thus producing megaloblastic cells in addition to neurological impairment (Gibson, 1990). In that sense, megaloblastic and pernicious anemias can be morphologically identical, however, pernicious anemia can also be non-megaloblastic, exhibiting only neurological symptoms which are manifested as losses in sensation, loss of lower limb motor power from myelin degeneration in the spinal cord, therefore resulting in disturbed gait. Although the preferred treatment for megaloblastic pernicious anemia is monthly 100 μg intramuscular (i.m) injections of vitamin B12, megaloblastic anemia can also be overcome with large doses of folate; synthetic folic acid (pteroylglutamic acid) does not require cobalamin as a cofactor as it is already in its reduced active THFA form. In contrast, large doses of dietary folate will do nothing to correct the neurological abnormalities if there is B12 deficiency, since inactive folate requires B12 to be activated to THFA. Because the inactive methyl-tetrahydrofolate requires homocystein in order to become demethylated and active, it is understandable that a folate deficiency will cause the buildup of homocysteine (Hcy) **(Figure 9.4)** in the blood, whereas the increase of both homocysteine and methylmalonic acid (MMA) **(Figure 9.5)** is usually indicative of a vitamin B12 deficiency (Snow, 1999). This is illustrated in the case report described by Stabler (2013) in which a 57 year old woman presented with serum MMA equal to 3600 nmol/L and a serum Hcy 49.1 mcmol/L, both values significantly greater than normal—serum MMA that is normal is < 400 pmol/L, and normal Hcy is <14mcmol/L. Despite a serum Hcy indicative of a possible folate deficiency, the MCV was normal at 96fL. Even though the serum B12 was not < 74pmol/L it was nevertheless suboptimal at 151 pmol/L The absence of megaloblastosis in combination with a normal hematocrit of 42% precludes a normal MCV derived from microcytic anemia countering a megaloblastic anemia (Stabler, 2013).

The enzyme methionine synthetase (Figure 9.4) receives a methyl group from the donor, 5-methyl–THFA, and transfers it to cobalamin for the generation of methyl cobalamin (Figure 9.4). The latter becomes the methyl donor to homocysteine for the production of methionine and THFA. The activity of methionine synthetase requires adequate amounts of cobalamin.

A dietary folate deficiency therefore implies a poor availability of methyl-THFA and thus a decreased availability of methyl groups; the consequence is a buildup of homocysteine. It can also be inferred that a B12 deficiency would prevent the methyl group transfer from occurring even though there may be abundant methyl THFA; the consequence here is very little methyl THFA changing into the more active THFA, again causing homocysteine concentrations in the blood to increase. It is essential to clearly point out that folate deficiency alone cannot result in neurological disorders; there must be B12 deficiency, however a B12 deficiency can cause both neurological degeneration and megaloblastosis. Folic acid supplementation would bypass this problem. Since it is already biologically active, the synthetic folic acid would not require vitamin B12 to gain the active

form. Thus, neurological abnormalities would occur in the absence of an MCV >100 fl.

Cobalamin is also a needed co-factor in the conversion of methyl-malonyl-coenzyme A (CoA) to succinyl-CoA (Figure 9.5). Hence, in a Cbl deficiency state, methyl-malonyl-CoA and its hydrolysis product, methyl malonic acid (MMA) will increase; the latter is a useful diagnostic marker.

9.8 ETIOLOGY AND PATHOPHYSIOLOGY OF FOLATE DEFICIENCY.

The primary cause of deficiency is a poor diet resulting from the poor intake of green leafy vegetables and milk, alcoholism and chronic TPN or excessive cooking of vegetables.

Secondary causes of folate deficiency are associated with the following conditions:

i- <u>inadequate absorption</u>: malabsorption syndromes, blind loop syndrome, drugs such as oral contraceptives, barbiturates, sycloserine, phenytoin, primidone).

ii- <u>inadequate utilization</u>: folate antagonists, B12 deficiency, scurvy, excessive alcohol intake, bacterial overgrowth in the intestine, drug induced: anticonvulsants, oral contraceptive, sulfasalazine, methotrexate, triamterene.

iii- <u>increase requirements</u>: pregnancy, infancy, malignancy, increased metabolism, increased hematopoiesis.

iv- <u>increased excretion</u>: In liver disease there may be increased excretion of bile which is B12- dependent.

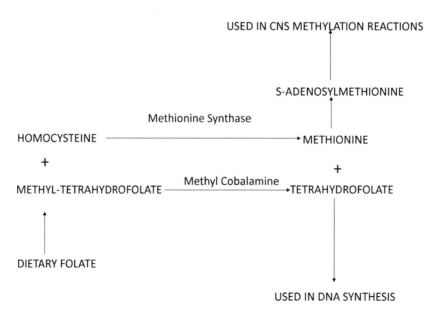

Figure 9.4 Synthesis of methionine from homocysteine

(Adapted from Snow, CF. 1999, Archive Intern Med; 159: 1289-1298)

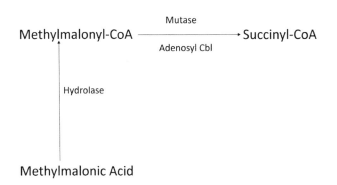

Figure 9.5 Conversion of methylmalonyl-CoA to succinyl-CoA

9.9 DIAGNOSTIC APPROACHES TO B-12 AND FOLATE DEFICIENCY.

A strategic approach should always be about getting the right information in order to make a decision on the kind of treatment that is needed. To do so, the clinician must take into account the sensitivity of the test, the cost and turnover time to run a particular test in addition to the value of the knowledge that can be derived from the test. In keeping with such a rationale, it is then advisable to think in terms of tests which can detect the earliest signs of a deficiency, especially if there are insufficient physical symptoms to confirm a diagnosis. Second, use a broad test, which can capture several problems and then proceed to a more specific test. The first step would be to establish the existence of macrocytosis and then attempt to determine if it is megaloblastic in nature.

The second step consists in a series of biochemical tests that can be used to confirm B12 and folate deficiencies; these are listed below. In terms of a practical clinical approach to diagnosing such deficiencies, only but a few are frequently used as they turn out to be very useful especially in cases when serum values fall below certain acceptable cut-off limits. The following markers can be used to monitor folate and cobalamin (Cbl) status:

1. **Serum folate: reflects recent folate intake** (< 3ug/L is lower cut-off limit indicative of an acute low folate status).
   a. Chronically low concentrations for longer than 1 month reflect a high likelihood of depleted folate stores
   b. Hemolysis may cause high serum folate
   c. Liver damage & renal failure equates to high folate levels.
   d. Contraceptives + smoking equates to low folate
   e. Alcohol intake can cause short term decreases in serum folate.
   f. Serum folate tends to increase in patients with Cbl deficiency. The impairment of methionine synthetase pathway leads to an increase of the inactive MTHFA, which is the principal form of serum in the blood (Gibson, 1990).

2. **Erythrocyte folate: reflect body stores** (<160 ng/mL is indicative of deficiency), however for an accurate interpretation it is important to consider the following:
   a. Not specific to folate deficiency, as values also decrease in B12 deficiency. In fact 60% of patients with pernicious anemia have low RBC folate (Snow, 1999; Gibson, 1990).
   b. Important to assay for serum B12 in addition to erythrocyte folate
   c. Erythrocyte values increase in conditions involving hemorrhage or hemolysis, as the reticulocyte count tends to increase, and also in cases of Fe-deficiency anemia. The reticulocytes contain higher concentrations of folate compared to the older erythrocytes (Gibson, 1990).
   d. There is a possibility of Fe-deficiency masking a folate deficiency.
   e. Erythrocyte folate tends to be less sensitive to short term variances in diet intake and therefore is more reflective of storage and status.

3. **Red cell indices**
   a. MCV: Elevated in folate deficiency and sometimes in B12 deficiency
   b. MCH: normal or slightly elevated: Cells are laden with hemoglobin but there are fewer cells.

4. **Serum Methylmalonic Acid**. Elevated values tend to mostly reflect Cbl deficiency however in 12% of cases folate deficiency is also reported. In cases of normal serum MMA, Cbl deficiency is rarely reported.

5. **Serum Homocysteine**. Elevated serum Hcy is invariably associated with Cbl and folate deficiencies. In the instance of normal Hcy, there is a small likelihood of either Cbl or folate deficiencies.

6. **S-Hcy, S-MMA and S-Folate**: Rather than rely on only one marker, there is greater diagnostic value in referring to a combination of three markers. The table below (Table 9.2) illustrates the diagnostic strengths in using these three markers.

TABLE 9.2 Evaluation of patients with hematological abnormalities and normal serum Cbl

Serum folate	Serum MMA	Serum Hcy	Interpretation
Normal	Normal	Normal	Neither Cbl or folate deficiency is likely
Normal	Normal	Elevated	Possible Cbl deficiency
Normal	Elevated	Normal	Possible Cbl deficiency
Normal	Elevated	Elevated	Probable Cbl deficiency
Low	Normal	Normal	Possible Folate deficiency
Low	Normal	Elevated	High probability of folate deficiency
Low	Elevated	Normal	Possible Cbl deficiency or mixed deficiency
Low	Elevated	Elevated	Cannot establish type of deficiency. Need to consider a therapeutic trial *

Adapted from Snow, CF. Archiv of Internal Med. 1999; 159: 1289-1298

* S-metabolite levels tend to normalize 7-14 d after nutritional replacement therapy

7. **Polymorphonuclear leukocyte lobe count**. The hypersegmentation of the neutrophils generally precedes the development of macrocytosis and is a main early feature of folate and B12 deficiencies. This test would become useful in attempting to confirm folate and B12 deficiency in a situation involving a macrocytosis that is masked by iron-deficiency anemia—red blood cells appear normocytic. In such a case the MCV would be normal but other indices would be suggesting low iron reserves. The paradoxical normal MCV, in this context, should cause the clinician to question the findings

Figure 9.6 Anemia Algorithm; Adapted from Gibson, 1990; Killip, et al. 2007; Snow, 1999.

9.10 PRACTICE PROBLEM SET IN ANEMIA.

The two next problem sets will give students the opportunity to look over several blood profiles representing various types of anemias. The questions are the same for all three profiles: First, what can you conclude from the profile at hand, and second, what other markers would you need to confirm the diagnosis.

9.10.1 Problem Set-1.

A woman age 20 presents with symptoms of tiredness and facial pallor.

The lab sends the physician the results of the blood test, who in turn reports them in the chart.

	Lab Values	Reference Values
Serum iron	0.62 mg/L	0.8 - 1.5 mg/L
TIBC	4.42 mg/L	3.0- 4.5 mg/L
Erythrocyte protoporphyrin	1.10 mg/L	0.4- 0.7 mg/L

What can you conclude from the blood values?

ANSWER: Serum Iron is low, which is consistent with iron deficiency anemia, chronic inflammation and pregnancy. Serum iron cut-off: < 0.60 mg/L, almost stage II iron deficient erythropoiesis (Gibson, 1990).

Erythrocyte protoporphyrin is elevated. This suggests a significant difference, which is consistently found in iron deficiency anemia and in a mucosal block defect; the latter prevents the release of iron from the reticulo-endothelial cells and despite the abundance of iron reserve in the body, there is a hindrance in the release of iron from the reticulo-endothelial cells of the liver, spleen and bone marrow, subsequently hindering the transport of iron to the erythrocyte and causing a rise in EP. The very high EP seen in this case should coincide with a transferrin saturation < 16% if it is Fe-deficiency anemia. The transferrin saturation is calculated (s-iron/TIBC) x 100 and found to be = (0.62/4.42) x 100 = 14%. In addition TIBC should increase in Fe-deficiency anemia.

TIBC: It is necessary to consider the TIBC as it remains within the normal range. This means the total number of free iron-binding sites on transferrin have not increased because more transferrin was not synthesized in response to depleted body iron reserves.

MOST LIKELY DIAGNOSIS: The evidence seems to point to a Fe-deficiency anemia. Facial pallor, elevated EP, and suboptimal transferrin saturation, which has dipped below the cut-off limit of 16%, indicate possible stages-2 or 3 iron depletion (Gibson, 1990). The problem is that TIBC, ideally higher than normal in iron-deficiency anemia, is within the normal range. Moreover, both EP and % transferrin saturation are also known to decline in anemia of chronic disease.

It would be advisable to order an MCV to assess whether there were microcytic cells. However, the determining marker will be ferritin as it will tend to not decline in anemia of chronic disease, but rather increase.

9.10.2 Problem Set-2

A male age 55 complains of general weakness, tiredness and abdominal pain (Gibson, 1990).

	Lab Values	Reference Values
Transferrin	1.240 g/L	> 2.00 g/L
Transferrin saturation	30 %	20 - 50 %
Plasma ferritin	12 mg/L	39.0 - 256.0 mg/L
Plasma iron	1.10 mg/L	0.8 - 1.5 mg/L

What can be concluded from the blood values?

ANSWER: The transferrin did not rise as is normally expected in iron deficiency. Rather the normal level suggests that the patient may be moderately protein deficient which causes a downward movement of transferrin concentrations (Gibson, 1990).

Transferrin saturation is within a normal range but does not invariable rule out a problem since normal values are also seen in anemia of chronic disease.

Serum ferritin is significantly low. Ferritin is secreted into the plasma from the reticulo-endothelial system and generally parallels the amount of storage iron. In chronic disease, the mucosal block defect results in an over synthesis of ferritin from the reticulo-endothelial system. The low values, observed in this case, suggest the absence of chronic disease and suspiciously points towards early iron depletion.

The serum iron is normal, but does not by itself provide any conclusive results because iron tends to greatly shift with diurnal rhythms.

This patient does appear to suffer from depleted iron stores—possible early stage of depletion leading to anemia—that have not shown up in other markers yet. This suggests the first stage of iron depletion. There is some evidence as well of visceral protein deficiency.

What additional markers would you need in order to confirm a diagnosis?

To conclude whether there is protein deficiency, request retinol binding protein (RBP) as it is NOT affected by iron-deficiency anemia and has a short half-life 12 hours. This protein is equally sensitive to protein depletion as thyroxin-binding pre-albumin (TBPA) (Gibson, 1990). The latter is too sensitive to minor stress. The dietitian should also complete a usual food assessment. The physician will want to order serum ferritin, as it will tend to increase in anemia of chronic disease but decline early on in Fe-deficiency anemia. To confirm iron deficiency anemia the physician can order the following tests:

To rule out acquired sideroblastic anemia, a hematologist should be consulted. The MCV tends to be elevated in acquired sideroblastic anemia. This kind of anemia can also present as microcytic and hypochromic, just like Fe-deficiency anemia. There tends to be high serum Fe, ferritin and saturation of transferrin. This is Not occurring in this case.

The physician should confirm that there is no blood loss by checking for a history of haemorrhoids, ulcer, and hiatus hernia. The doctor will want to also rule out a history of ulcerative colitis and colonic.

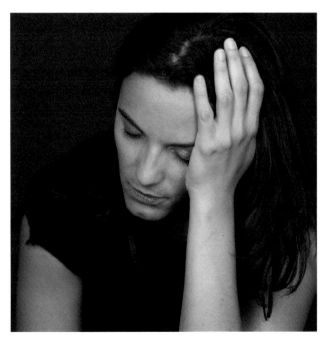

Figure 9.7 A Young 18 year-old woman, suffering from fatigue. © Adam Gregor/shutterstock.com

A physical examination would be the next step after reviewing the patient's history. Abdominal pain should raise some concerns, and will represent the needed incentive to look for GI occult blood in stool or melena. In the absence of any findings, it is worthwhile to proceed to an upper and lower endoscopy. Here again, a negative endoscopic finding is usually an incentive to move to Meckel's small bowel series and to a radioactive chromium fecal blood loss study.

Blood loss from non-GI sources such as lungs, renal, joints, skin should be the next logical avenue to rule out.

Malabsorption is the likely the last condition to rule out, by looking for abdominal distension and steatorrhea (fat in the stool), and inflammation of the intestinal lumen.

MOST LIKELY DIAGNOSIS: The low s-ferritin confirms early depletion of iron serves, while transferrin and transferrin saturation do not confirm anemia.

9.11 CASE STUDY—CHRONIC TIREDNESS

A. Case Title.

Chronic tiredness

Chief Complaint.

Katherine is an 18-year old emaciated and pale looking teenager girl who complains of low energy, difficulty concentrating, and being overly tired for the last 6 months. She claims to have lost 5 lbs in the last 6-8 months and to have increasing difficulties concentrating. She is in her freshman year at university and presents with abdominal pain in the left lower quadrant and complains of chronic tiredness.

C. Personal Information

Patient's first / last name	Katherine	Canon
Sex	Female	
Age	18 years	
Occupation	Freshman college student	
Marital status	Single, lives alone	
Number of children	none	

D. History of Present Illness

Katherine complains of poor appetite, tiredness, low energy, and decreased ability to concentrate for the last 6-8 months. Prior to this time she felt fine. She does not remember having similar symptoms previously.

E. Medications

She reports taking no medication currently. She took antibiotics a few years ago for an ear infection.

F. Vaccinations

Up to date

G. Past History

Katherine had low body weight as a teenager and has never been very active physically. She did not participate in sports during her childhood.

H. Surgeries

No surgeries reported

I. Personal & Social History

An 18-year-old girl, freshman in college
Lives alone for the past 1 year; the first time that she has lived away from home
Reports receiving high grades throughout her education
Has made a few friends but finds little time to socialize
Works weekends at a downtown bar

J. Family History

Katherine's father is an unemployed laborer with a long history of alcoholism. Her family has lived on social assistance for many years and receives frequent visits from social services. Her mother and father are alive.

K. Review of Other Systems

Poor appetite and frequent constipation, some mild abdominal pain in the left lower quadrant
Denies polyuria, polydypsia, and hyperphagia

PHYSICAL EXAMINATION

L. General Appearance.

No apparent symptoms of distress

Pleasant, well-groomed, emaciated, and pale-looking girl. Appears somewhat depressed. Patient appears young
for her age. There are signs of pallor in the face and conjunctiva and thinning hair, which are generally indicative
of Fe-deficiency.

M. Examination of Regions of the Body.

Region of Body	Examination Findings	Is Finding Normal? (Y/N)
Skin	Pallor, cold and extremely dry skin	N
Head, eyes, ENT	Pale conjunctiva, facial pallor, dry thinning hair	N
Neck	No palpable goiter	Y
Lymph nodes	No lymphadenopathy	Y
Thorax and lungs	Lungs clear bilaterally, no wheezing	Y
Cardiovascular	Regular rate and rhythm	Y
Abdomen	Soft, non-tender, bowel sounds present, no hepatosplenomegaly	Y
Peripheral vascular	Warm extremities	Y
Musculoskeletal	No muscle wasting in upper and lower extremities, no edema, no temporal muscle wasting, triceps skinfold is in 10-25th percentile	Y
Neurological	Cranial nerves II-XII intact, sensorium intact throughout, reflexes slightly decreased in upper and lower extremities	Y

N. Vital Signs.

Blood pressure,	130/70 mmHg, sitting
Pulse rate,	76 b.p.m. regular
Respiration rate,	14/min
Temperature	97.5 °F (36.4 °C)
Height,	5'5" (164.5 cm)
Height for age percentile (for children),	50-75th percentile
Weight	110 lbs (50 kg)
Weight for age percentile	25-50th percentile
Weight for height percentile (for children),	10-25th percentile

LABORATORY FINDINGS

LAB MARKERS	ACTUAL	NORMAL STD	INTERPRETATION
CBC (Complete blood count)			
Hemoglobin (Hgb)	9 g/dL	12-16 g/dL	Low
Hematocrit (Hct)	30%	38-46 %	Low
Red Blood Cell (RBC)	3.2million/mcL	4.2-5.4million/mcL	Low
MCV	41fl	84-99fl	Low
MCH	23pg	26-32pg	Low
BLOOD PROTEINS			
Serum Albumin	3.4g/dL	3.3-4.5g/dL	Normal
Retinol Binding Protein (RBP)	2.1g/dL	2.6-7.6mg/dL	Low
Serum Transferrin	195mg/dL	>200mg/dL	Mildly low
LIVER FUNCTION TESTS			
Alkaline Phosphatase	100 U/L	90-239 U/L	
Gamma-Glutamyl Transferase (GGT)	30 U/L	5-27 U/L	
Alanine Amino Transaminase (ASAT) also (SGPT)	19 U/L	9-24 U/L	
Amylase	95 SU/dL	60-180 SU/dL	
OTHER BLOOD MARKERS			
Erythrocyte			

Source: Gibson, 1990; Klusek-Hamilton (Eds), H. (1984)

Systems Review: Pain in the left lower quadrant suggests GI problems, possibly inflammatory bowel disease with some malabsorption. The patient presents as emaciated and depressed and has a high achiever profile typically seen among patients with anorexia nervosa; psychiatry should be consulted. The hematological profile shows abnormally low hemoglobin and hematocrit, thus intimating iron-deficiency anemia.

Overall she appears to have grown normally as indicated by the rating of her height which is between the 50-75th percentile. Her weight for height is between the 10-25th percentiles which is still considered normal. There is no sense from these values that the patient is severely underweight especially since patient claims to have lost only 5lbs in the last 6 months. This only represents only a 4% weight loss.

Review and Interpret Blood Biochemistry: RBP, hematocrit and hemoglobin are all suboptimal indicating possible iron deficiency anemia and protein malnutrition. Hepatic and pancreatic functions are normal.

Differential Diagnosis: Chronic infection, anorexia nervosa, inflammatory bowel disease, megaloblastic anemia, undernutrition, thyroid dysfunction and diabetes mellitus.

Likely Diagnosis: Iron deficiency anemia is likely because: s-Hb and Hct are suboptimal. The presence of facial pallor and pale conjunctiva are relatively strong physical symptoms. Menstruating women and those with poor dietary intakes are particularly susceptible. This is also a classical case typifying the first time away from home experience and the newness of cooking for self. Thalassemia is unlikely as there is no jaundice, splenomegaly and hepatic siderosis which are common symptoms. Moreover, it is more prevalent in African, Mediterranean, or Southeast-Asian women. Undernutrition should be considered here as there has been a loss of weight possibly tied to poor nutritional habits. The suboptimal RBP level further confirms that nutritional status may be less than ideal. The abdominal pain is assumed to be from constipation since there are no hepatic or pancreatic disorders that are apparent. The constipation can be confirmed with X-ray.

Recommendations: The patient's diet needs to improve, both in terms of quality (micronutrients including Fe) and total energy because of her recent weight loss. The American Medical Association recommends a repeat HGB or HCT after 4 weeks of iron supplementation to confirm iron-deficiency anemia. If HGB increases by >1 g/dL and HCT increases by >3%, iron-deficiency anemia is confirmed, and iron supplementation should be continued for 2 months before further evaluation. If these markers are unresponsive to iron supplementation, then a differential with mean corpuscular volume (MCV), RBC distribution width (RDW), and serum ferritin should be ordered. MCV will help diagnose megaloblastic anemia due to Vitamin B12 or folate deficiency. Diet should include high quality protein (>0.90 g/kg body weight) and adequate total energy (35 kcal/kg ideal body weight [54 kg]). Thus she should be consuming >45g protein and about1890 kcal per day. Weight gain should be slow thus allowing patient to better adapt to dietary recommendation and ensure long-term compliance. The patient needs to increase the amount of iron-rich foods in her diet. The American Medical Association recommends consumption of iron-rich foods and foods that enhance iron absorption, rather than iron supplementation, as the means of primary prevention and for the treatment of anemia. Patient should consume a high fiber diet. It is advisable to begin the day with a high fiber breakfast cereal such as raisin bran, shredded wheat, bran flakes or bran buds in combination with raisins, and other dried fruits such as apricots, cranberries and prunes. Most of the high fiber raisin bran cereals will contain between 10 and 50% of the DRI for iron. Some breakfast cereals such "TOTAL" will contain 100% of the DRI for iron in one serving. When combined with some kind of citrus juice or fruit such as orange or grapefruit, iron absorption is significantly enhanced. Often, diet in combination with iron supplements such as iron fumarate, gluconate or sulfate help replenish iron reserves more rapidly (Merck, 1987; Gibson, 1990; Bissonnette, 2014).

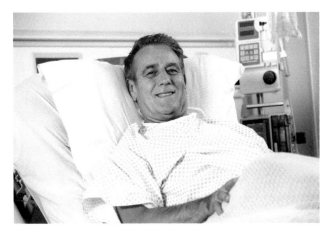

Figure 9.8 Man Suffering from Parathesias and Nystagmus © Monkey Business Images/shutterstock.com

9.12 CASE STUDY—PATIENT COMPLAINS
OF PARATHESIAS & NYSTAGMUS

A. Chief Complaint

Peripheral pins and needles paresthesias + spastic ataxia, intermittent diarrhea and fatigue

B. Description of main complaints

Jim LaRosa is a 43-year old Caucasian businessman, who lives alone. He has a five-year history of mild weight loss and anorexia. In the last year, he describes the anorexia as more pronounced and accompanied by nausea. In addition, he complains of feeling pins and needles and numbness in his legs, and a general lethargy that seems more pronounced over the last year. He describes feeling unsteady when standing as well as weakness in legs, arms, leg stiffness and some confusion. He has recently been experiencing spastic ataxia.

C. Personal Information

Patient's first / last name (fictional)	Jim	LaRosa
Sex (male/female)	Male	
Age (years + months for children)	43 years	2 months
Occupation	Businessman in pharmaceutical sales	
Marital status (single/married/separated/divorced**)**	Single and lives alone in an apartment	
Number of children	None	

D. History of Present Illness

J.L. complains of poor appetite, tiredness, lethargy, weight loss and episodes of vomiting and intermittent diarrhea over the last year. He has experienced pins-and –needles in his lower limbs, and finds that he has recently over the last year become unsteady on his feet. He also reports stiffness in her legs, especially near the end of the day. His work performance in the area of pharmaceutical sales has declined over the last year as well. He finds it difficult to concentrate long hours and becomes easily irritable. Prior to this time he reports feeling fine and being able to multi-task very easily.

E. Medications

He reports not being on any medication or nutritional supplements at the moment.

F. Vaccinations

He claims having received all childhood vaccinations

G. Past History

J.L has a history of inflammatory bowel disease, which necessitated the resection of 75% of his ileum 6 years ago. Prior to surgery he lost 10% of his initial weight. Following surgery he regained his weight with nutritional support involving supplemental feedings and vitamin and mineral supplements. Within 6 months he felt well enough to go back to work, although he experienced regular diarrhea/watery stool 3-4 x /week. Nevertheless, JL managed to maintain his weight stable up until 1 year ago. Since that time his appetite became poor and he began losing some weight..

H. Surgeries

Partial ileocolectomy 6 years ago involving 75% removal of the ileum.

I. Personal & Social History

J.L is a 43year-old male Caucasian living alone in Montreal for 7 years and working as a sales representative in the area of pharmaceutical sales, and is often working 60 hrs weeks. J.L. has been living alone since the age 20, and generally enjoys reading and cross-country skiing. He works out regularly at the gym since his surgery. He denies smoking and only occasionally drinks in social contexts.

J. Family History

Mother is a high school teacher and farther is a university professor in an MBA program. They live in Boston Massachusetts and are happily married. He has 2 younger brothers named Daniel and Jim, and one older sister, Joanne who are all busy in their different careers.

K. Review of Other Systems

G.I: Poor appetite. Some mild non-localized abdominal pain. HEENT: thyroid not enlarged Rectal: Occasional episodes of soft watery stool 3-4 times /week, but generally stools are formed and regular. Stool test for occult blood is negative. No rectal bleeding observed. Neurological: Alert, good memory. Evidence of ataxia, sensory loss of position and vibration sense in the lower extremities. In addition, there is a mild loss of reflex in legs and noticeable Babinski response.

PHYSICAL EXAMINATION

A. General Appearance.

No apparent distress symptoms.
Tired-looking but well-groomed man complains of fatigue, lethargy and spastic ataxia. He reports losing 6% of usual weight over the last year, which he attributes to poor appetite.

B. Vital Signs. Enter values in the boxes

Blood pressure,	130/90 mm Hg sitting
Pulse rate,	76 p.m regular
Respiration rate,	14 / min
Temperature,	97.5 °F (36.4 °C)
Height,	5' 9" (1.73 cm)
Triceps	7 mm
Height for age percentile	75th percentile
Present weight	154 lbs (70 kg)
Usual Weight,	164lbs (74.4 kg)
Usual weight for height (percentile)	25-50th percentile

Present weight for age percentile	25-50th percentile
Present weight for height percentile	10-25th percentile
Present triceps skinfold percentile	10-25th percentile

C. Examination of Regions of the Body.

Region of Body	Examination Findings	Is Finding Normal? (Y/N)	Supporting Materials
General	Pleasant well groomed man who presents with no noteworthy physical findings. Complains of fatigue, lethargy, spastic ataxia, and unsteadiness. Not in acute distress	**No**	The Merck Manual, Disorders of the Peripheral Nervous System, 1987
Skin	Skin color normal, warm to touch	**Yes**	Stallings, V. and Hark, L. 1996
Head, eyes, ENT	Absence of bi-temporal wasting,	**Yes**	Stallings, V. and Hark, L. 1996
Neck	No palpable goiter	**Yes**	
Lymph nodes	No lymphadenopathy	**Yes**	The Merck Manual, 1987 Pediatrics & genetics
Thorax and lungs	Lungs clear bilaterally, no wheezing	**Yes**	
Cardiovascular	Regular rate and rhythm	**Yes**	
Abdomen	Soft, non-tender, bowl sounds present, no hepatosplenomegaly, occasional constipation and diarrhea, generalized abdominal pain	**No**	Lichtenstein, GR. Mueller, DH. 1996 The Merck Manual Anemias, 1987
Genitalia and rectum	Soft pubic hair with full distribution, no perianal fistulas or rectal bleeding	**Yes**	The Merck Manual, Gynecology and obstetrics 1987, p: 1690-1691
Peripheral vascular	Warm extremities, feet and hands	**Yes**	The Merck Manual, Cardiovascular disorders
Musculoskeletal	No muscle wasting in upper and lower extremities. No edema. No temporal muscle wasting; evidence of spastic ataxia and peripheral muscle fatigue.	**No**	Stallings, V. and Hark, L. 1996 The Merck Manual, 1987,
Neurological	Cranial nerves II-XII intact, sensorium not intact throughout. Reflexes slightly decreased in lower extremities. Ataxia and moderate loss of propioceptive and vibratory sensations in the lower extremities. Babinski responses reported.	**No**	The Merck Manual, Neurological disorders. 1987, p:1432-1433

No.	Test name	Basic Result	Is Result Normal?	EXPLANATIONS
1	Hemoglobin	110 g/L	No	Non-specific indicator that also falls in B12 deficiency
2	Hematocrit	42%	Yes	Close to lower limit of normal
3	S-Ferritin	175 g/L	Yes	Indicates that iron reserve is normal and rules out Fe-deficiency anemia
4	S-albumin	43 g/L	Yes	
5	Spinal X-ray	No erosion, collapse or fracture	Yes	
6	S-glucose	4.0 umol/L	Yes	
7	WBC	9,000/uL	Yes	
8	Total lymphocytes	2.2 x10^9/L	Yes	
9	GGT	30 U/L	Yes	
10	Serum B-12	60 pmol/L	No	Values <74 pmol/L
11	T$_4$ RIA	110 nmol/L	Yes	
12	Abdominal Ultrasound	Normal	Yes	Pancreas not enlarged; no pseudocysts or cholelithiasis; and bile duct appears normal
13	Serum Amylase	130 U/dL	Yes	
14	MCV	98 fl	Yes	High normal
15	S-Folate	12 ng/ml (28 nmol/L) High	Yes	Values > 7nmol/L are considered normal
16	Endoscopy	Normal	Yes	No lesions or patchy ulcerations seen on mucosa. No fibrosis or edema observed. No sinus tracts or fistulas.

LABORATORY VALUES

Comments on Laboratory Findings:

Hemoglobin value is low however neurological signs are quite visible. Normally an iron supplement is given as a challenge, and if hemoglobin concentration rises after 4 weeks, this would confirm Fe-deficiency anemia. This cost efficient procedure is approved and supported by the AMA. In the present case, the patient presents with overt neurological symptoms and a partial ileal resection. The focus here is to measure serum B12 and if values are < 74 pmol/L in the presence of normal or elevated serum folate concentrations, then there is a reasonable basis for inferring B12 deficiency resulting in pernicious anemia. There is, therefore, impetus to promptly treat the neurological symptoms as if caused by pernicious anemia since the neurological disease may be irreversible should treatment be delayed. While treatment is being implemented, it's advisable to monitor the patient's CBC and red blood cell indices.

In this situation, the MCV is normal indicating no microcytosis or megaloblastosis. It is however important to indicate that although MCV may be normal, it could simply be the result of a combined microcytic anemia due to Fe-deficiency and megaloblastosis due to folate deficiency. There is therefore the need to check s-ferritin to confirm that Fe stores are adequate.

The spinal X-ray can be done afterwards to rule out spinal injury. This is a likely differential diagnosis as some of the neurological symptoms reported here overlap those of spinal compression. The abdominal pain reported by the patient necessitates an abdominal ultrasound in order to rule out liver and spleen abnormalities and the serum amylase to rule out pancreatitis. In addition, the endoscopy would be required to visualize and biopsy any abnormality of GI tract such as ulcers, filling defects and mass lesions. Poorly localized abdominal pain, intermittent diarrhea and anorexia are symptoms frequently reported by patients suffering from pernicious anemia.

A Review of Case Findings

LIKELY DIAGNOSIS	EXPLANATIONS	REFERENCES
Inflammatory Bowel Disease	This is a patient at high risk of a resurgence of inflammatory bowel disease since there is a history in this patient, which resulted in the partial resection of ileum 6 years ago. Only infrequent episodes of watery stools and no debilitating abdominal pains reported, however, he does report a poorly localized abdominal pain. Patients with inflammatory bowel disease report localized abdominal pain in the right lower quadrant. Patient has gained weight normally after ileum resection and maintained his usual expected weight up until 1 year ago. Referral to a gastroenterologist for an endoscopy followed by a barium contrast could be useful for the diagnosis of lesions, ulceration or inflammation of the GI tract.	The Merck Manual, Gastrointestinal Disorders, 1987 p: 711 The Merck Manual, Gastrointestinal disorders, 1987; p: 743; 797- 817
Undernutrition	Poor eating habits and suboptimal energy intake due to anorexia and the 6% weight loss over the last year raises suspicions. Poor absorption intimates a very good likelihood of poor nutritional status	Mann & Trustwell. The Essentials of Human Nutrition, 1998 p:271
Pernicious anemia	Resection of 75% of ileum could affect the re-absorption of bile and of intrinsic factor-B12 complex.	
Wernicke-Korsasyndromekoff syndrome	Not likely Thiamine deficiency resulting from poor food intake and abundant alcohol consumption. It presents as mental confusion, aphonia and confabulation resulting from acute hemorrhagic polioencephalitis. There is no such manifestation documented in the medical history.	Truswell & Milne, The Vitamins In: Essentials of Human Nutrition, 1998 p: 197
Guillaine-Barré Syndrome	Presents as a rapid acute idiopathic polyneuropathy with segmental demyelination. There are symptoms similar to pernicious anemia such paresthesias and ataxia. However, unlike pernicious anemia, Guillaine Barré characteristically causes the loss of deep tendon reflexes, in addition to cardiac arrhythmias and respiratory paralysis, which can become life threatening.	Merck Manual, 1987, Neurological disorders, p 1446

PHARMACEUTICAL TREATMENTS & RATIONALE

Intramuscular injections of vitamin B12 are necessary to correct the neurological symptoms that John has been experiencing. It is imperative that such injections begin as soon as possible because the neurological damage could become irreversible if treatment is delayed. It usually takes 18 months of intensive treatment to alleviate the neurological symptoms. After this time, he should be changed to a lifelong regimen of cyanocobalamin vitamin B12, 100-1000 micrograms IM injection once per month.

In cases were the diagnosis is debatable, the risk-benefit ratio still favors treatment with vitamin B12 injections until a neurological condition is identified. It is imperative not to delay as the neurological symptoms can be irreversible

This is because cobalamin treatment is non-toxic and folate has never been associated with neurological changes, thus folate treatment given concurrently with cobalamin is unlikely to be relevant especially since megaloblastosis is not identified.

While hematological signs can be corrected within 6 weeks, especially in the case of folic acid insufficiency due to B12 deficiency, it will take up to 18 months for neurological symptoms to subside. However, improvements in hematological and neurological symptoms have been reported after daily oral treatments (0.5 ug/d) over 3 to 5 months.

A multivitamin is strongly recommended for middle-aged men because their eating habits tend not to meet nutritional guidelines. John also works long hours and lives alone, which may make him especially prone to poor eating habits.

Moreover, high intake of antioxidants is recommended as it may decrease the risk of coronary heart disease, especially in men.

Iron-deficiency anemia is not an issue here.

Anti-diarrhea agent could be recommended if diarrhea persisted after the restriction of milk. The American Gastroenterological Association recommends Loperamide to reduce frequency of loose stool.

Antidepressants: SSRIs (e.g., fluoxetine, paroxetine, sertraline) are now commonly used in patients with IBS as they have low side effects and can be useful in IBS patients with either severe or less severe refractory symptoms of pain.

REFERENCES

1. Abuelo, JG et al (1992). Serum creatinine concentrations at the onset of uremia: higher levels in black males. Clin Nephrol. 37 (6): 303-7.
2. Ali, M.A.M (1976) The Hypochromic Anemias. Can. Fam. Physician 22: 1530
3. Allen, L.H. (2000). Anemia and Iron Deficiency: Effects on Pregnancy Outcomes. Am. J. Clin. Nutr. 71(5):1280-1284
4. Bergmann, AK et al (2010). Systematic molecular genetic analysis of congenital sideroblastic anemia: Evidence of genetic heterogeneity and identification of novel mutations. Pediatric Blood Cancer 54(2): 273-278. Retrieved May 27, 2014 from: http://www.ncbi.nlm.nih.gov/pubmed/19731322

5. de Benoist B et al., eds. (2008) Worldwide prevalence of anaemia 1993-2005. WHO Global Database on Anaemia Geneva, World Health Organization. Retrieved May 29, 2014 from: http://www.who.int/vmnis/anaemia/prevalence/summary/anaemia_data_status_t2/en/
6. Encyclopedia Britannica (2013). Reticuloendothelial system. Retrieved May 28, 2014 from: http://www.britannica.com/EBchecked/topic/499989/reticulo endothelial-system
7. Gallagher PG.(2011) Hemolytic anemias: red cell membrane and metabolic defects In: Goldman L, Schafer AI, eds.Cecil Medicine. 24th ed. Philadelphia, Pa: Saunders Elsevier;chap 164
8. Gonzalas-Casas, R. et al. (2009). Spectrum of Anemia Associated with Chronic Liver Disease. World J Gastroenterol. 15(37): 4653–4658. Retrieved June 3,

2014 from: http://www.ncbi.nlm.nih.gov/pmc/articles/ PMC2754513/

9. Killip, S. et al. (2007) Iron Deficiency Anemia. *Am Fam Physician*.75(5):671-678.

10. Klusek-Hamilton (Eds), H. (1984). Diagnostics: Nurses' Reference. Springhouse PA: Springhouse Corporation, 1133pp

11. Livingston, E.H. (2010). The Incidence of Bariatric Surgery has Plateaued in the U.S. Am. J. Surg. 200 (3): 378-85

12. Looker AC, et al. 1997 Prevalence of iron deficiency in the United States. JAMA. 277:973–6.

13. Merck (2013). The Merck Manual for Healthcare Professionals. Hematology & Oncology. Sideroblastic Anemias. Retrieved May 27, 2014 from: http://www.merckmanuals.com/professional/hematology_and_oncology/anemias_caused_by_deficient_erythropoiesis/sideroblastic_anemias.html?qt=anemias&alt=sh

14. Merck (2013B). The Merck Manual for Healthcare Professionals. Hematology & Oncology. Thalassemia. Retrieved May 28, 2014 from: http://www.merckmanuals.com/professional/hematology_and_oncology/anemias_caused_by_hemolysis/thalassemias.html?qt=thalassemia&alt=sh

15. Merck (2013C). The Merck Manual for Healthcare Professionals. Hematology & Oncology. Anemia of Chronic Disease. Retrieved May 28, 2014 from: http://www.merckmanuals.com/professional/hematology_and_oncology/anemias_caused_by_deficient_erythropoiesis/anemia_of_chronic_disease.html?qt=anemia of chronic disease&alt=sh

16. Merck (2013D). The Merck Manual of Diagnosis and Therapy. Genitourinary Disorders: Chronic Kidney Disease. Retrieved June 2, 2014 from: http://www.merckmanuals.com/professional/genitourinary_disorders/chronic_kidney_disease/chronic_kidney_disease.html?qt=uremia &alt=sh

17. Merck (2012). The Merck Manual of Diagnosis and Therapy. Endocrine and Metabolic Disorders: Hypothyroidism. Retrieved June 2, 2014 from: http://www.merckmanuals.com/professional/endocrine_and_metabolic_disorders/thyroid_disorders/hypothyroidism.html

18. Merck (1987). The Merck Manual of Diagnosis and Therapy. Hematology & Oncology: Anemias. Rahway, NJ: Merck & Co Inc: 1092-1194

19. Merck (1987B). The Merck Manual of Diagnosis and Therapy. Gastrointestinal Disorders: Pernicious Anemia. Rahway, NJ: Merck & Co Inc: 738-739

20. Picciano, MF (1999). Iron and folate supplementation: an effective intervention in adolescent females (Editorial). Am. J. Clin. Nutr. 69:1069–1070

21. Snow, C.F (1999). Laboratory Diagnosis of Vitamin B12 and Folate Deficiency. Archiv of Internal Med. 159: 1289-1298

22. Stabler, S.P. (2013). Vitamin B12 Deficiency. N Engl J Med 368:149-160

23. Strum, Judy M.; Gartner, Leslie P.; Hiatt, James L. (2007). Cell biology and histology. Hagerstwon, MD: Lippincott Williams & Wilkins. p.83

24. U.S. Department of Health & Human Services (DHHS, 2014)). National Heart, Lung and Blood Institute (NHLBI). Iron Deficiency Anemia. Retrieved June 3, 2014 from: http://www.nhlbi.nih.gov/health/health-topics/topics/ida/

25. U.S. Preventive Services Task Force (USPSTF1996). Screening for iron deficiency anemia – including iron prophylaxis. In: Guide to Clinical Preventive Services. 2nd ed. Baltimore, Md.: Williams & Wilkins:231–46

26. Weiss, G and Goodnough, L.T. (2005) Anemia of Chronic Disease. N Engl J Med; 352:1011-23.

27. Wiseman, DH et al. (2013). A novel syndrome of congenital sideroblastic anemia, B-cell immunodeficiency [~]. Blood 4;122(1): 112-23

28. WHO (2006). Guidelines on Food Fortification with Micronutrients. Lindsay Allen, Bruno de Benoist, Omar Dary, Richard Hurrell (Eds). 341pp

29. World Health Organization (WHO, 2002). The World Health Report 2002: Reducing risks, promoting healthy life. Geneva, WHO.

30. World Health Organization (WHO, 2001) WHO/NHD/ 01.3). Iron Deficiency Anemia: Assessment, Prevention and Control. A Guide for Program Mangers, Geneva.

INDEX

ABOUT THE AUTHOR

Dr. David Bissonnette is a registered dietitian (RD) and a member of both the Academy of Nutrition and Dietetics, and the Canadian Nutrition Society. He has close to 20 years of experience in the nutrition education of dietetic and nursing students. Having completed his doctoral work in Nutritional Biochemistry at the University of Toronto's Faculty of Medicine, Dr. Bissonnette held teaching and research positions at St-Francis Xavier University, in Nova Scotia, Canada and at McGill University's School of Dietetic & Human Nutrition, in Montreal, Canada. He is currently an associate professor of nutrition at Minnesota State University, Mankato, where he teaches and conducts research in the areas of nutritional support in critical care, antioxidant therapy in critical illness, muscle fatigue in malnutrition, and obesity. He also wrote and produced a DVD documentary on obesity titled: OBESITY IN AMERICA: A National Crisis which is distributed by Films for the Humanities and Sciences. He also authored a introductory textbook on nutrition for general education students, titled: IT'S ALL ABOUT NUTRITION: Saving the Health of Americans, which is published by University Press of America. Over the last two decades, Dr. Bissonnette has taught courses in introductory nutrition, nutrition for healthcare professionals, nutritional assessment, nutrition in sports and exercise, in addition to food-service and food production management. In 2014 Dr. Bissonnette and his research colleagues were awarded the highly prestigious Douglas R. Moore Presidential Lectureship Award.

Credits